The Spastic Forms of Cerebral Palsy

D1026477

DATE DUE

Adriano Ferrari · Giovanni Cioni

The Spastic Forms of Cerebral Palsy

A Guide to the Assessment of Adaptive Functions

Forewords by
Alain Berthoz
Pietro Pfanner

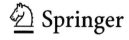 Springer

618.928
F375

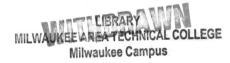
WITHDRAWN
LIBRARY
MILWAUKEE AREA TECHNICAL COLLEGE
Milwaukee Campus

Adriano Ferrari
Child Rehabilitation Unit
S. Maria Nuova Hospital
Department of Neuroscience
University of Modena and Reggio Emilia
Reggio Emilia, Italy

Giovanni Cioni
Department of Developmental Neuroscience
Stella Maris Scientific Institute
Division of Child Neurology and Psychiatry
University of Pisa
Pisa, Italy

This is a revised, enlarged and completely updated version of the Italian Edition published under the title
"Le forme spastiche della paralisi cerebrale infantile. Guida all'esplorazione delle funzioni adattive"
edited by A. Ferrari, G. Cioni
© Springer-Verlag Italia 2005
All rights reserved

Translation: Maurizio Boni and Vincent Corsentino, Italy

ISBN 978-88-470-1477-0   e-ISBN 978-88-470-1478-7

DOI 10.1007/978-88-470-1478-7

Springer Dordrecht Heidelberg London Milan New York

Library of Congress Control Number: 2009936779

© Springer-Verlag Italia 2010

This work is subject to copyright. All rights are reserved, whether the whole or part of the material is concerned, specifically the rights of translation, reprinting, reuse of illustrations, recitation, broadcasting, reproduction on microfilm or in any other way, and storage in data banks. Duplication of this publication or parts thereof is permitted only under the provisions of the Italian Copyright Law in its current version, and permission for use must always be obtained from Springer. Violations are liable to prosecution under the Italian Copyright Law.

The use of general descriptive names, registered names, trademarks, etc. in this publication does not imply, even in the absence of a specific statement, that such names are exempt from the relevant protective laws and regulations and therefore free for general use.

Product liability: The publishers cannot guarantee the accuracy of any information about dosage and application contained in this book. In every individual case the user must check such information by consulting the relevant literature.

Typesetting: Compostudio, Cernusco s/N (MI), Italy
Printing and binding: Arti Grafiche Nidasio, Assago (MI), Italy
Printed in Italy

Springer-Verlag Italia S.r.l, Via Decembrio 28, I-20137 Milan, Italy
Springer is part of Springer Science+Business Media (www.springer.com)

The publication of this volume, edited by Adriano Ferrari and Giovanni Cioni, is a major event for several reasons. Most importantly, it concerns an area of child pathology that has yet to be fully explored. In this context, the authors' efforts to compile their observations as well as those of other clinicians and to elaborate their theories have resulted in an essential step in the field of cerebral palsy (CP).

The originality of the book is its very clear focus, while at the same time the authors have encouraged the book's contributors to express their ideas and personal opinions. This leads sometimes to redundancy, but this is precisely one of the benefits of the book because the same problems are then exposed from different points of views. The reader is thus spared the normative attempts of many other pathology books, in which the complexity of a given disease is hidden by the authors' or editors' desire to impose a rigid taxonomy or epidemiology.

The chapters in the book offer a lively, up to date discussion about the mechanisms of CP as well as the possible approaches to the child with CP. This will be fruitful to the reader, whether he or she is involved in practical training and rehabilitation or in clinical practice. Furthermore, the book is a rich source of information for designers of rehabilitation equipments, basic research scientists, and those who are interested in the social consequences of this pathology (education, transportation, etc.).

A special feature of this book is that, in accordance with the originality of the Stella Maris Institute and its departments of Child Neurology and Psychiatry, it also includes chapters in which the psychiatric and psychosocial dimensions of CP are discussed.

This book is of interest not only because of the diversity of its approaches to CP, but also because it contains a number of extremely new ideas concerning the mechanisms of this condition. For instance, the possible involvement of top-down, cognitive, and perceptive factors in so-called motor deficits is extensively discussed. This is crucial because too often motor pathology is attributed only to low-level or muscular deficits. However, as frequently stated in the book, an understanding the relationship between cognitive, perceptive, and bottom-up sensory-motor factors still requires extensive research.

The consequences of this and related research will be important for the design of new rehabilitation methods; but they will also lead to "remediation" procedures, i.e., activities that allow the brain to discover and put into action as-yet-unexploited resources, alternative sensory-motor strategies, and new combinations of the elements of the motor repertoire – the brain is, after all, a clever and creative machine. This will also require that each individual with CP is given free rein to find his or her way to recuperation, or to a substitution of function.

The wide range of knowledge offered in this book will enable readers to consider the problem of "generalization". Today we see a rapidly developing market of training devices some of which are deceiving as the CP patient's capacities improve on the machine, but the improvements are not transferred to the many unexpected situations of daily life.

We owe the authors of this book our gratitude for inviting us to join in their efforts to better the life of so many bright and promising children.

Paris, September 2009   **Alain Berthoz**
Professor at the College de France
Member French Academy of Sciences
Associate member of American Academy of Arts and Sciences
and Royal Belgium and Bulgarian Academies of Medicine

Foreword

by P. Pfanner

It is with great pleasure that I present this book devoted to cerebral palsy, in which Adriano Ferrari and Giovanni Cioni have collected from their experiences and reflections the results of over a decade of productive collaboration in this field.

Its layout and contents mirror the expertise and background of the authors and their co-workers, and their original scientific approach.

Besides being a university professor in Child Neuropsychiatry, Giovanni Cioni is the director of the clinical department of an Italian scientific biomedical research institute, dedicated to child neurology, psychiatry, and rehabilitation, in which the research and clinical aspects of neurological and psychiatric disorders in childhood are treated.

Adriano Ferrari is the founder and director of an important specialized hospital center operating on a national level, that carries out multifaceted and innovative child rehabilitation program.

Progress in the rehabilitation field, a recent science that still needs to construct a framework in order to consolidate knowledge and experience, has to appropriately develop from the collaboration between clinics and rehabilitation, between purely neurobiological aspects of functioning and orthopedic ones of the locomotor apparatus, namely anatomy and pathology. However it must go further to also include important psychological aspects related to the motivation of the motor act and its emotional components, both of which inevitably play a crucial role in learning under pathological conditions.

In my opinion, the great medical and scientific contribution of Giovanni Cioni and Adriano Ferrari, expressed in this book, lies in their ability to integrate all these aspects in theoretical models and clinical procedures on cerebral palsy.

A look through the table of contents of this book will confirm my statements. The first part summarizes the history of cerebral palsy and describes how the understanding of this pathology has been modified over the years up to its present interpretation, which states palsy is a disorder that involves not only strictly motor functions, but also perceptual, cognitive, and emotional ones. This part also points out the recent contribution of neuroimaging, especially ultrasound and magnetic resonance, in visualizing and identifying brain lesions that cause cerebral palsy. Imaging, but also and especially careful observations of neonate's and young infant's movements, enables us to make diagnoses and prognoses starting from the first weeks of life, thus doing away with the ancient concept of the silent period.

The second, more extensive part of this book analyzes the adaptive functions of cerebral palsy patients, offering an extremely complete and integrated examination of the clinical aspects of these special children. This is followed by a section dealing with the classification of spastic forms of cerebral palsy. Here, the taxonomic proposal, which the authors have been working on for several years, is presented in an analytic format enhanced with designs and diagrams taken from the files of the Motion Analysis Laboratory in Pisa.

This classification proposal is innovative because it utilizes not only kinematic, but also multiple parameters in order to classify the various forms of cerebral palsy, and because it also gives suitable indications for prognosis and treatment. As with all proposals, also in this book, it is the intention of the authors to submit their model to the contributions and criticisms of the readers.

The book also comes with an interactive DVD on the different forms of cerebral palsy, prepared by the physiotherapists of Reggio Emilia and Pisa. It is particularly useful because it also contains exercises to assess learning.

This book therefore is full of the information and ideas of Giovanni Cioni and Adriano Ferrari and their co-workers, who have collaborated in drafting several chapters. However, as indicated by the authors themselves in their introduction, this is not a textbook in the classical sense, that is to say a comprehensive review of the literature and state of the art of the studied topic. The book instead reflects on the cultural and methodological approach and the original and very often provocative interpretation by the authors and their collaborators. It presents working hypotheses that in part must be confirmed through further research of evidence and verified by other groups, and one of the purposes of this text is to stimulate and promote additional useful and necessary scientific contributions.

I welcome and agree with the choice of the authors to search for the neurophysiopathological connection in every aspect of cerebral palsy, to more than merely present their quantitative data and clinical series collected over many years of work.

Springer has superbly edited and printed this work, praiseworthy of this well-known publishing house.

I would like to express once again my warmest congratulations to the authors. I am certain this book will be a great success among doctors, child neuropsychiatrists and physiatrists, therapists, and students specializing in these related fields.

Pisa, September 2009   **Pietro Pfanner**
                                           Former Professor of Child Neurology and Psychiatry
                                                                            University of Pisa

Preface

This book is the result of studies and reflections on cerebral palsy (CP) in children that the authors and their collaborators (medical doctors and therapists) from the Pisa and Reggio Emilia specialised centers have carried out in recent years. It addresses the main topics associated with the evaluation of adaptive functions in the spastic forms of CP (accepted definition and its modifications over the most recent decades, new taxonomic orientations, etiopathogenesis, semiotics, and the so-called associated impairments: visual, cognitive and behavioral).

The main goal of this book is not to relate or update the state of art of these topics, but to offer readily accessible information on the explored themes in order to encourage considerations and comparisons with the readers' experiences.

The topics are treated from a pathophysiological point of view that guides the authors' interpretations of the nature of the disease (functional diagnosis), the problems correlated with prognosis (such as the hypothesis of its natural history) and with rehabilitation (such as modification of the architecture of functions in adaptive terms). The text comes with a DVD of clinical cases which are subdivided according to classification criteria elaborated by the authors. These cases enhance the teaching usefulness of this book for people already working in this field (medical doctors, child neuropsychiatrists and physiatrists, rehabilitation therapists), for university students of physical and occupational therapy, and for residents in rehabilitation medicine, child neurology, and orthopedics. The reader, student, or professional interested in CP will find innovative ideas, proposals, remarks, and correlations resulting from the collective expertise of our two groups, to which the reader can compare his own personal ideas. For this reason, the book maintains the structure of personal notes, like a travel journal, offering the authors' interpretations and reflections, while referring to other scientific publications for detailed analyses of related clinical cases and comparisons with the viewpoints of other specialists. In this sense, every chapter represents an autonomous unit that can be studied separately. The statements presented in each chapter are frequently full of repercussions and, we hope, this will lead the reader to further reflections, comparisons, and, obviously, doubts and disagreements based on his own experiences. Also for this reason some concepts and references to the scientific literature and to primary authors are quoted in several chapters, as a common basis for specific topics.

The publication of this book would not have been possible without the effort and contribution of all the colleagues, medical doctors and therapists, of our specialised centres, and the collaboration of children and their parents. We would like to thank everyone for their cooperation.

Reggio Emilia and Pisa, September 2009   **Adriano Ferrari**
                                                          Giovanni Cioni

Contents

16   Forms of Hemiplegia
Giovanni Cioni, Giuseppina Sgandurra, Simonetta Muzzini,
Paola B. Paolicelli, Adriano Ferrari

List of Contributors

Silvia Alboresi
Child Rehabilitation Unit
S. Maria Nuova Hospital
Reggio Emilia

Ada Bancale
Department of Developmental
Neuroscience
Stella Maris Scientific Institute
Pisa

Vittorio Belmonti
Department of Developmental
Neuroscience
Stella Maris Scientific Institute
Pisa

Daniela Brizzolara
Department of Developmental
Neuroscience
Stella Maris Scientific Institute
Division of Child Neurology and
Psychiatry
University of Pisa
Pisa

Paola Brovedani
Department of Developmental
Neuroscience
Stella Maris Scientific Institute
Pisa

Giovanni Cioni
Department of Developmental
Neuroscience
Stella Maris Scientific Institute
Division of Child Neurology and
Psychiatry
University of Pisa
Pisa

Adriano Ferrari
Child Rehabilitation Unit
S. Maria Nuova Hospital
Department of Neuroscience
University of Modena and Reggio Emilia
Reggio Emilia

Alberto Ferrari
Department of Electronics,
Computer Sciences and Systems
Engineering Faculty
University of Bologna
Bologna

Giovanni Ferretti
Department of Developmental
Neuroscience
Stella Maris Scientific Institute
Pisa

Andrea Guzzetta
Department of Developmental
Neuroscience
Stella Maris Scientific Institute
Pisa

Roberta Leonetti
Child Neuropsychiatry Unit
Local Health Service
Carpi (Modena)

Manuela Lodesani
Child Rehabilitation Unit
S. Maria Nuova Hospital
Reggio Emilia

Sandra Maestro
Department of Developmental
Neuroscience
Stella Maris Scientific Institute
Pisa

Gabriele Masi
Department of Developmental
Neuroscience
Stella Maris Scientific Institute
Pisa

Simonetta Muzzini
Child Rehabilitation Unit
S. Maria Nuova Hospital
Reggio Emilia

Paola B. Paolicelli
Department of Developmental
Neuroscience
Stella Maris Scientific Institute
Pisa

Rosita Pascale
Department of Developmental
Neuroscience
Stella Maris Scientific Institute
Pisa

Silvia Perazza
Department of Developmental
Neuroscience
Stella Maris Scientific Institute
Pisa

Federico Posteraro
Neurological Rehabilitation and
Severe Acquired Brain Lesion Unit
Auxilium Vitae
Volterra (Pisa)

Silvia Sassi
Child Rehabilitation Unit
S. Maria Nuova Hospital
Reggio Emilia

Giuseppina Sgandurra
Department of Developmental
Neuroscience
Stella Maris Scientific Institute
S. Anna School of Advanced Studies
Pisa

Francesca Tinelli
Department of Developmental
Neuroscience
Stella Maris Scientific Institute
Pisa

DVD by

Giulia Borelli
Child Neuropsychiatry Unit
Local Health Service
Scandiano (Reggio Emilia)

Michele Coluccini
Department of Developmental
Neuroscience
Stella Maris Scientific Institute
Pisa

Maria Rita Conti
School of Physiotherapy
Medical Faculty
University of Modena and Reggio Emilia
Reggio Emilia

Franca Duchini
Department of Developmental
Neuroscience
Stella Maris Scientific Institute
Pisa

Maria Cristina Filippi
Child Rehabilitation Unit
S. Maria Nuova Hospital
Reggio Emilia

Annarosa Maoret
Child Rehabilitation Unit
S. Maria Nuova Hospital
Reggio Emilia

Antonella Ovi
Child Rehabilitataion Unit
S. Maria Nuova Hospital
Reggio Emilia

Maddalena Romei
Child Rehabilitation Unit
S. Maria Nuova Hospital
Reggio Emilia

Angelika Schneider
Child Rehabilitation Unit
S. Maria Nuova Hospital
Reggio Emilia

Elisa Sicola
Department of Developmental
Neuroscience
Stella Maris Scientific Institute
Pisa

PART I
Nature of the Defect

Cerebral Palsy Detection: from John Little to the Present

G. Cioni, P.B. Paolicelli

As for many essential aspects of human life, William Shakespeare wrote an outstanding description of a person affected by cerebral palsy (CP), through the words uttered by the Duke of Gloucester, future King Richard III, by which he hints at his condition as being related to prematurity and respiratory disorders.

> *"I, that am curtail'd of this fair proportion, cheated of feature by dissembling nature, deform'd, unfinish'd, sent before my time into this breathing world, scarce half made up, and that so lamely and unfashionable that dogs bark at me, as I halt by them"*
>
> (William Shakespeare, Richard III)

Historical documents report how the existence of children with movement disorders was already known at the time of the Sumerians, and certainly Hippocrates was aware of this disease (Ingram, 1955 and 1964, for a review of historical medical literature). However, the first detections and descriptions of CP certainly date back to the Victorian age.

In the mid 19th century, within the range of the widespread and severe motor disorders related to poliomyelitis, a new clinical picture was detected, that differed both in symptoms and etiopathogenesis. This clinical picture, in contrast with the peripheral paralysis typical of poliomyelitis, was referred to as of infantile "cerebral" palsy. The term infantile, rather than just expressing an etiopathogenetic feature, was employed to define an epidemiological aspect, differentiating the early or even connatal motor disorders in children from the post-apoplectic disorders of adult and elderly patients.

Sir John Little was the first to describe this disease, even though he did not employ the term "cerebral palsy" in his famous work of 1862. Little was an English orthopedics, affected by a palsy resulting from poliomyelitis, who studied the surgical interventions for Achilles' tendon stretching that were starting to be performed at that time, and even underwent the operation himself. He especially investigated deformities developing in individuals with generalized spasticity. In 1861, he published a report of his experience based on 20 years of clinical investigations on this type of disorder, supported by a rich data collection on possible correlations between pregnancy or delivery disorders and the resulting alterations of the physical and psychological development of children presenting with articular deformities. Little maintained that both spasticity and deformities were caused by asphyxia and cerebral hemorrhage secondary to delivery distress. A new nosological entity was then defined and named "Little's Disease".

Two other authors need to be mentioned who were later active researchers in the same field. William Osler, in his book "The cerebral palsy of children" (1889), did not provide a definition of CP, but described the clinical features of 151 children with CP and grouped them according to their assumed etiology, trying to interpret the physiopathological mechanisms of the cerebral lesion (damage location).

> *"By dividing the motor path into an upper cortico-spinal segment extending from the cerebral cortex to the grey matter of the cord and a lower spino-muscular, extending from the ganglia of the anterior horns to the motorial end plates, the palsies that I propose to consider have their anatomical seat in the former and may result from a destructive lesion of the motor centers or of the pyramidal tract, in hemisphere, internal capsule, cris or pons"*
> (Osler, 1887)

Sigmund Freud, in his "Die infantile Cerebrallahmung" (Infantile cerebral palsy), written in 1897, investigated the causes of these motor disorders, ascribing, in contrast with Little, more importance to pre-term birth and to intrauterine development disorders than to distress suffered during delivery. It is interesting to notice how, in the same work, Freud points at the inadequacy of the nosological entity of "CP" as a purely clinical category, related neither to a precise and single etiology nor to a precise and single anatomo-pathological picture. He then concludes by incorrectly predicting that this definition would soon be abandoned and replaced by different and more precise ones.

> *"The term infantile cerebral paralysis heading this treatise is a nomen proprium. It characterizes not merely what is implied in the combination of words, ie paralysis in childhood due to cerebral causes (as a result of cerebral affection), but what already has been applied over a long period of time to pathological conditions in which paralysis is overshadowed or replaced by muscular rigidity or spontaneous muscular twitching".*
> *"I actually advocate that this term be applied even to cases in which paralysis is completely absent or where the disease consists merely of a periodic recurrence of convulsions (epilepsy)". "Thus, infantile cerebral paralysis is merely a contrived term of our nosographic classification, a label referring to a group of pathological cases. It should not be defined, but should be explained by references to actual cases. It would be desirable to replace this term by another not conveying such a definite, inadequate image; this would then render the above assertions superfluous".*
> *"I have inserted this digression on the nosographic system in order to point out that the term infantile cerebral paralysis merely represents a clinically-based picture of disease. As the following pages will show, it is neither equated to a pathologico-anatomical not to an etiological entity. It is therefore probable that even clinically the*

term can only claim the value of a temporary entity that may soon be abandoned in favour of certain more coherent and possibly etiologically well-determined disease picture"
Freud, 1897 (transl. Russin LA, University of Miami Press, 1968)

In the first part of the 19th century until the Second World War, the interest in the investigation of spastic disorders in children remained quite low. Very few were also the attempts to establish rehabilitation programs, which were received with little enthusiasm. In the same period, orthopedic surgery gained more popularity due to the improvement of the neurotomy technique, used as specific procedure for the treatment of contractures. Surgery was positively received because it allowed physicians to immediately measure the results achieved, even though initial improvements were then followed by more severe disadvantages in the long term.

Physiotherapy in CP individuals was introduced in the USA by the work of Jennie Colby, a physical therapist who had a special interest in massotherapy, from which derived, in a fully empirical way, most of the exercises used in her proposed treatment for individuals affected by spastic paralysis. Physiotherapy practices proposed by Colby were then included in the intervention program applied by the rehabilitation clinic for children with CP, founded at the beginning of the 20th century in Boston by Bronson Crothers (Crothers and Paine, 1959). With a wholly innovative concept, the intervention program devoted special attention, along with motor treatment, also to the psychological aspects and the mental health of disabled individuals.

A broader view on the issues related to CP was then given by Winthrop Phelps (1950), an orthopedic surgeon who, in 1930, founded in Maryland the first community for the rehabilitation of disabled individuals, based on a multidisciplinary intervention model involving the close cooperation of different professionals.

Immediately after the Second World War, medical research revived the interest in this field, with the rapid creation of many specialties and a renewed focus on disabled children and their social and environmental context. Advances in obstetrician assistance techniques and more sophisticated instruments of neonatal intensive care significantly reduced overall mortality, but also allowed the survival of a larger number of individuals at risk. This rapidly led to the investigation of new and more appropriate working methods in different professional fields. Progress achieved in the investigation of genetic and metabolic diseases and their consequences on the central nervous system allowed a redefinition of many clinical pictures that were previously classified under the still nonspecific diagnostic label of CP. The specific etiology of some clinical pictures was also defined, such as the frequent association of choreoathetosis, deafness, and sight palsy, with a condition of hyperbilirubinemia involving infants with hemolytic disease. At the same time, public opinion started to become more aware and more sensitive to the issues of disabled people.

In this background, in 1947, the American Academy for Cerebral Palsy (AACP) was founded. Conceived as a multidisciplinary professional association aimed at promoting research in the field of infant disability, AACP gathered the most important clinical disciplines and their corresponding activities of motor therapy, psychopedagogy and psychology. The founders of AACP represented different clinical specializations, including neurology, pediatrics and psychiatry. Phelps was the first Chairman.

What had been conceived as a small forum for debate, by the 1950s marked the dawn of the growing interest in infant disability. This resulted in a rapid expansion of knowledge, but also in an unavoidable confusion on the definition and interpretation of CP, and, above all, on the ways to classify its extremely diversified symptoms (Minear et al. 1954). In 1957, driven by the need to clarify the terminology used in different parts of the world, but also aiming at raising consensus about the classification, of CP, an AACP conference was held. A definition, which is still very popular today, resulted from the conference, according to which CP must be considered as "*a permanent but not unchangeable disorder of posture and motion, due to a cerebral defect or non-progressive lesion, which took place before the brain had completed the main morphofunctional maturation processes; the motor disorder is prevalent but not exclusive, and may vary in type and severity*".

With the same objective, in England, Ronnie Mac Keith and coworkers created the "Little Club" (Mac Keith et al. 1959), which, after many meetings, in 1964 published, edited by Martin Bax, a definition of CP which still has the widest international consensus, according to which "*cerebral palsy is a posture and motion disorder, due to a defect or a lesion of the immature brain. For practical aims, we need to exclude from cerebral palsy those disorders of posture and motion which are 1) short-term, 2) due to a progressive disease, 3) exclusively due to mental retardation*".

Some authors also tried to rewrite and update this definition, with few substantial changes, such as Mutch et al (1992), who defined CP as "*an umbrella term covering a number of syndromes with motor deficiency, non progressive, but often changing, secondary to brain lesions or anomalies appearing in the early stages of brain development*".

It is partly surprising that the definition of CP remained quite unchanged for 40 years, even after the enormous progress achieved in imaging and other detection techniques, as well as in overall clinical nosography. Its strength maybe resides in its simplicity and in the fact that it is function-based. However, this does not imply that this definition is exempt from important limitations, both theoretical and practical (Dan and Cheron, 2004; chapters 2 and 11 of this book).

Among such limitations, the difficulty in tracing precise borders between normal and pathological motor development can be mentioned, with a concept of "normality" that seems more ideal and statistical than real (Latash and Anson, 1996), or the borders between certain types of motor control difficulties and awkwardness and of CP. Another issue is whether or not to exclude from the diagnosis of CP some children with progressive metabolic genetic syndromes with extremely slow progression, who are mostly classified as being affected by CP if not assessed by very expert clinicians. Another element of criticism is the exclusion from the definition of perceptive, cognitive, and behavioral aspects which, together with others, are often prevalent in determining the disability in the child.

In order to solve some of these issues, an international multidisciplinary team met in Bethesda (MD, USA) in July 2004. A revised definition was then produced by the Executive Committee of the team and published in 2006 (Rosenbaun et al. 2007).

> *"Cerebral palsy (CP) describes a group of disorders of the development of movement and posture, causing activity limitation, that are attributed to non-progressive disturbances that occurred in the developing fetal or infant brain. The motor disorders of cerebral palsy are often accompanied by disturbances of sensation, cognition, communication, perception, and/or behavior, and/or by a seizure disorder"*
> (Rosenbaum et al. 2007)

In this definition non-motor signs (perceptual, cognitive, epileptic) are now mentioned, but still as "accompanying" signs. Moreover, in line with the ICF approach, the importance of the assessment of activity limitation is acknowledged; people without activity limitation should not be included in the definition of CP. Despite progress, there are still limitations and unsolved critical points also in this attempt, as pointed out by Morris (2006) and in chapters 2 and 11.

Together with the work on the definition of CP, a growing number of proposals of new rehabilitation treatment methods were made, based on the increasing awareness of the close interactions between motor and psychological aspects in CP. The approach of these techniques was not aimed at recovering a maximum instrumental effectiveness, but at achieving the complete empowerment potential of the disabled person. The focus was shifted from exercises targeted at the recovery of single muscles to a more global approach on the control of posture and motion.

At the same time, a larger number of care and treatment centers were created, ensuring an increasingly specialized care service. Together with the simultaneous involvement of different clinical, psychological and psychopedagogical specialties, strong commitment was also devoted to the creation of special educational programs and social services for the support of families. The common aim was that of creating the optimal conditions to promote the individual maturation process regarding all the domains of development, to allow the patient to achieve the maximum level of independence.

The change in the approach to the disease and the implementation of early treatment inevitably implied a change in the type of problems to be faced. In the last decades, indeed, it has become more and more difficult to observe chronic clinical pictures with already stabilized and scarcely changeable multiple deficiencies. The path followed over the years was similar to the one that takes place every time interest is raised in a new type of disease: at first, the investigation is directed towards the most apparent and difficult cases, those that are usually easier to detect. The more causes that become known, the more earlier clinical signs of the disease that can be identified, allowing adequate treatment in a short time. By doing so, interest is shifted towards milder disease forms, with a complete change in the symptomatological background of the disease. This has also happened in CP, for which, in slightly more than a century, a complete revolution has occurred, not only in the interpretation of this clinical entity, but also in its clinical expression and in its natural history.

Initially conceived as an orthopedic deficiency of neurological origin, it was shortly recognized as a pathological condition involving more functional systems and, as such, requiring the concurrent attention of different specialists and care services. More recently,

1

it has started to be more and more considered as a complex developmental disorder, a disability that becomes increasingly evident during the growth of the individual, which, for this reason, deserves to receive early detection and treatment. In such a way, this disease, initially considered as orthopedic by Little, has become today the prototype of infant developmental disability.

Many issues are obviously still to be addressed, starting from the classification of CP.

Historical Models for the Classification of Cerebral Palsy

The large amount of criticism and the different proposals that were submitted over the years to the definition of CP reflected, and still reflect today, the uncertainty about the actual pathological features of this disease, due to symptom heterogeneity and to doubts related to its pathogenesis. Referring to the diagnosis, the term CP has the evident limitation of making no reference to etiology, physiopathology, clinical severity, or prognosis, to the extent that many researchers often expressed the need to abandon it.

Classifying and subdividing children with CP in different classes or categories of the same type may have other objectives that need to be considered to assess the validity and the effectiveness of a classification. In the case of CP, among such objectives could be listed epidemiological studies aimed at monitoring CP subtypes whose incidence could change over time, but also aimed at assessing the effectiveness of interventions or of other elements. As later stated, the judgment on the validity and on the usefulness of a classification is closely related to the aims by which the classification has been conceived and applied.

The continuous evolution of the concept of CP, together with the wide difference of clinical pictures, has led to the creation of different classification models. However, to-date none of these proposals has been fully able to evidence the multifaceted clinical expressions of the disorder, due to the impossibility to identify a single classification criterion that could be used as reference to subdivide and describe the different aspects of the disease in its evolution.

The first attempts at a classification date back to anatomopathologists, who tried to correlate the different forms of CP with the essentially inflammatory or hemorrhagic etiology of cerebral lesions. Indeed, for a long time, the different clinical syndromes were considered as being closely interrelated to cerebral lesions with a specific (vascular or infective) etiology. However, the limitation of this type of correlation was already pointed out by Freud, who, in his studies, underlined how the complexity of the transformation processes of cerebral lesions makes the nature of the primary lesion event poorly recognizable over time. The very scarce opportunities to perform anatomical investigations in individuals with CP make this type of classification mainly of theoretical interest.

Later, the prevailing aim became that of making a systematical classification of the different forms of CP according to the clinical criteria derived from traditional neurological semiotics, mainly based on the assessment of muscular tone anomalies and on the detection of reflex responses.

The main traditional classifications, with the same focus of the Little Club model of 1959, are based on muscle tone anomalies (hypertonia, dystonia, etc) as well as on the type of the prevailing neurological symptom (ataxia, choreoathetosis, etc) and on its somatic location (diplegia, tetraplegia, hemiplegia, etc). Even with some variations, all classifications following this approach are quite similar. The most popular are those by Ingram (1955, 1964), Crothers and Paine (1959), Michaelis and Edebol-Tysk (1989), the Australian school (Stanley et al. 2000; Evans et al. 1989) and, as the most widely recognized in Europe, the classification made by the Swedish school (Hagberg et al. 1975) and the classification by SCPE - Surveillance of Cerebral Palsy in Europe (2000). Some of these classifications include the "atonic" form, not included in others. The main diagnostic categories reported by these models are described as follows.

Traditional Clinical Syndromes

Spastic Tetraparesis

In tetraparesis, tone and motion disorders are usually severe, rarely symmetrical, "equally" involving upper and lower limbs, and generally becoming apparent from birth. Posture-motor development is severe delayed; the prognosis for autonomous walking and manipulation is adverse. Visual disorders (visual agnosia, gaze palsy, strabismus, reduction of visual acuity, etc) and hearing disorders are frequent. Epilepsy is very often present, usually in a secondary generalized form (infantile spasms, Lennox-Gastaut syndrome, etc). Mental failure is often associated, consequent both to the cortical neuropathological damage and to the early motor disorder, impairing the acquisition of the fundamental stages of physical development. Consequent to spasticity, patients suffer from widespread muscle contractures and from articular and skeletal position deformities. The most frequent anatomical lesions, also detectable *in vivo* through neuroimages and especially through magnetic resonance imaging (MRI), are represented by diffuse periventricular leukomalacia or by multicystic damage with severe cerebral atrophy.

Spastic Diplegia

In spastic diplegia, tone and motion disorders involve all four limbs, with more severe involvement of the lower limbs. This is the typical clinical picture of severe pre-term children, with high incidence of periventricular leukomalacia. The type of motor damage is caused by the proximity of the malacic lesions to the course of the cortico-spinal pathways to the lower part of the body. Hypertonia, mostly involving sural triceps and hip adductors, rarely becomes apparent before the third-fourth month after birth, and sometimes even later. Traditionally (but this term is no longer accepted, see chapter 3), the clinical history includes a "silent period" taking place after the acute stage of the cerebral damage and before tone disorders and motor development retardation become evident. Upper limb motricity is quite preserved; the prognosis for walking, even without walking supports, is usually favorable. Cranial nerve involvement is frequent, as well as strabismus. Intelligence and speech development are usually not impaired. Epilepsy is rare. Muscle contractures and articular deformities of the lower limbs are frequent.

Spastic Hemiplegia

Muscle tone and voluntary motion disorders only affect one body side. Involvement can be more marked in the upper or the lower limb, often mainly distal but sometimes also proximal. The prognosis for autonomous walking is almost always favorable. Patients often present with convulsion discharges, expressions of partial epilepsy. Alterations of the body pattern and of the praxic and gnosic organization are frequent. The development of intelligence can be impaired; when the paretic side corresponds to the dominant hemisphere, a retardation in speech development may be apparent. Muscle contractures and articular deformities usually develop in the paretic side, even at an early stage; muscle and bone trophysm is usually reduced. The anatomical and neuroradiological correlate is mostly represented by isolated poroencephalic cysts, lesions of the internal capsule, or even periventricular lesions, also bilateral, or by more diffuse damage of a cerebral hemisphere.

Ataxic Form

It is by far the rarest form of CP. Motion coordination disorders (tremors, dysmmetry, adiadocokinesia, etc) and balance disorders (ataxia) prevail. In the first months of life, it is characterized by the presence of a marked hypotonia, usually persisting even later in life; psychomotor development is usually delayed; often a cerebellar ocular nystagmus is present. Sometimes, it can be associated with symptoms of pyramidal origin. Speech is characterized by delayed development, sometimes even severe, and words are scanned. Mental deficiency is often present. From the anatomical point of view, these forms are associated with cerebellar damage and/or damage to cerebellar downstream pathways, usually due to malformative alterations, with structural growth defects, or with infectious diseases. Seldom it may derive from perinatal hypoxic-ischemic hemorrhagic damage.

Dystonic Form

Motor disorders result from an extrapyramidal system dysfunction, followed by a tone regulation alteration. Underlying muscular tone is reduced in rest conditions, while in conditions of stimulation and motor constraint it consistently increases, leading to postures that are fully overlapping to those observed in spastic syndromes. Rapid and non-coordinated involuntary hyperkinetic syndromes are constantly present, especially in the face and mouth. Pyramidal type clinical signs are sometimes associated (mixed forms). The continuous variability of tone also impacts mouth-speech muscles, resulting in an impaired voice emission, with very fast and often incomprehensible speech. Cognitive development is seldom impaired. At the encephalic level, the lesion is thought to be in the basal nuclei; when severe, it can be identified as the so-called "status marmoratus". Once mostly associated with neonatal jaundice due to mother-fetus incompatibility, this form of CP mostly represents the outcome of a severe perinatal asphyxia in term infants.

Athetosic (or Choreo-Athetosic) Form

Also in this form, symptoms are consequent to extrapyramidal system dysfunction, with the prevalent location in the caudate and putamen. The clinical picture is characterized by hypotonia and by the presence of slow, arrhythmic and continuous polypoidal movements, usually occurring from the first months after birth, and often by rapid, proximal, choreic movements involving the face, the tongue, and the distal part of the limbs. Pyramidal symptoms may coexist. Usually, the development of intelligence is not strongly impaired, and speech is dysarthric. When it is caused by hyperbilirubinemia, it is often associated with perceptive deafness.

Limitations of Traditional Classifications and Perspectives

The above-described traditional classification, which is still largely recognized and applied at the international level, presents some limitations that need to be evidenced to allow its correct application to clinical practice.

Indeed, if such categories may be useful in the systematical classification of clinical pictures, they are not so useful in early disorder diagnosis and classification. They do not consider an important element of CP: changes occurring during development. For this reason, an infant with a mainly hypotonic CP must be shifted into another category when, as it is often the case, a picture of spasticity occurs. Another important issue is represented by the difficulty in drawing useful prognostic elements from these classification models.

Unquestionably, these classifications are useful for epidemiological studies, allowing the assessment of incidence disorder and the comparison among different case studies. These types of studies also have an important social consequence, allowing the planning activity of those clinical structures in charge of early detection and care.

However, each classification, especially if employed for epidemiological objectives, but also for other objectives, must necessarily meet a number of criteria, among which is reliability, that is, the reproducibility of its results among different observers and among subsequent evaluations by the same observer, simplicity of use, and validity, i.e. the effectiveness in differentiating among individuals belonging to different groups. According to these parameters, the network SCPE - Surveillance of Cerebral Palsy in Europe (2000) - bringing together 14 centers in 8 countries, stated that the experience related to the application of these traditional classifications is not exempt from criticism. The large variability in the classification of children in the above mentioned categories, as evidenced in targeted research, has led SCPE experts to propose a simplified classification, abolishing the distinction between diplegia and tetraplegia and differentiating only between bilateral versus unilateral spastic forms (Colver and Sethumadhavan, 2002). A further recommendation of this group was also to devise specific training for health care professionals working in CP epidemiological projects. To that aim, an interactive DVD was prepared to teach health care professionals how to classify cases of CP.

The need of a classification methodology taking into account functional skills acquired by the child, rather than just focusing on the distribution or on the location of the motor disorder, is now perceived also at the international level. The Canadian group CanChild, author of the famous test on gross motor functions of children (GMFM, Gross Motor Function Measure), proposed a classification system (GMFCS, Gross Motor Function Classification System) based on the level of gross motor competence (sitting position, upright standing position, walking, etc) achieved by children of different age groups with CP (Palisano et al. 1997, 2000). It is an extremely useful tool to assess the measurement of disability and the level of autonomy achieved by the child, but it does not offer insight into the way a specific perceptive-motor function is organized and, therefore, it does not provide prognostic and rehabilitation orientation.

More recently, similar classification systems were proposed based on manipulation function, i.e. BFMFC (Bimanual Fine Manipulation Functional Classification) (Beckung and Hagberg, 2002), and MACS (Manual Ability Classification System) (Eliasson et al. 2006). They present similar advantages and drawbacks as GMFCS. SCPE proposed to add to all traditional diagnostic categories a double functional score by the application of GMFCS and BFMFC, along with a report about the etiological basis of the lesion and its main "associated" disorders, sensor disorders, cognitive disorders, epilepsy, etc.

Advances both in imaging technology and in quantitative motor assessments are challenging Freud's 100- year-old statement that correlations between neuroanatomy findings and clinical presentation in CP were weak. MRI can be used to detect structural impairments of the brain (Accardo et al. 2004) and to approximate the timing at which the brain was damaged (Krägeloh-Mann 2004). Correlations are emerging between the timing and location of the lesion and functional, cognitive, and sensory impairments.

The American Academy of Neurology has recommended obtaining neuroimaging findings for all children with CP whenever feasible. However, the goal of categorizing all patients on the basis of specific radiographic findings will require more development before implementation (Rosenbaum et al. 2006).

A thoroughly different approach, aimed at solving the problem of early detection and of prognosis, is the one based on the qualitative assessment of motor patterns in children with CP. An example of this classification model is offered by the work of Milani Comparetti (1978). The classification suggested by the author, derived from motor studies, refers to the dominant and stereotyped pathological patterns which may have an early impact on the motricity of the child with cerebral lesions. The detection and the careful assessment of these patters, according to the Author, would allow early detection and prognosis. The identification of different pathological categories (regression syndrome, diarchy I, diarchy II, etc) is therefore based on the presence/dominance of specific abnormal motor patterns (fetal patterns, extension pattern, startle, etc). Although it is a useful tool for early detection and prognosis, this classification presents different limitations, among which is the lack of indications for the rehabilitation treatment. Similar in many respects to the classification by Milani Comparetti is the classification pattern proposed by Michele Bottos, recently reviewed by himself (2002) and also including some elements drawn by the proposal by Ferrari.

An ideal model for the classification of CP, which could be useful both for prognosis and for the rehabilitation treatment (organization, results assessment), should be based on the identification of the physiopathological disorder determining the motor disorder in affected children. Of course, such disorders cannot be reduced only to spasticity or to the presence of "primitive reflexes" but have to be conceived as motor control defects. This more modern approach to the nature of the defect in CP (see chapter 4 and chapter 5) has largely been influenced by the updated neurophysiological reference models for motor control, normality, the main motor disorders of children (Shumway-Cook and Woollacott, 1995; Crenna, 1998; Cioni and Paolicelli, 1999; Fedrizzi, 2003). In this perspective, according to some authors (Ferrari, current text; Dan and Cheron, 2004) there are different groups of children in each of the traditional forms of CP (diplegia, tetraplegia, etc) that share stable strategies of motor control. For example, children with spastic diplegia, all of them with walking capacity, presenting with similar lesions at MRI and characterized by similar physiological processes (hypoxic-ischemic damage in prematurity), may conceal different strategies for motor control in walking (Ferrari et al. chapter 15; Dan and Cheron, 2004; Rodda et al. 2004). The most modern instruments for the recording and the off-line analysis of children's motor performances (videotape recording, 3D movement analysis and others) offer outstanding opportunities to formulate and validate classification assumptions based on these models.

An example of this novel approach to the definition and the classification of CP is offered by the model suggested for quite some time by Adriano Ferrari (Ferrari, 1990), largely covered by this text, which lays its foundations in considering CP not as an alteration of muscle tone or as a set of pathological motor patterns but as a problem of functional organization of the child in his interaction with the surrounding environment. The organization mode is related not only with the motor disorder but also with the cognitive, perceptive and motivation problems, which are interrelated to a certain extent. In this perspective, to prevent it from being fragmented and scattered, as well as to offer prognostic and rehabilitation elements, the classification must necessarily take into consideration all the mentioned aspects.

Conclusions

An extremely challenging time in the field of CP is underway, with the likely possibility to achieve, after more than one century, the aim set out by Freud about overcoming the concept of CP as a vague entity in favor of "more coherent and etiologically more well-determined" clinical pictures. For epidemiological objectives, traditional classifications may still maintain their validity, taking into account the suggestions deriving from the most advanced experiences of the experts in the field, such as the SCPE group. Certainly, the degree of disability will have to be assessed through tools with different levels of complexity, depending on the aims of the classification. Probably, the most modern neuroimaging techniques will allow the differentiating of categories of children with similar lesion nature and reorganization.

Certainly, the main interest of the rehabilitation professional is focused on classification approaches based on homogeneous deficiencies of motor control that are more strictly related to prognosis and treatment.

All these approaches, from the more traditional to the more modern, must follow the above described recommendation regarding reliability, simplicity and repeatability.

References

Accardo J, Kammann H, Hoon AH Jr (2004) Neuroimaging in cerebral palsy. Journal of Pediatrics 145:S19–27.

Bax MCO (1964) Terminology and classification of cerebral palsy. Dev Med Child Neurol 6:295-307

Beckung E, Hagberg E (2002) Neuroimpairments, activity limitations, and participation restrictions in children with cerebral palsy. Dev Med Child Neurol 44:309-316

Bottos M (2002) Paralisi cerebrale infantile: dalla guarigione all'autonomia. Piccin Editore, Padova

Cioni G, Paolicelli P (1999) Sviluppo fisico e motorio. In: Camaioni L (ed) Manuale di psicologia dello sviluppo (2a ed). Il Mulino Editore, pp 17-76

Colver AF, Sethumadhavan T (2003) The term diplegia should be abandoned. Arch Dis Child 88:286-290

Crenna P (1998) Spasticity and "spastic" gait in children with cerebral palsy. Neurosc Biobehav Rev 22:571-578

Crothers B, Paine R (1959) The natural history of cerebral palsy. Harvard University Press, Cambridge

Dan B, Cheron G (2004) Reconstructing cerebral palsy. J Ped Neurology 2:57-64

Denhoff E, Robnault IP (1960) Cerebral palsy and related disorders. McGraw Hill, NY

Eliasson AC, Krumlinde-Sundholm L, Rosblad B et al (2006) The Manual Ability Classification System (MACS) for children with cerebral palsy: scale development and evidence of validity and reliability. Developmental Medicine and Child Neurology 48:549-554.

Evans PM, Johnson A, Mutch L, Alberman E (1989) A standard form for recording clinical findings in children with a motor defect. Dev Med Child Neurol 31:119-129

Fedrizzi E (2003) I disordini dello sviluppo motorio. Piccin Padova

Ferrari A (1990) Interpretive dimensions of infantile cerebral paralysis. In: Papini M, Pasquinelli A, Gidoni EA (eds) Development, handicap, rehabilitation practice and theory. Excepta Medica, International Congress Series 902, Amsterdam, pp 193-204

Freud S (1897) Die infantile Cerebrallahmung. In: Nothnagel J (ed) Spezialle pathologie und therapie. Band IX, Th. III. Vienna Holder

Hagberg B (1989) Nosology and classification of cerebral palsy. Giornale di Neuropsichiatrica dell'Età Evolutiva 4:12-17

Hagberg B, Hagberg G, Olow I (1975) The changing panorama of cerebral palsy in Sweden 1954-1970. I. Analysis of general changes. Acta Paediatr Scand 64:187

Ingram TTS (1955) A study of cerebral palsy in the childhood population of Edinburgh. Arch Dis Child 30:85-98

Ingram TTS (1964) Paediatric Aspects of Cerebral Palsy. Livingstone

Krägeloh-Mann I (2004) Imaging of early brain injury and cortical plasticity. Experimental Neurology 190:S84-90

Latash ML, Anson JG (1996) What are "normal movements" in atypical populations? Behav Brian Sci 19:55-106

Little Club Clinics (1959) Memorandum on terminology and classification of cerebral palsy. Cerebral Palsy Bull 1/5:27

Little J (1861) On the influence of abnormal parturition, difficult labours, premature birth, and asphyxia neonatorum on the mental and physical condition of the child, especially in relation to deformities. Trans Obstet Soc London 3:293

Mac Keith RC, Mackenzie ICK, Polani PE (1959) Definition of Cerebral Palsy. Cerebral Palsy Bulletin 5:23

Mac Keith RC, Mackenzie ICK, Polani PE (1959) The Little Club: memorandum on terminology and classification of cerebral palsy. Cerebral Palsy Bulletin 5:27-35

Michaelis R, Edebol-Tysk K (1989) New aetiopathological and nosological aspects of cerebral palsy syndromes. Giorn Neuropsic Età Evolutiva Suppl 4:25-30

Milani Comparetti A (1978) Classification des infirmités motrices cérébrales. Médicine et Hygiène 36:2024-2029

Minear WL, Binkley E, Snow WB (1954) Report: Nomenclature and Classification Committee presented before American Academy for Cerebral Palsy. Paediatrics 1956:841-852

Morris C (2007) Definition and classification of cerebral palsy: a historical perspective. Dev Med Child Neurol Suppl 109:3-7

Mutch L, Alberman E, Hagberg B et al (1992) Cerebral palsy epidemiology: where are we now and where are we going? Dev Med Child Neurol 34:547-551

Osler W (1889) The Cerebral Palsies of children. Mac Keith Press, London

Palisano R, Rosenbaum P, Walter S (1997) Development and reliability of a system to classify gross motor function in children with cerebral palsy. Dev Med Child Neurol 39:214-223

Palisano RJ, Hanna Steven E, Rosenbaum PJ et al (2000) Validation of a model of Gross Motor Function for children with cerebral palsy. Physical Therapy 10:974-985

Phelps W (1950) Etiology and diagnostic classification of cerebral palsy. Nervous Child 7:10

Rodda JM, Graham HK, Carson L et al (2004) Sagittal gait patterns in spastic diplegia. J Bone Joint Surg 86:251-258

Rosenbaum P, Paneth N, Leviton A et al (2007) A report: the definition and classification of cerebral palsy April 2006. Dev Med Child Neurol Suppl 109:8-14. Erratum in: Dev Med Child Neurol Suppl 49(6):480

Shumway-Cook, A, Woollacott M (1995) Motor control: theory and practical applications. MD: Williams and Wilkins, Baltimore

Stanley F, Blair E, Alberman E (2000) Cerebral Palsies: epidemiology and causal pathways. clinics in developmental medicine No. 151. Mac Keith Press, London

Surveillance of Cerebral Palsy in Europe (2000) Surveillance of cerebral palsy in Europe: a collaboration of cerebral palsy registers. Dev Med Child Neurol 42:816-24

Guide to the Interpretation of Cerebral Palsy

2

A. Ferrari, S. Alboresi

Definition of Cerebral Palsy

The term cerebral palsy in English, paralisi cerebrale infantile in Italian, infirmité motrice cérébrale in French, paralisis cerebral in Spanish and Zerebral Bewegung Störung in German defines a *"persistent but not unchangeable disorder of posture and motion, due to an organic and not progressive alteration of the cerebral function, determined by pre-, peri- and post natal causes, before its growth and development are completed"* (Bax, 1964; Spastic Society Berlin, 1966, Edinburgh, 1969).

> *"Cerebral palsy describes a group of disorders of the development of movement and posture, causing activity limitation, that are attributed to non-progressive disturbances that occurred in the developing foetal or infant brain. The motor disorders of cerebral palsy are often accompanied by disturbances of sensation, cognition, communication, perception, and/or behavior, and/or by a seizure disorder"*
> (Bax, Goldstein, Rosenbaum et al. 2005)

The word **disorder** refers to a situation, i.e. a final state, and not to a disease, which instead can improve or worsen and in theory can also be overcome. So actually a CP child can be considered neither a sick person nor a healthy individual. The adjective **persistent** reinforces the concept of disorder as a stable and definitive situation, therefore not evolving (to express this concept, the term fixed encephalopathy is also used), while the expression **not unchangeable** partly weakens this concept by showing that motor and non-motor disorders provoked by CP can however improve or worsen, spontaneously by itself or through treatment. These changes can be related to the competence of the central nervous system (CNS) and to the structural conditions of the locomotion apparatus (LA). Improvements are possible due to the plasticity of the CNS, its compensatory capabilities, and, above all, the possibility to learn through experience. With regard to worsening, it is necessary to note that, although the damage does not itself evolve, environmental demands on the CNS become more and more challenging over time, consequently worsening the

2

disability due to the deficiencies carried over from the past. The lack of a certain function in fact will subsequently hinder the acquisition of further functions related to it (Sabbadini et al. 1982).

By **posture** (from Latin, ponere situs) we refer to a mutual relation in a specific instant between the segments composing the body (to be intended as an articulated solid, therefore moldable) to be assessed according to the coordinates of the surrounding space (geocentric coding according to Berthoz, 1997). The word **motion** indicates a displacement in space and time of one or more body segments or of the body as a whole, hence the passage from one posture to another. "*Motion can be considered as a sequence of postures. It can be achieved only after reaching a short or long term posture adjustment, before and during its execution*" (Jackson, 1874). However, posture is not a passive state, it is not only a "frozen" movement (Denny Brown, 1966). It is a preparation to move, an internal simulation of motor sequence features generally aimed at an action (Berthoz, 1997). It means being prepared to act: "readiness to move" (Bernstein, 1967).

The expression **alteration of cerebral function** underlines that palsy provokes the inability of the whole CNS, rather than the deficiency of one or more single organs, apparatuses or structures that compose it (hemispheres, cerebellum, brainstem, etc.). "*No function is located in only one cerebral structure, but all functions result from the cooperation of specific structures creating pathways in which neuron activity circulates in a sequential way accomplishing the operations belonging to each structure*" (Berthoz, 1997). Therefore the word **cerebral** has to be interpreted, in a holistic way, as a synonym of CNS instead of a synonym of brain (a system, as an operating coalition among different organs, systems and structures, is always greater than and different from the sum of the singular individual parts that compose it). It will be later described that a significant correlation among damage site, type, timing and degree with the nature and severity of the consequent palsy is only partially possible.

The expression **growth and development of the nervous system**, which refers to the adjective "cerebral" rather than to the noun "function", means that palsy in children differs from palsy in adults, being characterized by a lack of function acquisition instead of the loss of already acquired functions. However, the expression remains ambiguous, since it does not define which functions it refers to, although it is usually attributed to motor functions (posture control, locomotion, and manipulation).

The international definition of CP does not cover the full meaning of "palsy" and "cerebral", which deserve a more detailed and in-depth specific analysis.

Palsy: from a Neurological to a Rehabilitative Diagnosis

When detecting a new CP case, the first task of the rehabilitation physician is to translate to the parents the concept of lesion (loss of CNS anatomic and physiologic integrity) into the concept of palsy (alteration of produced functions). The therapeutic proposals to modify palsy (physiotherapy, antispastic drugs, orthosis and devices, functional surgery, etc.) will be accepted and agreed upon, and the achieved results will be evaluated and positively judged, in proportion to in what way and how much the idea of "palsy" has been conveyed and understood.

Neurological semeiotics describes the defect and locates the deficiency in terms of *objective signs* and *subjective symptoms* (hypertonic, dystonic, flaccid, tetraplegic, diplegic, hemiplegic, etc.) and approximately judges their *severity* according to a descriptive and empirical criterion (very severe, severe, moderate, mild, slight, etc). Sometimes it makes use of *etiology*: Little's disease with regard to premature infant diplegia; other times it favors *pathogenesis*: Phelps' syndrome, the athetoid tetraplegia with deafness which represents the consequence of severe nuclear icterus, etc.

Neurological diagnosis considers palsy as the sum of the defects which are present in the child's motor repertoire (spasticity, clonus, Babinski, scissor pattern, etc.); however it does not sufficiently clarify their nature. It is therefore important to be able to assess, beside the repertoire of *defects*, also the *resources* that are still available, be they related to the individual or to the context he lives in, and their *applicability,* since rehabilitation treatment is precisely based on exploiting resources rather than eliminating defects. "Therapy" can neither cancel CP symptoms or signs nor hide or disguise them (inhibit pathological reflexes, making hemiparetic patients' motricity symmetrical, etc.), nor can it solve the so-called "developmental delay". Instead, it will have to bring out the capabilities of the person considering his specific defects and residual abilities within his living environment, i.e. his physical environment as well as the social and cultural context (environmental treatment according to Pierro et al. 1984).

"It is therefore necessary to adopt a more global approach towards the child and his continuous interaction with the surrounding environment and the problems it poses, creating a dynamic balance between the child's personal resources and the most adequate (and most effective) tools to be able to activate and enhance them. The evoked function, therefore, can modify the acting subject and his interaction with the environment, if looked at from a cognitive point of view. In this sense, motor damage has to be seen as a direct or indirect pathology involving the planning of cognitive functions. There is an attempt to restore the pragmatic and communicative value of the individual-environment relation by stimulating and reinforcing the growth of the inner Self" (Caffo, 2003).

The easiest way to make parents understand the problem of palsy is to introduce it as a problem related to **muscles**. It could be a problem of *weakness*: the muscles are unable to support the head, they are too weak to straighten the trunk, extend the knees, etc. Or, it could be a problem due to *excessive power*: the muscles are too vigorous and they unbalance their antagonists, like those which result in clench fists, cross thighs (scissor pattern), tiptoe walking (talipes equinus), etc. If CP is presented as a problem related to muscle weakness, parents will probably focus on exercising, meaning "a lot" of physical exercise, massage, "shocks" (electrotherapy), progressive training (also in gyms, with weights, and "machines" for adolescents and young adults), as well as muscle transfer proposed by orthopedic surgery similar to poliomyelitis, and so on. Conversely, if the CP problem is related to excessive strength, together with massage (with de-contracting purpose instead of toning and trophic aim), more or less reliable -motor relaxation techniques will be seen as more important, as well as muscle stretching maneuvers, chemical inhibition of spasticity with systemic, zonal or focal drugs (like tizandine, dantrolene, baclofen, botulinum toxin, alcohol, phenol, etc.), serial inhibiting casts, progressive correction orthoses, surgical penalization (tendon release, aponeurectomies, more or less balanced selective myotomies, etc.).

However, it is difficult to explain how, in the same child, the same muscle can be simultaneously too weak at one end and too strong at the other: rectus femoris might be too weak as a knee extensor and too strong as a hip flexor, hamstrings might be too weak as thigh extensors and too strong as knee flexors and so on.

Progress could be achieved by trying to explain palsy not in terms of strength, but in terms of **contraction**. It is useful to remember that the term "spastic" (a particular type of muscle contraction) has for a long time been employed to refer to the whole category of CP patients. However, a definition of muscle contraction is essential, since there are many types of contraction disorders: they could be related to an excessive recruitment of motor units (MU) (quantity error) or to an excessively prolonged contraction, that is to say the inability to voluntarily relax muscles (duration error, which Dupré defined as paratonia in 1907); or there can be a timing error, an error related to the quality of contraction (tonic or phasic), determining early and excessive tiring; or there could be an error in the association of activated muscles (co-contraction); or a tendency to preserve imposed position (defined by Dupré as catalexia in 1907), or a lack of passivity due to overreaction to stretching, proportional to execution speed (the main meaning of spasticity), etc.

If parents understand that their spastic child's problem is mainly related to muscle spasticity, the request for anti spastic therapy will justify: the use of myorelaxing drugs, administered orally, with continuous intratechal infusion, with local infiltration, etc.; the surgical severing of efferent motor pathways (neurotomies); interruption of the spinal afferent loop which is responsible for the vicious circle generating spasticity (rhizotomy, radicellotomy, etc); the interruption of the activity of uninhibited central structures generating spasticity (stereotaxis); and the stimulation of cerebral areas which control inhibiting substances (deep brain stimulation), etc.

Another aspect of contraction alteration is represented by **muscle tone** disorders. Once again in this case it remains difficult to explain to parents what palsy is. First of all it is necessary to explain what tone we are talking about: do we mean the tone related to the single muscle that remains contracted also when it should be relaxed since it is "at rest", or the tone related to all muscles involved in maintaining that stable relation between segments that we named posture, that is to say **postural tone**? (see chapter 13).

The first option (muscle tone) can explain why we can see a child who is hypotonic in the trunk and hypertonic in the limbs, hypotonic in the ventral area and hypertonic in the dorsal one, hypotonic in flexion patterns and hypertonic in extension ones. Conversely, the second option (posture tone) explains the condition of a child who is hypotonic while lying still on the floor or when being held and suddenly becomes hypertonic if he has to stand up or is forced to move. As stated by Wallon (1949), the tonic function is not just a quantity equation between hypotonia and hypertonia, but it reflects through its fluctuations the harmony or lack of harmony in relation to the external environment. In all these uncertain cases, the word **dystonic** is used too often, since it refers to any tone variation; it ends up being too general and superficial and a synonym of CP itself.

Therapeutic modalities aimed at correcting tone disorders are extremely confusing: in

Interpretive model of different events that are usually classified by the term spasticit	
Excess-related mistakes	*Deficit-related mistakes*
> Recruiting intensity (excessive strength)	> Length of contraction (inability to relax)
> Recruiting speed (spasm)	> Timing error (delayed de-contraction)
> Recruiting extension (irradiation)	> Overreaction to stretching
> Space-time combination (pathological pattern)	> Early tiring
> Recruiting connection (associate movement)	> Reduced endurance (exhaustibility)
> Anomalous association (co-contraction)	
> Tonic or phasic character	
> Hyper-reflexia	
> Dyskinesia	
> Mirror movements	
> Pathological synkinesis	
> Catalexia	
> Primitive support reaction	
> Freezing, simplification	
> Myotactic crutch of hemiplegia	
> Perceptive defense (second skin)	
> Adaptive solution (exploitation of pathological synergy)	

or out of water? Supported or contrasted? Heavier or lighter? Stronger or weaker? On singular parts or globally? On foot or by horse? etc.

It is now clear how a vision which is overly focused on muscles, strength, contraction and tone is insufficient to explain to parents the real nature of CP.

It could be more adequate to conceive palsy as a **movement** problem, but only by defining which elements alter it (measure, form or content).

It might indeed be a problem of *measure*: on the one hand the "spastic" child who does not move enough, while on the other hand the "dyskinetic" one who moves too much. Physiotherapy should therefore both restore lost movement (physical motion) and correct it (change its form and remove defects). But it is difficult to explain how, in the same "spastic" child, besides the problem of not moving enough there is also inability to stop moving and stay still (postural control), or how, in the rich repertoire of the "dyskinetic" child, some movements which are fundamental to action, since they are related to orientation, direction, balance and defense, can be noticeably lacking.

It could be a problem connected to *motion pattern*, as Milani Comparetti has always stated (1978). In CP, the type of palsy can be recognized by competing patterns (i.e. first and second diarchy, see chapter 13), and its severity is indicated by their aggressiveness and stereotype (i.e. tetraplegia with antigravity defense in flexion, see chapter 13). Physiotherapy therefore should first of all deal with motion pattern. The "spastic" child should increase his repertoire by progressively acquiring new motor modules (greater ability to change), while the "dyskinetic" child should extract invariability rules from his variability, to make his actions more effective.

It could be a problem related to the *content* of motor activity, that is to say the relation between the chosen goal and the motor tool adopted to achieve it. Hence, palsy could involve not just tools but also aims (palsy as poverty of contents and rigidity of adopted strategies). The poverty of the CP child is not just a matter of motor behavior, but also involves the cognitive, emotional and relational areas. It is not just an inability to move but more precisely an inability to act.

In CP, palsy can contain all these elements and can be interpreted as a problem related to motion alteration, in terms of measure, form and content.

Time dimension does not fit into this interpretation: palsy is not just inability to act in space, but above all it is immobility in time, the unsurpassable delay and eternal promise of a future unachievable because it has already gone by. Time is the dimension of change, the true essence of growth. The lack of change measures palsy severity (time without change). If time could be stopped, maybe no goal would become unreachable. It is not a coincidence that the first expression used to announce CP in infants is "**psychomotor delay**". "*Until some years ago, according to psychiatric nosography, the word "delay" entailed the prediction of possible recovery. This concept has changed during the years, and "delay" has become a general synonym of function inadequacy. This change has been favored by the fact that the expression "delay" is more easily accepted because it contains and evokes the idea, the hope, or the ambiguity of recovery. However, for the same reason, delay has not been well defined, especially with reference to prognosis, considering the complexity of development dynamics and plasticity that characterizes the developmental age. In this regard, let us point out that the word "delay" mainly constitutes the concept of level, stage or phase, therefore refers more to the disorder quantity and not to the quality, it does not give importance to strategy analysis and adaptation modalities, hence it does not adequately refer to variability and development discontinuity [...] The word "psychomotor" has acquired particular importance due to the influence of a vision that rightly correlates the expressions "psychomotricity" and "psychomotor" to a synthesis and over all to the entire set of functions, repeating that "psychomotricity" includes motor, cognitive and relational aspects. The expression "psychomotor" delay becomes, at a "psychomotor" age, a synonym of global developmental delay: it does not refer to a function but to an age and a development stage, where multiple problems (encephalic kinetic pathologies, cognitive deficits, communication disorders, conditions of poor stimulation or giving up) become evident through motor expression*" (Camerini and De Panfilis, 2003).

Therefore, it becomes necessary to think more generally about the meaning of motion.

Motion is the first and most important tool possessed by the child to adapt (that is to say to become adequate) to the environment in which he lives and, at the same time, to progressively be able to adapt this environment to meet his specific needs. "*Adapting to the*

*new environment is indeed the first form of learning that the child has to face after birth".
(Bottos, 2003). "Contact with the external world, the fact of living immersed in the
surrounding world, from which he receives and to which he is obliged to give, is one of the
essential conditions for growth. Growing means building Self, different and renewed each
day, building the external world, which is richer and richer because it is continuously
better known and experienced in different ways, building and refining knowledge tools ..."*
(Sabbadini, 1978, 1995).

In CP, palsy means being contemporarily inadequate for the surrounding environment
and unable to act on this in order to adapt to it. Palsy therapy should therefore be intended
as building in the child the ability to adapt to the environment and to adapt it to himself
(development and recovery of adaptive functions), and as an intervention on the environment to make it more adequate to a poorly adaptable individual (elimination of physical,
social and cultural barriers).

Interpreting palsy as an interaction problem between the individual and the environment rather than as a problem related to posture and motion represents a completely innovative perspective. In CP, palsy cannot be seen or interpreted as a loss, a limitation, a stop,
a stiffening, an obstacle, or a constraint but as a response attempt to satisfy both the internal
need to be adequate and the external need to adapt to the immediate environment, created
by a child whose nervous system has been irremediably damaged. Palsy is an answer but
not a definitive one, it is not the end of a process but it is the start of a never ending process
that we have to define necessarily as development, since it is the result of the individual's
adaptation, within his pathology, to his specific environment (Ferrari, 1990a). Developmental age is a period of time where no condition is stable, not even the palsy.

But are we absolutely sure that motor disorder is the main cause for altered interaction
between individual and the environment in CP? What is the role of the **perceptive
problem**?

The motor action is designed to serve a specific purpose, according to the characteristics of the task to be carried out and the result to be achieved, but also according to sensitive and sensorial information that needs to be collected (a finger exploring temperature is
not the same as that that appreciates texture, or that touches an edge, or that presses a
computer button, etc). The ability to make a correct movement depends on the integrity of
the sensations that are needed to guide the execution of the action (see chapter 5). Lack of
attention and negligence testify to the inability to use a limb, which would potentially be
able to move, due to a poor perceptive support. There could be a difficulty in peripheral
collection and transfer to the information center (sensations), or there could be a problem
related to their recognition and comparison (perceptions), or their subsequent processing
(representations). However, also in a "peripheral" patient, the prognosis for the recovery of
a plegic limb is directly more connected to the problem of preserving sensitivity rather
than producing motion. But if it is true that a correct movement supposes a correct perception, it is also true that a correct perception can only be achieved through the performance
of a correct and specialized movement. Perception and movement are therefore the two
sides of the same coin, which are united by the motor control concept (Gibson, 1966; Lee
et al. 1997). However, perception cannot only be interpreted as information selection,
recognition and processing, that is as perceptive attention, but also in the opposite way, as

perceptive tolerance. For each type of perception it is possible in fact to identify a measure, which is specific for each individual, over which the collected information can become unbearable. Muscle tone variation cannot result from an alteration of motor control, but it can rather be a sign of a perceptive disorder: fear of space and depth, kinesthetic discomfort produced by motion (actively generated or passively sustained) sense of vertigo, awareness of instability, etc. (see chapter 14).

Cerebral

The use of the word "cerebral" is inappropriate for two reasons: first of all because the lesion does not only and always affect the brain, but it can also affect and impair other structures (cerebellum, brainstem, etc.), and secondly because the word recalls the idea of structure, while instead it should be attributed to the concept of system. The lesion of an organ can be limited and isolated but it cannot be overcome. The lesion of a system can allow a different functioning modality of the system itself (IT concept of network), but it affects all the consisting parts. "*The organization of motor ability is not a function related to more or less rigid patterns involving neuronal cortex circuits, but the interaction between different structures of the CNS, inside which there are afferent impulses coming from other levels*" (Brodal et al., 1962).

If, on the one hand, there can be alternative solutions, functional substitutions, and adjustments that make the individual able to build the function "despite" the lesion (plasticity), on the other hand we must recognize that no system function will remain undamaged by the consequences of the lesion. Therefore, CP rehabilitation cannot be anything but "global". It is important to highlight that the therapeutic project has to be all encompassing in itself and not just an intervention performed by a single therapist, or, even worse, an adopted therapeutic technique, which instead needs to be analytical, selective, and targeted in order to be effective.

Rehabilitation does not have to deal with the lesion as the loss of a more or less important or large part of an organ or system, which can be at least partially compensated by the activation of reserve or substitution structures (neuronal growth, dendritogenesis, synaptogenesis, etc). In CP, in fact, palsy means a different functioning of the entire system (computational error), due to a foreseeable internal coherence (self-organization), underlying the so-called "natural history" of any clinical form.

We have to accept the fact that a child is a living system and that each experience, event, and change will become a part of him and can never be canceled. The therapy will only be superimposed on the system to guide it to a better and more effective functioning (changeability, streamlining) but, in any case, without ever managing to achieve some degree of normality.

Defects analysis (**lesions**) will have to be countered by resources avaliability (**functions**). First of all, resources have to be linked to the person and interpreted not only as what has remained (residual potential) as opposed to what has been irremediably lost, but rather as the continuous commitment by the individual to adapt himself to the environment and to adapt the physical and social world in which he is living to himself (environmental rehabilitation according to Pierro et al. 1984). Therefore, the individual's resources do not have to be limited to the world of modules, combinations, and motor sequences, that is to the repertoire that physiotherapy should expand and correct, but they should also be extended to the individual's needs, dreams, rights and duties, necessities, and desires.

The traditional concept of CP as a **palsy of development** (defect analysis) theoretically has to be replaced with the notion of **development of palsy** (Ferrari, 1990b), i.e., as the product of the relationship that the individual however tries to dynamically build with the surrounding environment (resource semeiotics). *"Each individual, during his onthogenic development, through the interaction with the external world, builds his own representation of the world that is made up of facts and relations among facts, that are hierarchically organized according to an increasing complexity, corresponding to behavior strategies that allow him to survive in the best possible way"* (Starita, 1987). Hence, development is the expression of a dynamic interaction between biological maturation and environment (Camerini and De Panfilis, 2003).

Child CP

The term cerebral palsy does not only refer to an age, but it also describes the specificity of child palsy as a lack of function acquisition (compared to the usual age of appearance), as opposed to adult palsy as loss of already-acquired functions. In this sense, breast-feeding age and infancy seem to be the deadlines for CP.

During the construction of adaptive functions, precise **development deadlines** can be recognized. Within these deadlines the child has to become aware of his needs and of the rules related to the mechanisms and processes needed to comply with them. *"Functional deadlines are dates within which different developmental competences, that are individual, neuromotor, cognitive, emotional, environmental, technical, family-related and social, must come together to develop those functions which are critical for the development, for example walking. The lack of even one of this requisites at its appointment deadline can be sufficient to block a motor competence that otherwise would be potentially ready"* (Papini and Allori, 1999).

Growing up while respecting the deadlines means to be able to face and solve specific problems (needs, desires) once they become significant for the individual.

The influence of the environment on the CNS during extrauterine life has been well documented for a long time. Nervous system functions, especially adaptive ones, although produced by genetically programmed structures, need contact with the environment in order to develop and stabilize (epigenesis according to Changeaux, 1983). In the case of the CNS lesion, to accomplish potentially "undamaged" functions and to "recover" the affected ones (plasticity) this epigenetic process becomes even more relevant. The genetic characteristics of the structure will not be available forever to meet those of the environment in order to fix a certain function; but, as shown by Cowan (1973), CNS development is also made up of processes for the removal and the re-attribution to different goals of what was potentially available but had not been used. Quite simply, the function allows the CNS to save the structure only if it is activated within a determined period of time (date or critical period, meant as time of structure "fertility"). *"The process of function differentiation results to be closely related not only to CNS maturation development, but also to its integrity and to the experiences (environmental variable) of the individual"* (Stella and Biolcati, 2003). In rehabilitation, it must be clearly understood that some functions can be proposed to the child only within specific periods of time (in time) and that development is not just a sequence of chronological acquisitions, regardless of *why* (needs and desires), *when* (importance of the experience), and *how* (influence of models and environment).

> *"The intervention of gravity in motion organization occurs during particular development moments. For example, if the action of gravity is modified in young rats, a significant delay in locomotion development is observed. Therefore, there is a critical period for motricity, at around ten days after birth, during which the nervous system needs gravity as a reference to organize movement co-ordination"* (Berthoz, 1997).
>
> "Wiesel and Hubel (1969) *showed that in new-born kittens, that do not usually open their eyes until the 10th day of life, if the period of eyelid closure is experimentally extended, the retina, already connected to the visual cortex by a detailed topography on the basis of adult's configuration, becomes un-organized and experiences permanent regression"*

Only those functions acquired within determined periods (met deadlines) become part of the individual's identity and therefore become impossible to renounce. In children with CP, identity development is not always necessarily simultaneous with motor development. This is why the rehabilitation of CP children requires a completely different approach from the rehabilitation of adults with neural damage and, in terms of methodology, justifies the existence of "windows of opportunity" beyond which the re-educational treatment of the function loses its intrinsic meaning.

> *"....Functional activities/abilities do not follow a fixed hierarchical order (milestones), but they change according to the individual's age range. For example, walking is an important goal between 0 and 2 years of age and between 3 and 5 years, and it can still be so between 6 and 8 in some specific situations, while it is not so important later on (outside time limit). Conversely, being able to autonomously use a manual or electric wheelchair instead becomes a important developmental progress. This device can be proposed to patient already between 3 and 5 years of age, if walking prognosis reveals negative"*
>
> *The continuation of re-educational treatment is to be considered as unjustified if, after a reasonable period of time, no significant modification has occurred (outside time limit....)*
>
> Guidelines for the rehabilitation of children affected by cerebral palsy, 2005

In CP, together with the space dimension, defining the nature and size of the deficit (posture and gesture disorder, perceptive organization disturbance, conceptual deficiency, etc.), there is a time dimension that explains how and why the individual's ability to modify himself reduces according to age, while his adaptation to disability progressively increases. From a **primary damage** of organs, systems, and CNS structures directly related to the lesion site, there is a shift to a **secondary damage** represented by a missing acquisition of motor, cognitive, communicative, and relational competences (also from a morphological point of view: during the first stages of cortical development, the lesion of a cortical area provokes defects in the neuronal maturation of other areas, since they have no trophic support from the damaged area's connections), and then a **third damage** or LA pathology occurs (weakness, fatigue, instability, ROM limitation, bone deformity, etc.), which further contributes to reducing the choice of freedom provided by CP to the individual's CNS (**developmental disability**) (see chapter 12).

References

Bax M (1964) Terminology and classification of cerebral palsy. Dev Med Child Neurol 6: 295-97

Bax M, Goldstein M, Rosenbaum P et al (2005) Proposed definition and classification of cerebral palsy. Dev Med Child Neurol 47:571-6

Bernstein NA (1967) The coordination and regulation of movement. Pergamon Press, New York

Berthoz A (1997) Le sens du mouvement. Odile Jacob Edition, Paris. English edition: Berthoz A (2000) The brain's sense of movement. Harvard University Press, Cambridge, Ma

Bottos M (2003) Paralisi cerebrale infantile. Dalla "guarigione all'autonomia". Diagnosi e proposte riabilitative. Piccin editore, Padova

Brodal A, Pompeiano O, Walburg F (1962) The vestibular nuclei and their connections, anatomy and functional correlations. The William Ramsay Henderson Trust, Oliver and Boyd, Edinburgh London

Camerini GB, De Panfilis C (2003) Psicomotricità dello sviluppo. Carocci Faber editore, Roma

Changeaux JP (1983) L'homme neuronal. Librarie Arthème Fayard

Cowan W (1973) Neuronal death as a regulative mechanism in the control of cell number in the nervous system. In: Rockstein M (ed) Developmental and aging in the nervous system. Academy Press, New York, pp 19-41

Denny-Brown D (1966) The cerebral control of movement. Sherrington Lectures VIII, Liverpool University Press

Ferrari A (1990a) Interpretative dimensions of infantile cerebral paralysis. In: Papini M, Pasquinelli A, Gidoni EA (eds) Development, handicap, rehabilitation: practice and theory. International Congress Series 902, Excepta Medica, Amsterdam, pp 193-204

Ferrari A (1990b) Presupposti per il trattamento rieducativo nelle sindromi spastiche della paralisi cerebrale infantile. Eur Med Phys 26:173-187

Ferrari A, Cioni G, Società Italiana di Medicina Fisica e Riabilitazione (SIMFER), Società Italiana di Neuropsichiatria dell'Infanzia e dell'Adolescenza (SINPIA) (2005) Guidelines for rehabilitation of children with cerebral palsy. Europa Medicophysica vol. 42 n. 3 pp 243-60

Gibson JJ (1966) The senses considered as perceptual system. Houghton Mifflin, Boston

Jackson JH (1874) On the nature of the duality of the brain. Med Press Circ 1, 19, 41, 63

Lee DN, von Hofsten C, Cotton E (1997) Perception in action approach to cerebral palsy. In: Connolly KJ, Forssberg H (eds) Neurophysiology and neuropsychology of motor development. Clinics in Dev Med 143/144 Mac Keith Press, Cambridge University Press, Cambridge, pp 257-285

Milani Comparetti A (1978) Classification des infirmités motrices cérébrales. Médicine et Hygiène 36:2024-2029

Papini M, Allori P (1999) Il progetto abilitativo nel bambino con disabilità. Giorn Neuropsich Età Evol 20:260-273

Pierro MM, Giannarelli P, Rampolli P (1984) Osservazione clinica e riabilitazione precoce. Del Cerro Editore, Pisa

Sabbadini G (1995) Manuale di neuropsicologia dell'età evolutiva. Feltrinelli editore, Bologna

Sabbadini G, Bonini P, Pezzarossa B, Pierro MM (1978) Paralisi cerebrale e condizioni affini. Il Pensiero Scientifico editore, Roma

Sabbadini G, Pierro MM, Ferrari A (1982) La riabilitazione in età evolutiva. Bulzoni editore, Roma

Starita A (1987) Metodi di intelligenza artificiale in rieducazione motoria. In: Leo T, Rizzolatti G (eds) Bioingegneria della Riabilitazione. Patron editore, Bologna, pp 225-239

Stella G, Biolcati C (2003) La valutazione neuropsicologica in bambini con danno neuromotorio. In: Bottos M (ed) Paralisi cerebrale infantile. Dalla "guarigione all'autonomia". Diagnosi e proposte riabilitative. Piccin editore, Padova, pp 53-61

Wallon H (1949) Les origines du caractère chez l'enfant. Presses Universitaires de France, Paris

Wiesel and Hubel (1970) The period of susceptibility to the physiological effects of unilateral eye closure in kittens. J Physiol 206 pp 418-436

PART II
Function Analysis

Functional Diagnosis in Infants and in Very Young Children: Early Predictive Signs

3

G. Cioni, A. Guzzetta, V. Belmonti

Introduction

The progress achieved in the last decades in Neonatal Intensive Care Units (NICU) has extensively modified the care of the infant at risk, and especially that of extremely low birth weight infants and of infants with other conditions of high neurological risk. Life expectancy has considerably increased for these children, but they still remain at risk for neurological damage caused by perinatal infections, hypoxic-ischemic damage, hemorrhagic insult, or by a combination of these factors. Compared to the effort produced to monitor functional indexes and respiratory or cardiovascular activities, there is a surprising lack of detailed information about the functional status of the central nervous system (CNS) of patients in neonatal intensive care. Often, even a general evaluation of the vigilance or the integrity of the infant's perceptual or motor system is lacking.

Some progress has been achieved in the last few years with the development of neuroimaging techniques. Computed tomography (CT scan) has allowed the detection of intracranial hemorrhages or severe hypoxic-ischemic damage. This is, however, quite an invasive technique due to its ionizing radiation, and it requires the transfer of infants, often in unstable conditions, from the NICU to the department of neuroradiology. The advent of cerebral ultrasonography (US) has allowed visualization of the hemorrhagic or hypoxic damage and monitoring at the patient's bedside. Moreover, this technique is safe, noninvasive, and relatively cheap (Govaert and De Vries, 1997, for a review). There are, however, limitations to the use of cerebral US, mainly related to the examiner's experience and to the low spatial resolution of this technique.

More recently, new neuroimaging techniques based on magnetic resonance imaging (MRI) have been applied to the infant's brain, allowing the exploration, with high spatial resolution, of different types of cerebral damage (Rutherford, 2002, for a review). Also for this technique, however, the transfer of the infant from the NICU is required; moreover, the equipment is extremely expensive and therefore not affordable for all centers.

It has to be remarked that even the most advanced neuroimaging techniques show only structural changes of the brain, thus not providing information on the functional

The Spastic Forms of Cerebral Palsy. Adriano Ferrari, Giovanni Cioni
© Springer-Verlag Italia 2010

status of the nervous system. For this and other reasons, a clinical assessment is always necessary.

Techniques for the Clinical Assessment of the Neonatal Nervous System

In newborns and infants, the clinical assessment is generally carried out through traditional neurological methods, largely based on out-dated models of CNS development. Nowadays, it is widely recognized that the human nervous system can express many complex and rapidly changing functions from as early as the first weeks of gestation. The fetal and neonatal nervous system is no longer seen as just a collection of reflexes, but as a complex organism producing a great deal of endogenously generated behaviors. This may partly explain why many clinicians are often convinced that the contribution of the neurological examination to the diagnosis and prognosis at these early stages of development is limited.

To be truly useful, new methods of neurological assessment should fulfill a series of basic requirements, clearly indicated by Prechtl (1990, 2001). Firstly, they should include items strictly related to the age-specific functional repertoire of the CNS, which changes very rapidly during the pre- and early post-natal periods, when new functions emerge and others undergo a regression. The concept of ontogenetic adaptation of the organism to the age-specific requirements of the environment (Oppenheimer, 1981) may account for such a rapid transformation of neural functions.

However, not all the age-specific functions of the infant's repertoire are suitable for clinical assessment. Diagnostic tools also need to be non-invasive and non-time-consuming. Both conditions are needed to allow repeated longitudinal observations, particularly of fragile individuals such as pre-term infants. Moreover, the reliability and prognostic value of these methods have to be carefully tested. New methods of functional evaluation of newborns and infants which fulfill these conditions may help in understanding the possible consequences of brain lesions, as detected by brain imaging techniques.

As previously mentioned, the assessment tools usually employed in clinical settings do not necessarily meet all the stated requirements. Some of them, though standing as milestones of modern infant neurology, are still influenced by considerations drawn from adult neurology and experiments on animal models. For instance, Saint-Anne Dargassies (1977) developed a pioneering examination protocol based on the evaluation of active and passive tone. Other methods were then proposed in the following decades, including items for muscle tone, postural-motor milestones and, in some cases, behavioral aspects.

The method proposed by Prechtl (1977) has been standardized and validated only for the examination of infants at term. It includes the extremely important concept of behavioral status, but many of its items are still based on muscle tone and responses integrated at a low-level in the CNS. Moreover, it is rather time-consuming and cannot be applied to pre-term infants.

The Neonatal Behavioral Assessment Scale (NBAS) is a technique developed by Brazelton (Brazelton and Nugent, 1973) for examining the behaviour of term infants during the first couple of months of age. Its conceptual basis is founded on the assumption that the newborn has active and specific responses to environmental stimulations, rather than passive behavior. NBAS involves the exploration of spontaneous neonatal behavior and the ability to modify the infant's behavioral functioning by means of facilitations by the examiner. Four functional systems are taken into account: autonomic nervous system regulation, motor activity organization, behavioral state organization, and social abilities. Each system interacts with the others and is influenced by the environment. The NBAS includes 28 behavioral items and 18 neurological items related to reflexes. On the basis of Brazelton's assessment of term infants, Als et al. (1982) standardized a behavioral scale for pre-term infants, the Assessment of Pre-term Infant Behavior (APIB), devised to be employed in NICU and for providing and monitoring individualized intervention program. These techniques are time-consuming and not easily applicable in clinical settings. Moreover, for the same test a high intra-individual day-to-day variability in the responses has been shown (Sameroff, 1978). Their main applications are in research and early intervention protocols.

Currently, the most recently updated and extensively validated method for the traditional neurological examination of pre-term and full-term newborn infants is the Hammersmith Neonatal Neurological Examination, first published by Dubowitz and Dubowitz (1981) and updated by Dubowitz et al. (1999). These authors adapted tests drawn from the previous works of Prechtl, Saint-Anne Dargassies, Parmelee and Michaelis (1971), and Brazelton, in a simplified and user-friendly format, also including items based on the concepts of Prechtl and co-workers on spontaneous motor activity (see below). The Hammersmith Neonatal Neurological Examination consists of 34 items organized in six sections: posture and tone, tone patterns, reflexes, movements, abnormal signs, behavior. The scoring sheet presents each item with a 5 (or less)-point scale, supplied, when possible, with diagrams and/or brief instructions. There is no normal range to refer to: instead, each item is simply graded from its minimum to its maximum response. Moreover, instead of using just a quantitative total score, the whole pattern of responses is recorded and assumed to reflect many different aspects of neurological function. Typical normal and abnormal patterns are extensively described in the manual (Dubowitz et al. 1999) and have proven easily recognizable and clinically useful for diagnosis and prognosis. For research purposes, an optimality score for full-term newborn infants was also calculated on the basis of the statistical distribution of the responses observed in a cohort of 224 low-risk term babies ranging from 6 to 48 hours of post-natal age (Dubowitz et al. 1999). The differences in responses at the same age between this population and that of infants born pre-term were described in another study (Mercuri et al. 2003). Moreover, significant correlations have been demonstrated between abnormal findings at the test, especially in the posture and tone section, and specific MRI alterations due to hypoxic-ischemic encephalopathy (Mercuri et al. 1999).

On the basis of the neonatal examination, the same authors also developed a protocol for use after the neonatal period in infants up to 24 months of age: the Hammersmith Infant Neurological Examination (Dubowitz et al. 1999). It is divided into three sections: the first one consists of 26 non-age-dependent items assessing cranial nerve function, posture, movements, tone and relexes; the second one provides a summary of motor milestones, where the cut-off between normal and abnormal responses is age-dependent;

finally, the third section comprises three simple behavioral items. An optimality score was obtained on a cohort of low-risk term infants assessed at 12 and 18 months of age (Haataja et al. 1999). Its prognostic value as to motor outcome has been found to be high both in pre-term infants born before 31 weeks of gestation (Frisone et al. 2002) and in term infants with hypoxic-ischemic encephalopathy (Haataja et al. 2001).

Although both the Hammersmith Neonatal Neurological Examination and the Hammersmith Infant Neurological Examination have been tested in several clinical and research settings, they also present some limitations. Most items are still correlated with muscle tone and reflexes and the distinction between normal and abnormal patterns may turn out, to some extent, to be rigid and schematic, hardly comprising the whole complexity of the infant's repertoire. Moreover, while several studies have reported statistically significant correlations between clinical findings and mid- and long term outcome, others have reported a relevant number of false positive and false negative results, especially among pre-term infants (Volpe, 2008, for a review of follow-up studies).

Neonatal Neurological Examination: a Novel Approach

A novel approach to neonatal neurological evaluation, based on the observation of fetal, neonatal, and infant spontaneous motor activity, was recently proposed by Prechtl (1990, 2001). The reasons for this choice derive from theoretical as well as practical considerations. First, it is known that both the fetus and the infant present with a high number of endogenously generated motor patterns, i.e., movements produced by central pattern generators located in different areas of the CNS and not necessarily triggered by an external input; second, there is strong evidence that spontaneous motor activity is an indicator of alterations occurring in the nervous systems, one that is more sensitive than the responses to sensory stimulations and reflexes.

Among the many distinct endogenously generated motor patterns appearing during the course of early human development (such as startles, twitches, stretches, yawning, breathing, and isolated limb movements), general movements (GMs), i.e. global movements involving all the body parts, have proven to be the most effective in the functional assessment of the young nervous system. In fact, GMs are complex, occur frequently, and last long enough to be observed and scored properly. According to the definition, they involve the whole body in a variable sequence of arm, leg, neck, and trunk movements. They wax and wane in intensity, force, and speed and have a gradual beginning and end. Rotations along the axis of the limbs and slight changes in the direction of movements make them fluent and elegant and create the impression of complexity and variability (Prechtl, 1990).

Normal and Abnormal GMs

The normal developmental course of GMs and its deviations (Figure 3.1) have been extensively described in several studies and correlated to a number of pathological conditions

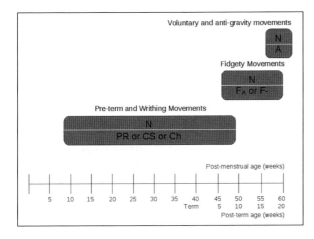

Fig. 3.1 Development of normal and abnormal general movements.
N, Normal; *A*, Abnormal; *PR*, Poor repertoire; *CS*, Cramped-synchronized; *Ch*, Chaotic; F_A, Abnormal fidgety movements; *F-*, Absence of fidgety movements

and events in the neonatal and infant period, as well as to the neurological outcome at toddler and school age (see below).

GMs emerge as early as 9 to 12 weeks post-natal age (de Vries et al. 1982) and continue after birth without substantially changing their form, irrespective of when birth occurs (Prechtl, 2001). A first, very gradual modification takes place during the whole fetal life or pre-term age, consisting in a progressive reduction of movement speed, jerkiness, and amplitude. While before term we speak of *pre-term* or *fetal GMs*, from term until about 6 to 9 weeks the expression *writhing movements* is used, indicating the typical writhing character of GMs at this age (Hopkins and Prechtl, 1984). Writhing movements are characterized by small to moderate amplitude and by slow to moderate speed, are typically ellipsoid in form, and describe trajectories that tend to lie close to the sagittal plane (Hopkins and Prechtl, 1984; Cioni et al. 1989; Prechtl et al. 1997b; Einspieler and Prechtl, 2004). A second, deeper change in form occurs at 6 to 9 weeks post-term age, when writhing movements gradually disappear and are replaced with *fidgety movements* (Hopkins and Prechtl, 1984; Prechtl et al. 1997a, b). Fidgety movements (FMs) are small movements of moderate speed and variable acceleration involving the neck, trunk, and limbs, occurring in all directions, and continual in the awake infant, except during fussing, crying, and focused attention (Prechtl et al. 1997a, b; Einspieler and Prechtl, 2004). They do not involve simultaneously all body parts, but typically migrate from one to the other, involving one or more segments at a time for a few seconds in an on-going flow of movement. The impression received by the observer is still that of complexity, fluency, and variability, as in the writhing period, though the form of movement is different. Various other motor patterns emerge and mingle with GMs in the fidgety period, such as wiggling-oscillating and saccadic arm movements, swipes, mutual manipulation of fingers, manipulation of clothing, reaching and touching, leg lifting, trunk rotation, and axial rolling (Hopkins and Prechtl, 1984; Einspieler and Prechtl, 2004). FMs gradually disappear from fifteen weeks post-term age onwards, but may still be present up to six months.

3

Studies performed in high-risk fetuses as well as in pre-term and full-term newborn infants with and without cerebral damage have shown that it is not the quantity of GMs but rather their quality that is a good indicator of neurological conditions (Prechtl, 1990). GMs of infants with cerebral impairment lack complexity, fluency, and variability. They can be slow and monotonous or rapid and chaotic, do not involve all spatial planes, nor all body parts, start and stop abruptly, and do not show the gradual fluctuation in amplitude, strength, and speed, that is always present in normal individuals. The 'global' visual perception of movement form (Gestalt perception) represents a powerful and reliable instrument for the analysis of such alterations. This approach to behavioral observation, initially suggested by the Nobel Prize winner Konrad Lorenz, allows the simultaneous consideration of a large number of details and their relationships in a much shorter time and with much more comprehensiveness than it would take for the separate analysis of each aspect at a time. By means of Gestalt observation, abnormal GMs can be recognized and classified as described below (see also Figure 3.1).

In the pre-term and the writhing periods, GMs may lose their complex and variable character and have therefore a *poor repertoire*, or be *cramped-synchronized,* or *chaotic.*

- *Poor repertoire*: the sequence of involvement of the different body parts is monotonous, movement components are few, repetitive, and not so complex as in normal GMs (Ferrari et al. 1990; Prechtl et al. 1997b). They can also appear more abrupt and jerkier than normal, but fluency is in general more spared than complexity and variability.
- *Cramped-synchronized*: GMs completely lack complexity, fluency, and variability; all limb and trunk muscles contract and relax almost simultaneously (Ferrari et al. 1990; Prechtl et al. 1997b).
- *Chaotic GMs*: movements of all limbs are of large amplitude and occur in a chaotic order without any fluency or smoothness. They consistently appeare to be abrupt (Bos at al. 1997; Ferrari et al. 1997). Chaotic GMs are rare and often evolve into cramped-synchronized GMs (Einspieler and Prechtl, 2004).

In the fidgety period, GMs are judged as abnormal if FMs are absent, or if they have an abnormal appearance.

- *Absence of fidgety movements* means that they are never observed from 9 to 20 weeks post-term.
- *Abnormal fidgety movements* look like normal ones but their amplitude, speed, and jerkiness are exaggerated (Prechtl et al. 1997a, b). Abnormal FMs are rare and their predictive value is low.

Other methods of GM assessment have been proposed (Touwen, 1990; Van Kranen-Mastenbroek et al. 1992, 1994; Kakebeeke et al. 1997, 1998). Among them, Hadders-Algra et al. (1997, 2004) introduced a new terminology and enlarged the categorization of the existing types of GM abnormalities. In particular, normal GMs are defined according to Prechtl's definition, while abnormal GMs are distinguished as "mildly" or "definitely" abnormal. According to the Authors' definition, "mildly abnormal GMs" lack fluency but still show some complexity and variation; they were correlated with the later development of behavioral disorders and minor neurological deficits (MND, see below).

GMs: the Assessment Procedure

A thorough description of the standardized assessment procedure of GMs can be found in Einspieler and Prechtl, 2004. As stated above, the assessment is based on visual Gestalt observation, as suggested by Konrad Lorenz for the global analysis of complex behaviors (Lorenz, 1971). This is a powerful but vulnerable instrument, and there are therefore some basic rules to follow in order to obtain a reliable and reproducible evaluation (Einspieler et al. 1997, 2005). Firstly, the standard observation should be recorded and not carried out directly at the bedside. Recording modality, timing and duration are described in the cited references. Importantly, the observer does not need to watch the whole session, as only three selected GM sequences are needed for scoring. Any attention to details should be avoided in order not to interfere with Gestalt perception. Although an experienced observer can reach a reliable judgement after just one to three minutes of optimal GM recording, an accurate evaluation should preferably be carried out on a set of properly selected record-ings, called an *individual developmental trajectory* (IDT). Three instances of abnormal IDTs are shown in Figures 3.2, 3.3 and 3.4 (see the next sections for the prognostic value of the patterns shown). An optimal IDT is made up of at least two to three recordings (of at least three GM sequences each) in the pre-term period, one or two at term or early post-term age, and at least one between 9 and 15 weeks post-term (Einspieler and Prechtl, 2004). Gestalt perception is also liable to observer weariness and calibration decay; therefore, it is advisable to take a break every 45 minutes and to re-calibrate Gestalt perception by watching a criterion standard normal recording from time to time (Einspieler et al. 1997).

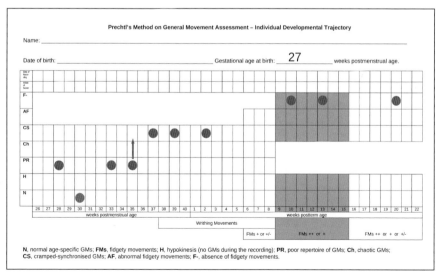

Fig. 3.2 Individual developmental trajectory of an infant born pre-term, small for gestational age (SGA), with severe postnatal respiratory distress. He initially presented with PR GMs, transiently improved towards normal GMs, and then worsened until the development of a predominant CS pattern (see below in the text for details), followed by an absence of FMs. The outcome was that of a spastic diplegia with severe learning difficulties

3

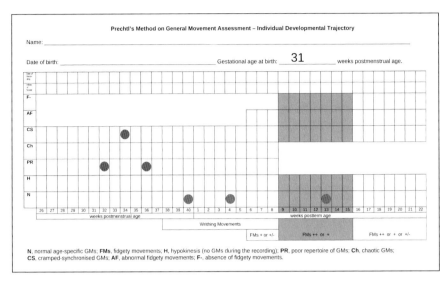

Fig. 3.3 Individual developmental trajectory of an infant born pre-term with peri-natal respiratory distress. He presented with PR GMs, evolving towards a transient CS pattern (see below in the text for details), then again to PR GMs, followed by normal writhing and fidgety movements. The outcome was normal

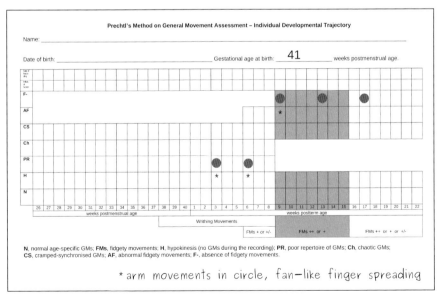

Fig. 3.4 Individual developmental trajectory of an infant born at term with birth asphyxia. She presented with PR GMs characterized by arm movements in a circle and exaggerated (fan-like) finger spreading as additional features (see the text for details), evolving towards an absence of fidgety movements. She later developed a dyskinetic tetraplegia

Being fully non-invasive, this method can even be applied to infants who are still in the incubator. GMs assessment is cheap, fast, and easy to perform. The interobserver agreement has proved to be very high, but only if the observers are trained and experienced enough (Einspieler et al. 1997). Evaluation of almost 9000 assessments performed by some 800 observers demonstrated that 83 percent of the assessments were fully correct, while the mere discrimination between normal and abnormal GMs was correct in 92 percent (Valentin et al. 2005). The average kappa (Cohen, 1969) in four studies on 108 infants assessed by 11 observers was 0.88 (for a review see Einspieler and Prechtl, 2004). Test-retest reliability for global judgement proved also to be extremely high (100 percent, Einspieler, 1994).

However, there are some limitations to the application of GMs observation to infants at high risk. Obviously, this technique cannot be applied to those infants who do not produce any movement, such as in cases of severe CNS depression or coma. Moreover, the standard observation procedure strictly requires properly timed and performed video-recordings, which are not always available. Video reviewing and GMs selection for assessment may be rather time-consuming. Recently, a new method of direct, camera-free observation of GMs was proposed and validated, proving useful in case videorecording is impossible (Guzzetta et al. 2007). Importantly, its agreement with the standard method was found to be rather high at fidgety age (correlation coefficient: 0.79) but much lower in the writhing period (correlation coefficient: 0.42), although false negative cases regarding the prediction of CP, were never seen.

In conclusion, Prechtl's method of GMs assessment seems to be a useful and complementary supplement to the traditional neurological examination in newborns and infants, and it can successfully replace it when it cannot be applied.

Semi-quantitative Assessment and Motor Optimality Scores

A semi-quantitative assessment of GM quality can be achieved by applying Prechtl's optimality concept (Prechtl, 1980). A score for optimal or non-optimal performance is given to every movement criterion, such as amplitude, speed, movement character, sequence, range in space, and onset and cessation of GMs. Two different optimality scoring lists have been reported: the first for pre-term and term age (Ferrari et al. 1990) and the second covering motor behavior, not only GMs, of 3- to 5-month-old infants (Bos et al. 2003; see Figure 3.5). The latter score is the sum of five components: 1) the presence and quality of FMs, 2) the presence and normality of other movement patterns, 3) the presence and normality of postural patterns, 4) the age-adequacy of the concurrent motor repertoire, 5) the quality of the concurrent motor repertoire. The presence and quality of FMs is always the most important feature and is weighted more than the other components.

A GM optimality score can be used for statistical calculations and comparisons with other measures, especially in research settings. GM optimality scoring should never be carried out prior to or together with the qualitative assessment of GMs by means of Gestalt observation, the latter being easily disrupted by detail analysis.

Assessment of Motor Repertoire - 3 to 5 Months
Christa Einspieler and Arie Bos, the GM Trust 2001

Name: ....

born: .... Postmenstrual Age: .... Birth weight: ....

Recording Date: .... Postterm Age: ....

Number of movement patterns observed: |_| normal (N) |_| abnormal (A)

N A	fidgety movements	N	hand-face contact	N A	legs lift, flexion at knees
N A	swiping movements	N	hand-mouth contact	N A	legs lift extension at knees
N A	wiggling-oscillating movem.	N	hand-hand contact	N	hand-knee contact
N A	saccadic arm movements	N	hand-hand manipulation	N A	arching
N A	kicking	N A	fiddling / clothes, blanket	N A	trunk rotation
N A	excitement bursts	N	reaching	N	axial rolling
A	'cha-cha-cha movements'	N A	foot-foot contact	N A	visual scanning
N A	smiles	N	foot-foot manipulation	N	hand regard
N A	mouth movements	N A	segmental movements arms	N	head anteflexion
N A	tongue movements	N A	segmental movements legs	A	arm movements in circles
N A	head rotation	A	segm: discrepancy arm-leg	A	almost no leg movements

Number of postural patterns observed: |_| normal (N) |_| abnormal (A)

N A	head in midline (20 °)	N	variable finger postures	A	hyperextension of the neck
N A	symmetrical	A	predominant fisting	A	hyperextension of trunk
N A	spontaneous ATNR absent or	A	finger spreading	A	extended arms/ on / above
	could be overcome	A	few finger postures		surface are predominant
A	body and limbs 'flat' on	A	synchronised opening and	A	extended legs / on / above
	surface		closing of the fingers		surface are predominant

Movement character (global score):

N	smooth and fluent	A	stiff	A	predominantly slow speed
A	jerky	A	cramped	A	predominantly fast speed
A	monotonous	A	synchronous	A	predomin. large amplitude
A	tremulous	A	cramped-synchronised	A	predomin. small amplitude

Motor Optimality List:

1.	Fidgety Movements	normal	❏	12
		abnormal	❏	4
	± + ++ P D	absent	❏	1
2.	Repertoire of	age-adequate	❏	4
	co-existent other movements	reduced	❏	2
		absent	❏	1
3.	Quality of other movements	N > A	❏	4
		N = A	❏	2
		N < A	❏	1
4.	Posture	N > A	❏	4
		N = A	❏	2
		N < A	❏	1
5.	Movement character	smooth and fluent	❏	4
		abnormal, not cramped-synchr.	❏	2
		cramped-synchronised	❏	1

Motor Optimality Score:
Maximum: 28; Minimum: 5

Fig. 3.5 Questionnaire for the assessment of the spontaneous motor repertoire of 3- to 5-month-old infants

GM Assessment and the Prognosis of Cerebral Palsy

The principal aims of neurological analyses in newborn and older infants are: to detect the presence of anomalies in neural functions, to monitor the natural history of neurological disorders, and to assess the effects of therapies. The neurological examination should also contribute to prognosis formulation, i.e. the mid- and long term prediction of the neuro-motor and psychological development of the infant with CNS structural or functional anomalies. Currently, extensive effort is devoted to the detection and prognosis of CP from the first weeks of life, due to the high incidence of this disorder in infants at risk, especially in extremely low birth weight infants. Moreover, early CP detection is extremely important in order to establish as early as possible a proper relationship with the family, as well as to start early treatment protocols and to assess their results. Perlman (1998) stated that there are no early markers of evolution towards CP in infants, but that diagnosis exclusively depends on the traditional neurological examination. The novel approach of infant evaluation based on GM observation, instead, seems to be very reliable for CP early detection and prognosis.

The first longitudinal study on the predictive value of the various abnormal GM patterns revealed cramped-synchronized (CS) GMs as highly predictive for spastic cerebral palsy (Ferrari et al. 1990). Later, in the to-date largest longitudinal study on GM assessment (Prechtl et al. 1997a), 130 infants were followed from birth to the age of two (Figure 3.6). The sample included both term and pre-term infants, subdivided into two categories of low and high risk according to the results of cranial ultrasound, which consisted of the whole spectrum from normal to abnormal findings due to hypoxic-ischemic lesions or haemorrhages. The study confirmed the significance of CS GMs: all infants who consistently showed CS GMs at repeated assessments later developed spastic cerebral palsy, which means that the specificity of consistent CS GMs was 100% (Prechtl et al. 1997a).

Another early marker for the later development of cerebral palsy is the absence of FMs between 9 and 15 weeks post-term age (Prechtl et al. 1997a). Absence of FMs can be preceded by CS GMs or, less frequently, by poor-repertoire GMs. In another study, transient CS GMs (i.e., not consistent through repeated assessments before and after term age) were associated with later cerebral palsy only if followed by an absence of FMs (Ferrari et al. 2002). The absence of fidgety type GMs has proven to be the most sensitive predictor of cerebral palsy, with a 95% sensitivity, its specificity being also very high (96%; Prechtl et al. 1997a).

Thus, both these events, namely, the persistence of the CS pattern and the absence of FMs, are highly specific markers for the subsequent evolution towards spastic CP (see also Figures 3.2 and 3.3 for two opposite, prototypical IDTs). However, in the above-mentioned largest longitudinal study (Prechtl et al. 1997a), two subjects who presented with normal FMs subsequently developed CP (both with a mild form of hemiplegia). Moreover, the results of this study did not allow the prediction of CP type and severity: the CS pattern and the absence of fidgety movements were present both in subjects who subsequently developed tetraplegia and in those who developed diplegia or hemiplegia. In the following sections, the prognosis of CP type and severity, as well as that of non-CP neurodevelopmental disorders, will be dealt with.

In conclusion, the predictive value of Prechtl's method of GM assessment for the prognosis of cerebral palsy has proven to be very high, overcoming the limits of the traditional neurological examination, especially, but not only, in pre-term infants (Ferrari et al. 1990; Cioni et al. 1997a, b). This holds true not only in large case studies, but also in individual

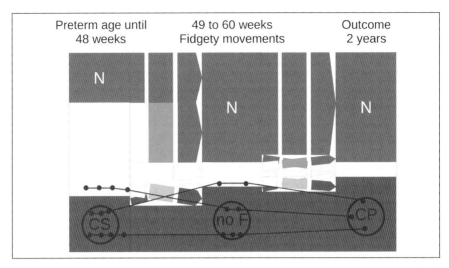

Fig. 3.6 Results of the neurological assessment the during pre-term period and until 48 weeks of post-natal age, the fidgety period (49-60 weeks of post-natal age) and the outcome, at least at 2 years, in 130 infants at high risk. Data from Prechtl et al. (1997). *N*, Normal; *PR*, Poor repertoire; *CS*, Cramped-synchronized; *AF*, Abnormal fidgety; *no F*, no fidgety; *MMR*, Mental and motor retardation; *CP*, Cerebral palsy (as a courtesy of C. Einspieler)

cases, especially when longitudinal assessments are performed. The quality of GMs is correlated with brain pathology, as detected by the proper neuroimaging techniques, such as repeated cranial US in the pre-term infant (Ferrari et al. 1990; Prechtl et al. 1997a; Bos et al. 1998a; Cioni et al. 2000) and MRI both in pre-term (Spittle et al. 2008; 2009) and full-term infants at risk for hypoxic-ischemic encephalopathy (Prechtl et al. 1993) or focal infarction (Guzzetta et al. 2003). GM quality is however more related to neurological function than to neuroimaging findings and can have a higher predictive value for later neurological outcome in certain conditions, showing, for instance, a higher sensitivity than neonatal MRI in very pre-term infants (Spittle, 2009), and overall higher sensitivity and specificity than cranial US (Prechtl et al. 1997a). As far as it concerns clinical investigations, the integrated use of GM observation and of traditional neurological examination seems to give the best results for the early prediction of cerebral palsy (Snider et al. 2008; Romeo et al. 2008), allowing the assessment of neurological impairment and functional limitations at a very early developmental stage (Palmer, 2004). The inclusion of GM assessment into organized follow-up programs and the developmental surveillance of infants at risk is definitely strongly recommended (Palmer, 2004).

Prognosis of Type and Severity of Cerebral Palsy

Several other studies investigated the ability to of GMs early predict, not only the presence of CP, but also its type and severity. The present section is mainly concerned with the prediction of the overall severity of CP, while the specific issues of the detection of unilateral and dyskinetic forms of CPs are dealt with in the following sections.

As already stated, consistent or predominant CS GMs have proven able to predict spastic CP from its very early stage of development, but the detection of this GM pattern can give even more information on the prognosis. Ferrari et al. (2002) studied 84 pre-term infants with cerebral lesions shown on cranial ultrasound. The motor outcome was assessed at least at the age of three and classified in agreement with the GMF-CS (Gross Motor Function Classification System, Palisano, 1997). GMs were recorded and assessed in a blind study from birth to 56 to 60 weeks post-natal age (Table 3.1). A traditional neurological examination was also performed. All infants with a consistent or predominant CS pattern (33 cases) developed CP. In case of transient CS GMs (8 cases), either the onset of mild CP (when FMs were absent) or normal development (when FMs were present, see for instance the IDT in Figure 3.3) were observed. Moreover, the earlier the onset of CS GMs, the worse the neurological outcome. In this study, GM observation showed an overall 100% sensitivity, and the specificity of the CS pattern ranged from 92.5% to 100%, much higher than that of a traditional neurological examination.

Another study (Cioni et al. 1997b) described other aspects of the early motor repertoire in individuals who later developed spastic diplegia (DP) and tetraplegia (TP). Serial video-recordings, made in the first weeks of life until the acquisition of walking with or without supporting devices, were retrospectively analyzed in a group of pre-term infants, 12 with DP and 12 with TP. Anoher 12 children at risk for neurological development, but without CP, were also assessed. Videotape assessment was carried out on the basis of quantity and quality criteria related to motor patterns, posture organization, and other characteristics. As expected, severe alterations of spontaneous motor activity were present from the first observations both in individuals with DP and in those with TP, but not in the control group. Moreover, already from the first months of life, relevant differences were noted in both motor and postural characteristics in the two groups with CP. Already from 8 weeks post-term age onward, DP children showed more frequent segmental movements of the

Table 3.1 Correlation between characteristics of cramped-synchronized GMs and neurological outcome

Cramped Synchronized General Movements	Neurological Outcome						
	Norm.	Severity of the Motor Deficit					
		ICP-I	ICP-II	ICP-III	ICP-IV	ICP-V	Total
Absent	36	7	-	-	-	-	43
Occasional	4	4	-	-	-	-	8
Predominant (start at ≥43 weeks)	-	4	3	1	-	2	10
Predominant (start at ≥43 weeks)	-	-	2	2	3	2	9
Consistent	-	-	-	3	5	6	14
Total	40	15	5	5	9	10	84

CP, cerebral palsy, classified according to the Gross Motor Function Classification System (Palisano et al. 1997); *Norm*, Normal (from Ferrari et al. 2002, modified).

3

upper limbs than TP ones. Segmental movements are flexion, extension, and rotation distal movements occurring either isolated or within the context of a GM but not as a part of an extension or flexion movement of the whole limb (Cioni et al. 2000). In addition, head control in supine and in a supported sitting position was better in DP than in TP subjects of the same age. These data confirm that a careful examination of the child's motor and postural patterns allows the early identificaion of markers of the evolution towards diplegic vs tetraplegic CP.

As far as it concerns CP severity, a recent study by Bruggink et al. (2009, in press) investigated the predictive value of the motor optimality score at fidgety age (see above) in relation to the level of self-mobility of CP children at school age. In this study, the abnormal quality of the concurrent motor repertoire was separately scored as monotonous, jerky, and/or cramped.

The assessment of the motor optimality score was carried out on the video-tapes of all children with a diagnosis of CP (n=37) who had been prospectively included in a total sample of 347 children. All of them underwent neurological examination between 6 and 12 years of age and were classified according to the GMF-CS (Palisano et al. 1997). Nine children had a unilateral form of CP, while the other 28 showed bilateral involvement. The distribution among the five levels of the GMF-CS was as follows: 32% were at level I, 8% at level II, 27% at level III, 11% at level IV, 22% at level V. The higher the motor optimality score of the infants, the better the GMF-CS level. Using a cut-off point of 9 and distinguishing, as to the outcome, children with low self-mobility (GMF-CS levels III to V) from those with high self-mobility (GMF-CS levels I to II), the positive and the negative predictive values of the optimality score were both 70%. Among the various single features of the motor repertoire, the absence of an age-adequate motor repertoire, a cramped quality of the motor repertoire, an abnormal kicking pattern, and a non-flat posture were all associated with lower levels of self-mobility.

GMs and Early Signs of Hemiplegia

Congenital hemiplegia, the most frequent type of CP in term infants, and the second one, after diplegia, in pre-term infants, is often detected only after the first year of life (see chapter 16). It is still debated whether such a delayed diagnosis is due to a late appearance of clinical signs or to a difficulty in the detection of already present signs.

From neonatal age onward, neuroimaging techniques such as US, CT, or MRI allow one to identify the cerebral lesions which can cause hemiplegia, in particular cerebral infarction. Therefore, it is now possible to perform prospective studies on the neurological development of these children. Two different studies on the observation of spontaneous motor activity for the prediction of hemiplegia have been carried out: one on pre-term infants with unilateral intraparenchymal echodensity (UIPE), which is the main feature of venous infarction (Cioni et al. 2000), and the other on full-term infants with cerebral infarction detected by MRI (Guzzetta et al. 2003).

Cioni et al. (2000) longitudinally assessed the quality of GMs in 16 pre-term infants with UIPE and in 16 controls, from birth until around 4 months post-term. Contextually,

Table 3.2 Side of prevalence of segmental movements in children with focal lesions on brain ultrasound

Case no.	UIPE Side	Pre-term Period 30-35 weeks of PNA	Term Period 38-42 weeks of PNA	Fidgety Period 49-56 weeks of PNA	Outcome at 2 years
1	LT			LT	RT Hemi
2	LT			LT	N
3	RT			RT	LT Hemi
4	LT			LT	RT Hemi
5	LT			LT	RT Hemi
6	LT			LT	RT Hemi
7	LT				Mild delay
8	RT			RT	LT Hemi
9	LT	RT		LT	Dipl (RT>LT)
10	RT	-		RT	LT Hemi
11	RT			RT	LT Hemi
12	LT	-	RT	LT	RT Hemi
13	LT	LT		LT	RT Hemi
14	LT			LT	RT Hemi
15	RT	-		LT	Mild delay
16	RT			RT	LT Hemi

PNA, post-natal age; *UIPE*, unilateral intraparenchymal echodensity; *RT*, right; *LT*, left; Hemi, hemiplegia; *Dipl*, diplegia; -, no observation (from Cioni et al. 2000, modified).

longitudinal neurological examinations were also performed (Table 3.2). At two years, 12 of the infants with cerebral lesions showed hemiplegia, and one had double hemiplegia (see chapter 15). From the first observation onwards, all infants with UIPE showed bilaterally abnormal GMs, and in those with unfavorable outcome FMs were absent. During the fidgety period (9-16 weeks post-term), all infants with subsequent hemiplegia showed an asymmetry of distal segmental movements, which were reduced or absent on the side contralateral to the lesion. Also the findings of the traditional neurological examination were abnormal for the large majority of subjects, although normal findings were recorded in some cases, especially during the pre-term period. Asymmetries were found at neurological examinations at term age in 9 of the infants with cerebral lesions and in 2 controls. These results suggest that unilateral brain lesions induce clear neurological signs, and abnormal GMs in particular, although these abnormalities are not initially asymmetrical. A reduction of segmental movements on one side of the body during the third month postterm is highly predictive of hemiplegia.

Similar results were obtained in another group of 11 term infants with neonatal cerebral infarction (Guzzetta et al. 2003). In all cases, FMs were predictive of neurological outcome, and the presence of early motor asymmetries, especially in segmental movements, at 3 - 6 and 9 - 16 weeks also turned out to be significantly associated with later signs of hemiplegia.

These results prove that the assessment of neurological function through the observation of GMs is a useful tool in the early detection of hemiplegia in individuals with unilat-

3

eral lesions on neuroimaging. Observation of GMs therefore allows clinical confirmation of the early prediction from neuroimaging. The detection of post-term GM asymmetries suggests a focal cerebral lesion requiring appropriate investigations. Finally, these clinical observations allow one to target adequate therapies to those infants at high risk for developing hemiplegia. The early detection of subjects who will subsequently develop hemiplegia may also lead to early treatment and therefore contribute to modify the natural history of this condition.

Early Markers of Dyskinetic Cerebral Palsy

As reported in the previous section, the main forms of spastic CP and the severity of the motor disorder can be predicted depending on the quality of GMs, especially by the presence and characteristics of the CS pattern in the first weeks post-term and subsequently by the absence of FMs, together with possible asymmetries of segmental movements.

The large, multi-center study by Prechtl et al. (1997a), reported that an individual who later developed dyskinetic CP presented with GM features different from those of the 48 individuals who developed spastic CP. During the first months post-term, and subsequently before the absence of FMs, the GMs of this infant lacked the normal complexity and variability, although they could never be considered as CS.

In a recent collaboration study, 12 individuals with the rare condition of dyskinetic CP were prospectively recruited and then compared for their early motor development with the same number of individuals presenting with spastic CP (Einspieler et al. 2002). From birth to five months post-term, all individuals underwent serial videotape recordings, and their spontaneous motor patterns, including GMs, were assessed in a double blind study. Infants who subsequently developed dyskinetic paralysis, shared the absence of FMs with those with later spastic CP. Until the second month of post-term life, dyskinetic infants presented with PR GMs associated with repeated and monotonous arm movements in a circle and a fan-like spreading of the fingers (see for instance the Individual developmental trajectory in Figure 3.4). These two abnormal movement patterns persisted at least until five months post-term, and were associated at fidgety age with a lack of limb movements towards the mid-line. In agreement with this study, the qualitative assessment of spontaneous motor activity allows the identification of subjects at high risk for dyskinetic CP already from the first weeks post-term, differentiating them from infants at risk for spastic CP. These results are extremely important from a clinical point of view, since these two types of CP require different treatments starting at their early stages.

GMs and Mild Neurological Impairment

Abnormal fidgety movements are less predictive for neurological outcome than the absence of fidgety movements (Prechtl et al. 1997a), but they have been discussed in the context of the development of mild neurological impairments.

Hadders-Algra and co-workers described how "mildly abnormal GMs" in infants aged

3 to 4 months were predictive for the development of minor neurological deficits (MND), attention deficit hyperactivity disorder, and the boisterous, disobedient behavior of 4- to 9-year-old children (Hadders-Algra and Groothuis, 1999; Hadders-Algra et al. 2004). Results from Bruggink et al. (2006) indicate that the quality of the early motor repertoire, in particular an abnormal quality of FMs and an abnormal quality of the concurrent motor repertoire at 11-16 weeks post-term, is associated with the development of complex MND at 7 to 11 years of age. The longest-lasting follow-up study to date (12 to 15 years) demonstrated that the GM quality was not predictive for complex MND at puberty age, but rather for fine manipulative disabilities at school age (Einspieler et al. 2007). Moreover, Bruggink et al. (2008) showed that the quality of FMs and the quality of the concurrent motor repertoire had independent prognostic value for MND at school age.

Early Detection of "Sense of Motion" Disorders

Although traditional definitions of CP do not include disorders of self-motion perception, the relevance of this aspect for a better understanding of postural and motor disorders cannot be underestimated (see chapter 5). Modern concepts in the field of motor control development, both in CP and in other developmental disorders, strengthen the key role of perception, not just for motor and postural adjustments but also for anticipatory motor control. The kind of perception we are dealing with, the one most relevant to motor control in CP subjects, has been called "sense of motion" (Berthoz, 1997), and can be considered as the result of the integration of multiple sensory information (proprioceptive, vestibular, visual, acoustic etc.) into coherent spatial references for posture and movement. The issues of sensory integration and of the use multiple spatial reference frames in the context of cognitive and motor tasks have been extensively investigated in normal and brain damaged adults but seldom in children and even more rarely in CP.

To date, some clinical contributions support the important role of sense of motion disorders for the understanding of pathophysiological factors determining motor impairment in some children with CP (see chapter 5). The inability of many children with CP to achieve an adaptive control of posture cannot be explained only on the basis of their motor deficiencies. Indeed, these children can show, in specific circumstances, rather good postural abilities, e.g., in sitting and standing, but they then turn out to be strongly dependent on certain perceptual and cognitive conditions, in particular on certain visual features of the surroundings and on the awareness of the presence of an adult or of a close support. Sometimes, these children seem able to perceive sensory information correctly, but unable to tune perceptual indexes in relation to anticipatory motor control, thus failing in using spatial information for voluntary movement. Such difficulties may last for years and in some cases can never be overcome. These individuals seem to present a more "perceptual" than "motor" disorder (see chapter 14). The recognition of perceptual disorders as the main component of the fucntional impairment in a child with CP, is extremely important for the prognosis of the final motor disorder, its severity, and the timing of his/her most significant motor milestones. Finally, the presence of disorders related to the sense of motion should lead to specific treatment programs.

Preliminary results of a prospective study (Paolicelli and Bianchini, 2002) seem to indicate that the observation of spontaneous motor behaviors in the first months post-term can be an important source of information for the early detection of sense of motion disorders. The authors selected a group of 29 children who later developed spastic tetraplegia or diplegia, from a sample of pre-term infants with brain abnormalities on US who regularly underwent videotape recordings in the first months of life at intervals of 6 months, until at least the age of four. Observers blind to the final outcome assessed the recordings taken at 2 and 12 months of age as well a corresponding set of tapes of pre-term infants with normal outcome. The presence and severity of perceptual disorders were revealed by a reduced capacity of the infant to treat and process perceptual information (indicated by startle reactions, frequent blinking and postural freezing as a defense from emotional stress and as low-threshold, consistent responses to sudden acoustic, tactile or proprioceptive stimulations) and later by a strong and persistent dependence from perceptual indexes for posture control (e.g., a constant need for visual cues, close support and external reference, a persistent lack of automated control, etc).

The main results of this study are reported in Table 3.3. Children who presented with severe perceptual disorders already at 2 to 6 months post-term, maintained a similar degree of severity also afterwards. The same children developed more severe motor disorders at subsequent stages of development, as indicated by the GMFCS score (Palisano et al. 1997). Postural and motor milestones, such as sitting position, walking with supporting devices, and independent walking, were also achieved much later by these children than by the others, or even never. Such perceptual disorders were never seen in controls.

Conclusions

As shown in the reported studies, the observation of the quality of GMs is an extremely sensitive and specific technique for assessing the infant, neurological condition's before and shortly after discharge from the neonatal intensive care unit. It can be adopted to detect CNS abnormalities, to monitor the natural history of the neurological disorder, to formulate long-term prognosis, and also to assess the effects of treatment.

Differently from other more sophisticated instrumental diagnostic tools, this method uses visual Gestalt perception to detect alterations of movement complexity, fluency and variability, and for this reason it is often considered as liable to subjectivity. However, as clearly indicated by Prechtl (2001), the visual analysis of an EEG or of MRI scans, is also based on Gestalt perception. Moreover, the inter-rater agreement of GM assessment has been found to be very high, with an average kappa (Cohen, 1969) of 0.88.

This technique has proven particularly useful for the early prediction of cerebral palsy. CP early detection is extremely important in order to perform in-depth longitudinal observations, and for early treatment program. This aspect is very important for the improvement of functional prognosis, and for the prevention of physical and mental complications. CP is a disorder that involves subjects often presenting with different symptoms and different natural histories, therefore requiring different treatments from the very beginning.

Table 3.3 Correlations between early signs of "sense of motion" disorders and the severity of motor impairment (from Paolicelli and Bianchini, 2002, modified)

Case n.	ICP type	Perceptual disorders	GMFCS	Sitting position	Walking with support devices	Autonomous walking
	(Hagberg et al. 1975)	(Ferrari, 2007)	(Palisano et al. 1997)	Months	Months	Months
1	DP	-	1	16	30	36
2	DP	-	1	8	12	28
3	DP	-	1	8	12	18
4	DP	-	1	16	20	30
5	DP	-	1	9	20	30
6	DP	-	1	11	15	19
7	DP	+	1	9	21	22
8	DP	+	1	9	20	25
9	DP	+	1	10	15	18
10	DP	+	1	18	22	32
11	TP	++	5	/	/	/
12	TP	++	5	/	/	/
13	TP	++	3	36	54	/
14	DP	++	2	18	42	66
15	DP	++	3	13	84	/
16	DP	++	3	16	84	156
17	DP	++	2	/	48	96
18	TP	++	3	21	80	/
19	TP	++	5	/	/	/
20	DP	+++	2	18	30	72
21	TP	+++	5	/	/	/
22	TP	+++	5	/	/	/
23	DP	+++	3	19	/	/
24	TP	+++	4	84	/	/
25	TP	+++	5	/	/	/
26	TP	+++	4	72	/	/
27	TP	+++	4	/	/	/
28	TP	+++	4	48	/	/
29	TP	+++	3	48	108	/

GMFCS, Gross Motor Function Classification System; TP, Tetraplegia; DP, Diplegia

Knowledge about the natural history of the different forms of CP, from the first weeks post-term, is necessary to assess the results of traditional and novel treatments and to formulate new treatment guidelines (Cioni, 2002). However, for many different reasons, the early detection of CP is still quite difficult to achieve even today. Different authors claim that individuals with CP experience a silent period in the first stages of their lives, in which neurological signs are unclear or absent: a diagnosis of CP, and especially of its specific type, would therefore be reliable only after a few months. The quality assessment of spontaneous motor activity, integrated by the observation of some aspects of perceptual disorders, represents a useful tool to identify individuals at high risk for CP already in the

3

first stages of their lives. Moreover, this technique can even discriminate among the early signs of the different types of CP. This aspect has a relevant clinical value, since these infants have different prognoses and require different treatment program.

References

Als H, Lester BM, Tronick EZ, Brazelton TB (1982) Toward a research instrument for the assessment of pre-term infants' behavior (APIB). In: Fitzgerald H, Lester M, Yooman MW, editors. Theory and Research in Behavioral Pediatrics. New York: Plenum Press, pp. 35-132

Berthoz A (1997) Le sens du mouvement. Odile Jacob Edition, Paris. English edition: Berthoz A (2000) The brain's sense of movement. Harvard University Press, Cambridge, Ma

Bos AF, Martijn A, Okken A, Prechtl HFR (1998a) Quality of general movements in pre-term infants with transient periventricular echodensities. Acta Pediatrica 87:328-335

Bos AF, Martijn A, van Asperen RM et al (1998b) Qualitative assessment of general movements in high risk pre-term infants with chronic lung disease requiring dexamethasone therapy. Journal of Pediatrics 132:300-306

Bos AF, van Loon AJ, Hadders-Algra M et al (1997) Spontaneous motility in pre-term, small-for-gestational age infants. II. Qualitative aspects. Early Human Development 50(1):131-147

Brazelton TB, Nugent JK (1973) Neonatal behavioral assessment scale. CDM London: 2nd Edition Mac Keith Press 137

Bruggink JLM, Cioni G, Einspieler C et al (2009) The early motor repertoire is related to the level of self mobility in children with cerebral palsy at school age. Developmental Medicine and Child Neurology, Mar 20 Epub

Bruggink JLM, Einspieler C, Butcher PR et al (2006) Can mild neurological abnormalities at 7 to 11 years be predicted from the motor repertoire at early age in pre-term infants? PAS 3570:310 (Abstract)

Bruggink JLM, Einspieler C, Butcher PR et al (2008) The quality of the early motor repertoire in pre-term infants predicts minor neurological dysfunction at school age. Journal of Pediatrics 153(1):32-39

Cioni G (2002) Natural history and treatment of disabilities. Developmental Medicine and Child Neurology 44:651

Cioni G, Bos AF, Einspieler C et al (2000) Early neurological signs in pre-term infants with unilateral intraparenchymal echodensity. Neuropediatrics 31:240-251

Cioni G, Ferrari F, Einspieler C et al (1997) Comparison between observation of spontaneous movements and neurological examination in pre-term infants. Journal of Pediatrics 130:704-711

Cioni G, Ferrari F, Prechtl HF (1989) Posture and spontaneous motility in fullterm infants. Early Human Development 18(4):247-262

Cioni G, Paolicelli PB, Rapisardi G et al (1997) Early natural history of spastic diplegia and tetraplegia. European Journal of Pediatric Neurology 1:33

Cioni G, Prechtl HFR, F Ferrari et al (1997) Which better predicts later outcome in fullterm infants: quality of general movements or neurological examination? Early Human Development 50:71-85

Dubowitz LMS, Dubowitz V, Mercuri E (1999) The neurological assessment of the pre-term and fullterm newborn infant. CDM London: 2nd Edition Mac Keith Press 148

Einspieler C, Cioni G, Paolicelli PB et al (2002) The early markers for later dyskinetic cerebral palsy are different from those for spastic cerebral palsy. Neuropediatrics 33:73-78

Einspieler C, Marschik PB, Milioti S et al (2007) Are abnormal fidgety movements an early marker for complex minor neurological dysfunction at puberty? Early Human Development 83(8):521-525

Einspieler C, Prechtl HFR (2004) Prechtl's Method on the Qualitative Assessment of general movements in pre-term, term and young infants. Clinics in Developmental Medicine 167. Mac Keith Press, London

Einspieler C, Prechtl HFR, Ferrari F et al (1997) The qualitative assessment of general movements in pre-term, term and young infants - a review of the methodology. Early Human Development 50:47-60

Einspieler C, Prechtl HFR, van Eykern L, de Roos B (1994) Observation of movements during sleep in ALTE and apnoeic infants. Early Human Development 40:39-50

Ferrari F, Cioni G, Einspieler C et al (2002) Cramped synchronized general movements in pre-term infants as an early marker for cerebral palsy. Archives of Pediatrics & Adolescent Medicine 156(5):460-467

Ferrari F, Cioni G, Prechtl HFR (1990) Qualitative changes of general movements in pre-term infants with brain lesions. Early Human Development 23:193-231

Ferrari F, Prechtl HFR, Cioni G et al (1997) Posture, spontaneous movements, and behavioral state organisation in infants affected by brain malformations. Early Human Development 50(1):87-113

Frisone MF, Mercuri E, Laroche S et al (2002) Prognostic value of the neurologic optimality score at 9 and 18 months in pre-term infants born before 31 weeks' gestation. Journal of Pediatrics 140:57-60

Govaert P, de Vries LS (1997) An atlas of neonatal brain sonography. CDM London: Mac Keith Press 141-142

Guzzetta A, Belmonti V, Battini R et al (2007) Does the assessment of general movements without video observation reliably predict neurological outcome? European Journal of Paediatric Neurology 11(6):362-367

Guzzetta A, Mercuri E, Rapisardi G et al (2003) General movements detect early signs of hemiplegia in term infants with neonatal cerebral infarction. Neuropediatrics 34:61-66

Haataja L, Mercuri E, Guzzetta A et al (2001) Neurologic examination in infants with hypoxic-ischemic encephalopathy at age 9 to 14 months: use of optimality scores and correlation with magnetic resonance imaging findings. Journal of Pediatrics 138:332-337

Haataja L, Mercuri E, Regev R et al (1999) Optimality score for the neurologic examination of the infant at 12 and 18 months of age. Journal of Pediatrics 135:153-161

Hopkins B, Prechtl HFR (1984) A qualitative approach to the development of movements during early infants. In: Prechtl HFR (ed) Continuity of neural functions from prenatal to postnatal life. CDM Blackwell Oxford: 94, pp.179-197

Mercuri E, Guzzetta A, Haataja L et al (1999) Neonatal neurological examination in infants with hypoxic ischaemic encephalopathy: correlation with MRI findings. Neuropediatrics 30(2) 83-89

Mercuri E, Guzzetta A, Laroche S et al (2003) Neurologic examination of pre-term infants at term age: comparison with term infants. Journal of Pediatrics 142:647-655

Oppenheimer RW (1981) Ontogenetic adaptations and regressive processes in the development of the nervous system and behavior: a neuroembryological perspective. In: Connolly KJ, Prechtl HFR (eds) Maturation and development, biological and psychological perspectives. CDM London, 77/78, Heinemann Medical Books

Palisano R, Rosenbaum P, Walter S et al (1997) Development and reliability of a system to classify gross motor function in children with cerebral palsy. Dev Med Child Neurology 39:214-223

Paolicelli PB, Bianchini E (2002) Perceptual disorders in children with cerebral palsy: implication for prognosis and treatment. Dev Med Child Neurology 44:9

3

Perlman JM (1998) White matter injury in the pre-term infant: an important determination of abnormal neurodevelopmental outcome. Early Human Development 53:99-120

Prechtl HFR (1977) The neurological examination of the fullterm newborn infant. 2nd Edition. Clinics in Developmental Medicine 63. London: Heinemann

Prechtl HFR (1980) The optimality concept. Early Human Development 4:201-205

Prechtl HFR (1990) Qualitative changes of spontaneous movements in pre-term infants are a marker of neurological dysfunction. Early Human Development 23:151-158

Prechtl HFR (1997b) State of the art of a new functional assessment of the young nervous system. An early predictor of cerebral palsy. Early Human Development 50(1):1-11

Prechtl HFR (2001) General movement assessment as a method of developmental neurology: new paradigms and their consequences. The 1999 Ronnie MacKeith lecture. Dev Med Child Neurology 43:836-842

Prechtl HFR, Einspieler C, Cioni G et al (1997a) An early marker for neurological deficits after perinatal brain lesions. The Lancet 339:1361-1363

Prechtl HFR, Ferrari F, Cioni G (1993) Predictive value of general movements in asphyxiated full-term infants. Early Human Development 35:91-120

Rutherford M (2002) MRI of the neonatal brain. Saunders, London

Saint-Anne Dargassies S (1977) Neurological development in the fullterm and pre-term infants. Elsevier, Amsterdam

Sameroff AJ (1978) Summary and conclusion: the future of newborn assessment. In: Sameroff AJ (ed) Monographs of the Society for Research in Child Development: Organization and Stability of Newborn Behavior Assessment Scale 43, pp.102-123

Spittle AJ, Boyd RN, Inder TE, Doyle LW (2009) Predicting motor development in very pre-term infants at 12 months' corrected age: the role of qualitative magnetic resonance imaging and general movements assessments. Pediatrics 123(2): 512-517

Spittle AJ, Brown NC, Doyle LW et al (2008) Quality of general movements is related to white matter pathology in very pre-term infants. Pediatrics 121(5):1184-1189

Volpe JJ (2008) Neurology of the newborn, 5th Ed. Saunders, Philadelphia

Motor Defects

4

A. Ferrari

Motor defects are usually considered as the core of cerebral palsy (CP). Although we know that often this is not the only existing problem, and that sometimes it is not even the most important, we think it is necessary to start the analysis of the disorders provoked by this complex disease by dealing with the disorders of posture and movement (gesture).

The observation-assessment of motor behavior in children with CP can be tackled in two opposite ways: zooming out from details to general or zooming in. Physiatrists and physiotherapists prefer the first option, maybe because it is closer to therapy planning. instead, child neurologists and pediatricians prefer the second one, maybe because it is more congruent with "global" care of the child and his family. In this chapter, we chose the first option (zooming out from details to general), because this is the easiest and most predictive way especially in young children and in those situations in which we are asked for the first time to express our opinion on a new case of CP and its motor prognosis.

We analyze the level of motor modules (first level or mean level), followed by the level of praxias (second level or level of modalities), and finally the action level (third level or level of aims). To facilitate understanding, we will take as a general example what happens in writing, associating the first level to grammar, the second to syntax, and the third to semantics.

Jeannerod (2006) distinguishes between a higher level (*planning*) with a supervision task, where representation should be accessible and modifiable by consciousness, an intermediate level (*programming*), organized into modules and not accessible by consciousness, which chooses the best strategy to carry out the action by putting into practice the global instructions received at the higher level, and a lower level (*accomplishment*) which complies with the strategies chosen at the intermediate level to achieve the aim set at the higher level. The higher level is linked to conceptual and linguistic factors and supervises the ideal aspects of praxic activity. It is often impaired in case of cognitive deficiency and it is directly proportional to its severity. The second level is more strictly linked to specific neuropsychological dysfunctions (dyspractognosia) that are related to motor function. The third level is primitively altered in neuromuscular pathology.

The Spastic Forms of Cerebral Palsy. Adriano Ferrari, Giovanni Cioni
© Springer-Verlag Italia 2010

4

Modules
> Module repertoire (alphabet letters)
> Combinations (letter "h" and letter "q")
> Competitive interaction (capital letters and small letters)
> Vowels (postures) and consonants (gestures)
> Pathological patterns (letters of a foreign alphabet)
> Functional use of residual motor repertoire
> Internal and exter

Praxias
> Group of coordinated movements aimed at a specific result
> Formulas

Actions
> Movements that are cognitively organized to achieve an aim
> Synergies and strategies
> Competence: capacity, ability, passion
> Context framing
> Consonance

First Level: Motor Modules

The analysis of motor repertoire in the child with CP can start with the observation and assessment of the motor modules that are still present in his spontaneous production. Modules are the individual preformed motor elements that compose the motricity alphabet. Alone, they have no individual meaning (they are simple units without any meaning), but when appropriately combined, as it happens with alphabet letters or language phonemes, they can produce the postures and gestures of any motor activity, that is to say the words of movement (complex units with a meaning).

Repertoire analysis can provide quantitative data (entities of motor production) and qualitative data (variability and type of movement).

The *quantitative aspect* is the easiest to observe. Often parents reporting that the child moves one hand less than the other, or the lower limbs less than the upper ones, can direct the clinician towards a diagnosis of CP. It can be easily stated that the severity of a child's cerebral palsy is directly proportional to his "poorer" and "more stereotyped" movements. This is at least what happens with spastic syndromes. In dyskinetic syndromes, which can however present with an onset characterized by a long-term impoverishment of motor production (see chapter 13), it is the qualitative data that strike the parents' attention: the child moves, but in an unusual and different way. He sometimes moves too much, or in jerks, and alternates periods of excessive motor production with reduced or even absent motor activity.

In case of dyskinesia, the wide range of movements may even surprise the clinician, if the analysis was only limited to the assessment of quantity data.

In spastic syndromes, extremely poor and stereotyped motor modules characterize the most severe *tetraplegic forms*, like the apostural form and the stiff form with antigravity defense in flexion, which is also defined as the akinetic form (see chapter 13). With reference to tetraplegia with quadruped antigravity and to tetraplegia with biped antigravity, we observe an increase in the patient's motor repertoire, both in the number of motor modules that are still present, and in their variability and accessibility.

Children with *diplegic forms* show a much wider motor repertoire than tetraplegic ones. Sometimes the repertoire is so wide that controlling it becomes one of the many problems of these forms of CP (see chapter 15).

With reference to *hemiplegic forms*, it might seem obvious to say that the motor repertoire of the affected side is quantitatively inferior to that of the unaffected one. However, it is not always the case. Of course, there are qualitative differences (variety and form of motor modules) between the two sides, but some forms of hemiplegia, like early malformative (see chapter 16), do not show significant quantitative differences in motor production, at least in the lower limbs. This may justify a slight delay in diagnosis.

The *qualitative aspect* aims at assessing the range of existing motor modules and their form, therefore at considering if the alphabet of motricity is present with all its letters, also those which are less frequently used. The first mode of evaluation consists in recognizing some motor modules that, if present, can reassure parents about the motor prognosis in the long term. Wrist supination with flexed elbow (looking at the hand palm) and isolated foot eversion with extended knee (see test for selective control of foot dorsiflexion proposed by Berweck and Heinen, 2003) are largely applied and have raised a broad consensus. Their prognostic usefulness lies in the fact that they oppose the more frequent and known expressions of the CP pathological pattern (clenched fist, flexed wrist, pronated forearm, talipes equinus-valgus or equinus-varus, etc.). Milani Comparetti (1971) used to call them "gracious movements" (see chapter 11), considering them as expressions of the patient's **freedom of choice**. They usually are single segment gestures, mainly distal, allowing the selection of the direction and to change intensity and range. In agreement with Milani Comparetti, we can state that generally the following movements have a positive prognosis: spontaneous or voluntarily evoked (upon request), isolated, specialized or progressively adaptable, changeable with experience and easily converted into automated activities. Conversely, the following movements are to be considered as negative indicators from a prognostic point of view: reflex movements, especially if induced from the outside, movements that are repetitive and stereotyped, poorly adaptable and easy to be generalized, therefore widely spread and global. The consequences deriving from the selection of a "therapy" method for CP rehabilitation are easy to understand.

To explain why specific **combinations** of motor modules acquire a prognostic meaning, it is sufficient to think about the association of some alphabet letters and about the function of capital letters as compared to small letters in writing.

4

Movements with negative prognostic value	Movements with positive prognostic value
> Reflex	> Spontaneous
> Induced (upon stimulation)	> Voluntary (upon request)
> Generalized (global, widespread)	> Isolated (segmented)
> Stereotyped	> Specialized
> Repetitive and unchangeable	> Differentiated (changeable with experience)
> Poorly adaptable	> Progressively adaptable

In language, the letter "h" is only associated to specific vowels and consonants. The letter "q" is even more specialized, as it can only be combined with the letter "u". From the motor point of view, it is different to produce foot dorsal flexion together with knee and hip flexion (triple flexion) rather than to associate it to an extending knee (phase inversion), or to close the fist to grasp something while the elbow is extending and the hand is moving away far from the trunk, rather than closing the fist while shoulder, elbow, wrist, and fingers are flexing. CP is characterized by a rigidity of combination constraints and it is therefore more severe if freedom of choice (possibility to associate different modules, implying independence from primitive and pathological patterns, reflexes, reactions, primary motor schemes, secondary automatisms, etc.), and **redundancy** (etymologically overabundance) are low. Redundancy, in CP, means richness of alterative solutions (or motor equivalence, see later on) allowing the child to carry out the same task with the same result. The forced association of flexion, adduction, and internal rotation of the thigh, very common in spastic syndromes, is a clear example. In dyskinetic syndromes, the problem appears in the opposite way: the freedom of choice can be so wide that even modules that normally should not combine among themselves end up doing so (**illogical combinations**), like wrist flexion and finger extension, arm internal rotation and forearm supination, etc. The results are grotesque, unpredictable and bizarre movements. In these syndromes, redundancy results are so high that patients do not manage to repeat the same movement twice in the same way, with severe consequences on their learning capacity and gesture automation.

The example of capital and small letters helps us to understand the **competitive interaction** mentioned by Milani Comparetti (1965), that is to say the mechanism by which a motor module manages to organize functional movements. In written language, capital letters indicate the beginning of a new sentence, report the presence of a name, or stress the importance of a certain word. In the motor repertoire, all the modules that are combined to form a specific gesture have to be able to mutually interact and integrate, respecting the integrity of the module that is organizing the functional activity of that moment. For example, to manipulate an object it is necessary to combine the modules related to grasping, releasing, pursuing, avoiding, keeping, assessing the distance, etc. But if grasping turns out to be too predominant as compared to releasing, we will not be able to tune the grasping strength and delicately release the object. Conversely, if avoiding dominates pursuing it will not be possible to catch a moving object, or if keeping dominates assessing the distance, we will not be able to accelerate an object, as happens when we launch something, etc. In CP there are too many capital letters. It is sufficient to notice that in many spastic forms the impossibility to grasp derives from the fact that the thumb is caught and clenched by the other fingers and therefore the hand, closed in a fist, is not able to open because it is engaged in grasping itself. Intensity modulation and range regulation result from a wide combination of motor modules, in which between white and black (grasping and releasing, laying down and lifting, pushing and pulling, etc) there are many nuances of gray.

According to Milani Comparetti (1978), some forms of CP may display a diarchic character (fight between two tyrants) in the competitive interaction between the motor modules organizing the related activity:

- *Reaching-avoiding* (reaching reaction, turning the hand "towards", being attracted by, pointing at ... opposite to the reaction of assessing the distance from, avoiding, repulsing). They induce opposite movements towards the same objective by the same person. The reaching reaction includes a surprise reaction, a visual association based on the desire to grasp and explore the object (when the patient sees the object, he bends the head, opens his mouth, stretches the tongue, presents hypersalivation and sialorrhea, pulls his upper limbs forward, getting them ready to grasp with the hands with research movements). This reaction increases if the research is carried out without visual control, and is reduced when sight comes along, testifying to the organizing influence of epicritical tactile sensitivity (see chapter 5). The avoiding reaction starts as soon as the object is touched and it is characterized by removal of gaze, which is oriented elsewhere; the hand moves away from the object or the foot touches the floor (fluttering).

- *Grasping – releasing*. They strongly influence the ability to manipulate objects in order to appropriately explore them. To assess the child's grasping reaction, it is necessary to distinguish between two abilities: grasp organizing antigravity reaction in flexion, and grasp organizing praxic activity. The infant, raised by his hands (pulling up to sit maneuver), remains grasped and achieves the sitting position. This grasp organizes the antigravity reaction: the child lifts through the flexion of upper limbs on wrist, elbow, and shoulder. If the child is held from the head to cancel the effect of gravity on the body axis, as demonstrated by Grenier (1981), grasp disappears and the child manages to appropriately move the hands by grasping the object and moving it from one hand to the other. This second grasp, free from postural tasks, represents the manipulation organizing principle together with the release capacity (releasing). Praxic grasping is indeed the reaction allowing the hand to adjust itself to the object aiming at the following exploration: the hand approaches the object and orients, prepares, adapts and stabilizes itself during the entire duration of its task. And then again, guided by a realizing reaction, it opens, frees itself, detaches and assesses distance. In healthy infants these two principles organizing manipulation do not develop at the same time, since the capacity to grasp anticipates and dominates for a while over the capacity to realize. In CP these two reactions are often conflicting: usually, in spastic syndromes the grasping reaction prevails (as if the object was trapped in the child's fingers, and the child does not manage to release it), while in dyskinetic syndromes the realizing reaction prevails, therefore making it difficult for the patient to keep an object in his hand and maintain the limb in position. Among the compensation strategies adopted by dyskinetic individuals, it is possible to mention that based on holding and grasping the object tighter than needed, not to lose it, with a subsequent excessive realizing reaction, almost like a mannerism or caricature of the requested movement. Obviously, the reference to modules as organizers of a voluntary activity during a certain stage of development cannot be pushed beyond certain limits. Manipulating an object is not the following or piling up of elementary modules combined into reflex reactions, but it is something more and different that, regardless of the module and reflex rules, is able to form the endless number of variables composing a normal performance. A high influence of reflex reactions on the explored activity detects the pathological organization of CP, and the more severe the palsy, the more these aspects are clear. Obviously, this does not mean that a CP child literally "lives as a prisoner" of his own reflexes.

- *Support – escape*. They justify the conflict between the desire to lean and transfer the load, and the need to get free from the weight and move away from the ground as soon as possible.
- *Asymmetric right – left tonic neck reflex* (east-west conflict) with subsequent difficulties in trying to perform manipulative tasks on the median line and especially to perform bimanual activities, unless a hip posture is applied, by reinforcing grasping and making the grasp distal, with the head adequately rotated on the opposite side and the gaze obliquely oriented towards the object. Usually, patients who suffer from this conflict manage to reach their maximum manipulative ability by exploiting asymmetry, detaching the hand from the body axis (extended elbow instead of flexed elbow). With these individuals, it is necessary to make reference not just to neck reflexes but also to the conflict of the whole tonic activity (lumbar reflexes, labyrinthine reflexes, Galant, Juanico Perez, etc.) of one side as compared to the opposite one, and to the competition between rightward and leftward rotatory-derotatory upright reactions.
- *Extension pattern – flexion pattern*, that is to say "hypertonia" and "hypotonia", excessive support and astasia reaction, opisthotonus and aposturality, generally under the influence of head movements. They characterize the first diarchy by Milani Comparetti (1978), which can be recognized in tetraparesis with biped antigravity (see chapter 13).
- *Propulsive reaction – startle* (pseudo Moro). They characterize the second diarchy by Milani Comparetti (1978), which refers to tetraparesis with quadruped antigravity (see chapter 13).

While combinations represent a space association of motor modules, **sequences** represent their time association. Combinations and sequences together form the **motor scheme** or pattern (space-time configuration of movement). Also in sequences, CP presents with characteristic errors on which motor prognosis can be based. For example, it is different to organize the capacity to turn on one side starting from head flexion versus starting from head extension, or bipedal kicking by alternating complete sequences of flexion and extension instead of accidentally stopping at any intermediate position during movement, versus doing it with only one lower limb, keeping the other still. In general terms, combinations are related to **postures**, 3D movements, as Milani Comparetti (1971) would call them, and sequences are related to **gestures**, which are 4D movements, since they are related to space and time. Postures and gestures are associations of motor modules, like words are associations of vowels and consonants. We can imagine that, inside the word, vowels are the link that bonds letters, while consonants are the element that allows one word to be differentiated from the other. In the alphabet of the CP child's motricity, an excessive presence of vowels characterizes spastic syndromes, where ideally posture prevails over gesture, while an excessive presence of consonants characterizes dyskinetic syndromes, where gesture dominates over posture. We will see in chapter 12 that children's posture and gesture patterns allow us to classify the different forms of CP consistently with its international classification: posture and movement disorder (Bax et al. 2005).

All these remarks about motricity alphabet would not be sufficient to let us detect CP in a young child, if we were not able to recognize the real main core of cerebral palsy, namely the presence of pathological patterns.

It is as if in our writing, letters of another alphabet get mixed with letters of the Latin alphabet, changing the shape of words and making them almost unreadable. If pathological patterns are more aggressive, suffocating any alternative to their expression, CP's prognosis will be more severe.

Apart from observing the quality and quantity of the child's motor repertoire, it is important to assess its **functional use**, that is to say judging which and how much of the preserved motor repertoire is accessible from the "inside" (pattern elicitability, see following text) and can be used for functional tasks. Especially in the most severe forms, it is easy to observe that the child uses only a part of the preserved motor repertoire and ends up impoverishing it while growing up. This is probably the reason why, during the first months of life, even the most affected patients show a certain freedom of choice that gives some hope of rehabilitation. Unfortunately, this freedom will not be present later on. The second and third level of CP motor deficiency analyzed in this chapter, and in particular perceptive defects (see chapter 5) and intentional defects (see chapter 9) will help us to understand this subject.

When, in CP patients, the motor repertoire and its functional use are far apart from each other, the original nature of physiotherapy has to be changed, and not be intended as the tool that "in some way" favors the production of movement in the child and corrects its form. In fact, by doing so, in all those individuals with problems of use, powering of the repertoire would aggravate palsy, forcing the patient to engage more in the selection and choice of modules, combinations and motor sequences to be used, namely the things he cannot do.

A second serious problem related to physiotherapy of these children is represented by the **"internal" access** to motor modules. The object of physiotherapy manipulation is traditionally the evocation of specific movement patterns (repertoire) through appropriate "facilitations" or "inhibitions". The possibility to access the patient's movement repertoire from "outside" has always been considered as a proof of the therapist's ability and of the efficacy of the chosen "method". Only seldom was it assessed if the same movement could be easily accessible also from the "inside" for a child who had become aware of it through therapy exercise. It is easy to demonstrate that in CP not all the patient's repertoire is accessible from the inside. Indeed, some movements remain not accessible and others are differently accessible in some postures, as if some specific positions opened windows allowing internal access, but which are kept strictly closed by others. Therefore, not everything that the therapist manages to obtain from the child and with the child will become a

4

transferable and interior ability that can later be owned and used by the child. The use of movements that are accessible from the outside, but not from the inside, through physiotherapy facilitation, although making the patient appear more free and able, is only an interesting experience, maybe an important emotion, but it will not be an available conduct for him. The motor performance induced by the therapist is in fact reduced with exercise and at the end of the treatment, the patient, without the range and variability of movement shown during therapy, is once again as poor as he was before, while his parents' hopes and expectations increase regarding the therapy and therapist's capacities. This is the main limit of the most skilled therapists: through their ability, in an appropriate setting, they show the child resources which would not be spontaneously accessible. But treatment cannot lead to "stable" improvements in the patient's capacities, and therefore this is not a real "therapy". Showing the child what he "can" do in certain conditions does not mean indicating to him what he "must" do. It is necessary to explain to parents that not everything that can be obtained from the child in certain situations, certain moments and with a certain person, will be preserved by the child as stable motor performance and spontaneously re-used as available conduct. This is why the "provision" of tools to the family and the caregivers of the community the child lives in will have to be related to his internal access and not to the external one provided by the therapist. Internal access, in a certain way, defines the borders of motor rehabilitation.

The brain is fed with pieces of information, but emotions make us feel alive.

Emotions reached in an artificial way, through performances whose access remains impossible, can increase the gap between what the child dreams of becoming and what he can really achieve, be, and have. Emotions that are unbearable for him can lead to refusal and renunciation (intentional palsy, see chapter 9). This is why it is so important that, during therapy, the child experiences success in what he is doing (developing his resources through internal access), so that his self-esteem increases, and therefore his awareness of his capacities improves. The child becomes depressed when he realizes that everybody around him knows what he should do and he is the only person who does not understand it: this increases his sense of incapacity and lack of power, his external refusal and internal renunciation. As a consequence, intentional palsy becomes more severe, and the main prerequisite of therapy is missing: the willingness to change.

Second Level: Praxias

While at the first level the deficiencies shown by the patient, such as his palsy, are related to the loss or alteration of motor modules, at the second level it is their preservation and their quantity that create a different type of problem. **Dyspraxia** is a disorder influencing the management of movements commonly used for daily activities (washing, dressing, tying shoe laces, using cutlery or other tools, etc) and to accomplish expressive gestures (those aimed at communication), be they linked to the use of an object, therefore transitive, or abstract and with a symbolic content, therefore intransitive. Dyspraxia produces an alteration of voluntary movement that is not to be attributed to palsy, sensory deficit, cerebellar disorder or intellectual deficiency. *"In ideative apraxia (the individual does not know what to do) the representation of the gesture to be accomplished is lost, while in ideomotor apraxia (the individual does not know how to do) the capacity to translate the motor sequence into an "operational program" is lost ... the dyspractic child has a reduced capacity to "represent" the object on which he has to act, the whole action and the sequences that compose it. He has difficulties in tidying up into series and coordinating the corresponding elementary movements to achieve an objective (programming). He has also difficulties in starting the related programmes, forecasting (anticipating) a certain result, controlling each sequence and the whole activity during action (feedback), comparing the obtained result with expectations"* (Sabbadini, 1995).

In theory, in CP, the presence of palsy should not allow us to legitimately talk about dyspraxia, since this disorder refers to the difficulties that an otherwise "normal" individual, or at least an individual "with normal motor perceptual abilities", encounters when carrying out some tasks that require a certain skill.

It is necessary to separate repertoire problems from problems related to utilization, if one aims to understand that renouncing the use of some motor modules that are still present in their repertoire is part of the development strategy adopted by CP individuals, especially those with tetraparesis. This idea was put forward by Sabbadini already in the 1970s (Sabbadini et al. 1978); he talked about dyspraxia as a "hidden" phenomenon of CP. A clarifying example is considering palsy as a fit-in toy still to be built. On the box cover we see the image of the object as it would look after assembling it. Let us suppose it is a pirate galleon. Inside the box there are many pieces, of different colors and shape. These pieces are the modules. There is also a sheet of paper, which contains the instructions on how to build the final product (executive planning).

The first level of the palsy is represented by the loss of some modules (the more that are lost, the more severe the palsy), by the defect of others that do not join or separate (combination limits), and finally by the inappropriate introduction inside the box of modules that are not related to our pirate ship, for example pieces belonging to another toy, maybe the firemen's truck (pathological patterns). It is easy to understand that, in terms of motor repertoire (first level), a higher degree of module absence and imperfection corresponds to a more severe form of palsy. Instead dyspraxia (second level) results from the mistakes and omissions related to the instruction sheet. In this case the preservation of a high number of modules hampers the patient's capacity to continue the building task. The puzzle is a game in which modules have to be fitted in, without explicit instructions (the implicit ones will have to be built by the player with time, relying on the module, color, drawing, dimensions, etc). In the absence of precise instructions, if the number of pieces to be gathered is higher, then the game will be more difficult. Dyspraxia expresses the condition of a child who does not know which pieces to choose and how to put them together. The only solution is to use just a few pieces to make a simplified construction, for example, just create a rescue boat with a sailor, a cannon and the pirates' black flag. In motor terms this could be identified as **posture freezing** and **gesture simplification**. This is what happens to those children with tetraparesis who show a richer motor repertoire when they are younger compared to what they manage to preserve and use just a few years later.

4

In severe dyspraxia, rehabilitation will have to suggest the operating models to be adopted, rather than evoke the missing motor modules.

This therapeutic conduct can allow the dyspraxic child to learn how to do certain things, but does not help him not to do them in an unsatisfactory and stereotyped way, with poor alternatives (lack of redundancy) and with a reduced capacity to represent the whole action and the composing sequences. He often stops between one step and the next, looking for instructions from the caregivers, or at least for confirmation of what he is doing. The lack of strategies and the stereotyped adopted behaviors do not allow him to move on from learning to acquisition, and from acquisition to progress (see chapter 11), transferring by analogy already-experimented solutions to new tasks. To maintain their capacity to do things, dyspraxic children need to repeat them frequently, respecting the **formulas** they have learnt. By doing so, they learn one thing at a time, in a certain way, and learn to do it only in that way, without experimenting with alternative solutions and without the possibility to decode what they have learnt and to transfer it to new abilities, new tasks, and new contexts.

In a few words, movement (posture and gesture) derives from the assembly of elementary motor modules according to a specific logic. This logic (praxia = planning) is to be meant as the sum of the instructions needed to pass from a project to a product, that is to say as the sequential organization (program) of the movements needed to accomplish a specific action. Broadening motor repertoire and achieving highly functional performance are associated to subtle modifications of space-time parameters of program and to the appearance of a new property: the capacity to separately tune the elementary components of the acquired program (capacity that depends on the training level), which therefore become less and less rigid, and which can better adapt to the changing environmental requirements. The experience, by favoring program that are more suitable to the objective and that use the most efficient and less tiring strategies, gradually reduces the executive variability of movements though a progressive restriction of freedom, transforming abilities into skills.

According to Gentilucci and Rizzolatti (1987), a vocabulary of modules encoding motor actions in each neuron is contained in the lower area 6 of monkeys. Other vocabularies are contained in other pre-motor areas and cortical associative areas. One of these is area 7 of the parietal lobe (Mountcastle et al. 1975). Finally, other cortical regions can be involved in the organization of the entire action. One of these could be localized in the frontal lobe. It has been demonstrated that in human beings frontal lobe lesions cause deficiencies during the performance of tasks requiring a sequence of operations. Patients, in task performance, omit some segments of the action and add other, meaningless ones, showing their inability to produce a whole action plan (Damasio, 1985).

The units or "words" of the vocabulary are represented by neuronal populations, each one indicating a particular motor action or a single aspect: some indicate an entire action in a generic way, often including more effectors (*what*), others specify *how* the action should be accomplished, some others *when*. The vocabulary would consist of potential movements (motor ideas) (Gentilucci and Rizzolatti, 1987). What is encoded is not just a movement parameter like strength or direction, but rather the relation between the agent performing the action and its object. This vocabulary contains different "words", each one consisting of a group of neurons that are related to different motor actions.

Third Level: Actions

To understand how the brain makes this selection, we have to reach the third level and mention motivation and action. In CP, palsy is first of all a conceptual disorder of cognitive, emotional, and relational organization, therefore an **action** problem. It is only secondarily a planning disorder (praxia) and a movement execution problem (motor performance).

> *"The motor response is the product of a synthesis that takes into consideration motor, cognitive and emotional aspects of the problem…"* (Anokhin, 1966)
>
> *"At the beginning, we find the act of willingness, a physical act, and then the transmission of this willingness, a nervous act, and then the muscle contraction, a muscular act, and finally the organ movement, which is a mechanic act"* (Marey quoted by Berthoz, 1997)
>
> *"From the point of view of psychic reflex range, all mental events end up in motor phenomena through which stimuli are processed. As regard as internal understanding, the voluntary conscious act converts into movement: the voluntary act is submitted to a motor extra-conscious act that provides the capacity to act"* (Jasper, 1959)
>
> *"If we analyze the time development of an action, we will see that it consists of motor segments, each one with a different objective. These segments are defined as motor actions. Each motor action is composed of a series of movements that, one after the other, allow to accomplish every motor action. To perform an action it is necessary to have information … finally, movements, last stage of action organization, presuppose a motor program … the motor program specifies movement parameters like speed, acceleration and strength. Movement is then shown through the sequential activation of different muscle groups"* (Keele, 1968)

According to Piaget (1936), action is a transformation of reality, since through actions the human organism interacts with the external environment by modifying it. Actions also lead to an internal transformation, as the individual, thinking about his own, action, modifies his own cognitive structures. The child knows the world through action, and the first type of world representation is related to the capacity to act (sensory-motor period). Action is a tool to acquire knowledge about the world, therefore having the same characteristics of thought. Both thought and action can actively transform reality. The child's development starts from real action, through interiorized action, up to the mentally operated action. *"All the child's intelligence is characterized by the interiorization of real actions into simply represented actions and operations. The latter are characterized by the reversibility of their composition"* (Piaget, 1936).

According to Bruner (1966), actions are characterized by the possibility to produce mental structures, which he defines as representations: actions are a way to create a representation, an encoding of reality. The first representation is executive and based on real actions; then it changes, and it is replaced by an iconic representation, that it to say by the objective form of images, until reaching a symbolic representation. In knowledge building, during cognitive development, there is no separation between thought and action, since thought is literally built starting from sensory-motor competences.

The motor system was previously conceived as a simple movement controller (Hennemann, 1984). Recent experimental neurophysiological results show, instead, that a consistent portion of the motor system is devoted to action control. Every single action is characterized by the presence of an **objective**. The same movements can be made to achieve different objectives. The presence of different objectives converts movements into different actions. It is not the movement, but rather the action which is at the basis of the motor system. For example, in area F5 (a particular area in the most rostral part of the premotor ventral cortex, or in area 6), some groups of neurons activate when the monkey grasps the objects, regardless of grasping them with the right hand, the left hand or the mouth. The movement of each part of the body is controlled by muscle groups that are very different. Therefore, neither muscles nor movements can be the common denominator at the basis for the activation of these neurons. The common denominator is represented by the objective of the actions (Fadiga et al. 2000).

If the action is a cognitively organized movement to achieve an objective, the "primum movens" leading to its accomplishment is represented by the awareness that the individual must have a specific need, or a desire to be attained, as well as a determination in finding an operating solution that satisfies him, in other words his **motivation**. "*In general, we can say that each action responds to a need. A need always testifies a lack of balance. A need emerges when something inside us or outside us, in our mental or physical structure has changed, or when our conduct has to be re-adapted due to this change. Eating or sleeping, playing or achieving our objectives are all satisfactions that re-establish balance between the new situation that has provoked the need, and our mental organization. Therefore, we could say that in every moment the action is imbalanced by the transformations internally or externally occurring in the world, and each new conduct is not just aimed at re-establishing the balance, but also at reaching a more stable balance*" (Piaget, 1936).

Without motivation there is no way to build actions and therefore to reach any motor ability, either spontaneously or through re-education activity. Very often, among the words that parents use to describe the character of a child with CP, is the adjective "lazy". Laziness expresses the child's lack of commitment to motor activity from which he probably does not draw enough satisfaction or pleasure, so that he is always ready to give up. That lack of intention is the third dimension of CP.

It is the cognitive aspect determining if the solution to a need or an "inspiring" desire is "good enough" to be accepted, or if it needs to be further improved. According to Eccles (1952), movement does not only represent the operating translation of intentionality, but rather it becomes knowledge heritage, enriching intentionality.

The creation of a **memory** allows the motor pattern to be repeated and further adapted, control strategies to be changed and improved to perfection. According to Schmidt (1988),

patterns consist of memorized relations (topological links) between the different sensory and motor components of the action. Memory allows for the prediction of the consequences of future actions by evoking the consequences of past ones, according to Berthoz (1997). The brain (hippocampus, prefrontal and parietal cortex) uses the memory of past experiences to mentally anticipate the possible results of the action it is about to perform.

One of the effects of knowing the existing relations between single events in an action sequence is the capacity to assess the action flow. Knowing that an event is simultaneously and unavoidably the consequence and the cause of another event is the ground of the ability to perform prevision and **anticipation** operations. Bernstein states that planning a motor action, regardless of the way it is encoded by the CNS, implies the recognition of situations that still have to occur. Seeing an object, for example, means automatically evoking a potential motor action, the idea of a movement towards the observed object (Fadiga et al. 2000). For this reason, it can be said that planning requires an exploration into the future (anticipation) about the most likely consequences of the action we want to perform. Beyond (modular theory according to Fodor 1983) or inside (connection theory according to Rumehaltr and Mc Clelland, 1996) these cognitive operations, there is a metacognitive ability, to be intended as the control on any attempt to solve the problem, the planning of any next move, the monitoring of action effectiveness and the testing, checking and evaluating the learning strategy. According to Bain quoted by Berthoz (1997), thinking means refraining from acting.

Exercise and repetition of the same performance allow the individual to differentiate and coordinate the preferential motor patterns until reaching their **automation**. Recent neuroradiological techniques have shown that, during motor learning, the vertebral cortex is only used at the beginning of the learning process, then progressively becomes less active. The activity related to repetition is in fact transferred to subcortical structures and the cerebellum to allow the cortex to face new problems and invent new solutions.

Movement **coordination** is the process allowing us to control the redundant freedom of the motion organ, converting it into a controllable system…. Briefly, coordination represents the organization of motor system control (Bernstein, 1967).

To improve movement control, the brain applies motor **synergies** (from Greek "sin", together, and "ergos", work), that is to say pre-wired sensory-motor patterns. Motor synergies are at the basis of movements: "*this concept was proposed by Bernstein to maintain the idea according which, since the CNS cannot control all the levels of freedom, evolution would have progressively select a repertoire of movements and postural reactions that involve muscle groups and body segments interacting to achieve a specific performance, coordinated in such a way that a single control activates the whole sequence*" (Berthoz, 1997).

Therefore, synergies are links between the different levels of freedom, and their use reflects CNS strategies: "*reducing to the minimum the number of motor parameters to be controlled*" (Morasso et al. 1987). "*Movement is organized from a repertoire of synergies composing the highest possible number of actions. By pre-cabling motor synergies it is possible to simplify neurocomputation*" (Berthoz, 1997). It has recently been discovered that projections related to the different parts of the body involved in a specific motor action, i.e. into a synergy, are topographically grouped (Rispal-Padel et al. 1982). The axons of corticospinal neurons are systematically subdivided at the spinal cord level, so that activation of just one of these neurons simultaneously induces the contraction of different muscle groups that are distributed on different parts of the body, hence determining a synergy. The connection between the cortical pyramidal neurons and the different muscles of a motor synergy is specifically related to the function and not to the aimed muscles. For the organization of a motor synergy, time is as important as activity distribution (Berthoz, 1997). Some synergies are genetically determined and are produced by central pattern generators (CPG); some others are learnt and need a relation with the environment to be applied (epigenesis according to Changeux, 1983). The genetic program is fully responsible for the formation of simple nervous circuits lying at the basis of innate behaviors (specific behavior modules), aimed at satisfying primary needs. These innate behaviors can be activated also in the absence of afferent stimuli, and can be modified through CPG tuning, which grounds their functioning. As for the development of learnt behaviors (adaptive functions), this requires a continuous comparison with the environment through experience. In this case, adopted solutions are a model of automatic coordination.

However, it is necessary to recognize that the number of possible solutions is not endless, but depends on the genetic asset of sensory-motor subsystems (Berthoz, 1997), and that an impaired CNS, just like an affected locomotion apparatus, only produces altered synergies.

The *strategy* is the selection of a particularly appropriate synergy or sequence of synergies, that compose a complex movement aimed at an objective, namely the motor action. Movements are therefore organized into synergic sequences that are the basis of behaviors, hence they compose the highest possible number of actions. Balance is a typical example of synergies being organized into strategies. It is not ensured by error detection and subsequent correction, but rather by an anticipation of the postural variations that are necessary to compensate the consequences of the gesture that is about to be produced (Babinski's synergies). The brain presents with selection mechanisms able to choose strategies, i.e. combinations of the different repertoire elements, which are more suitable to the situation faced and to the achievement of the aim of the action. To build actions, the CNS presents with a somatotopic organization of movements, which consists of motor cortical representations (Rizzolatti et al. 1996). In other words, the motor repertoire is organized into actions and not into elementary movements: *"In the CNS there are models of our body segments, deriving from the effect of gravity on our movements. Perception and action are therefore linked to the existence of these mysterious models, internal to the limb properties and to the physical world objects. The consequences of movement can be simulated and hence predicted by the brain by using these internal models ... The first movements made by the child and his first games would then be useful to learn new motor programmes and build new internal models. Their importance is therefore very clear, especially in the variability of the competences that will be induced. These competences will be induced in each child according to the internal models that he will be able to build ... The theory of the internal models of body mechanic properties is a way to understand the capacity of the brain to simulate reactions with the environment and anticipate them. In case of lesion or sensory conflict, the brain can invent new solutions to re-establish a certain functional adaptability"* (Berthoz, 1997).

Motor equivalence is a simple property of the brain allowing us to carry out the same performance by using different effectors. For example, we can write with a pencil, on a sheet of paper, the letter "O" of different sizes, but we can also write them with chalk on the blackboard or on the wall, trace them with our foot on the sand, or compose them by keeping the pencil in our mouth: movements will all have the same distribution of speed and angular acceleration, in accordance with the principle of motor equivalence. Despite the variability in dimensions and tools employed, all the letters will show the author's style. Therefore, the brain can choose different operating solutions to solve the same problem; in case of suspicion of CNS disorder, their range and variability (redundancy and differentiation) are a reliable indicator of good health. Motor equivalence is proof of the fact that the brain encodes a motor form (morphokinesis) in a very general way, to be able to immediately express it or put into practice through a series of muscle and movement combinations. At the basis of this property lies the central representation of the motor action that Anokhin (1966) called **engram**. According to Bernstein (1967), engram is what makes the physiognomy of the motor action resistant to the variables imposed by the physical world. The periphery can decide on the motor effectors, but the engram will not vary.

The motor project is deposited at the same time on different levels of the CNS: both the idea of the general development of action and its result are deposited at the level of the conscious cortex, while the mechanical characteristics of the action are represented, as well as the sequences that compose the action, the muscle combinations that are necessary to compose it, etc, at the various secondary cortical and subcortical levels. Obviously, these representations are not static and unchangeable, but they are in continuous transformation and dynamic adaptation. Representation is not only correlated to the external reality, as Anokhin would say, but also to the construction of the most suitable action, the single movements, and the corresponding motor and perceptive sequential feedback.

Action programming makes reference to a vocabulary of potential movements (motor synergies according to Bernstein, motor ideas according to Rizzolatti), which can or cannot be put into practice. The same structures are activated when the movement is accomplished as when it is simply imagined. *"The idea is that genetically-determined local synergies composing the sensory-motor repertoire of all species – like the different types of locomotion, ocular movements (saccadic, vestibular-ocular reflex, etc), sexual exhibitions, postures, and so on - are organized into behavioural strategies guided by global mechanisms. In superior animals and human beings, these strategies can be internally anticipated, chosen and simulated (imagined) before being put into practice, by using the same structures as action ... The brain is an inventive simulator that is able to work as a reality emulator ... perception is a simulation of the action"* (Berthoz, 1997).

This CNS property can be exploited for learning objectives both in the sport field (**mental training** or motor imagery) and in the re-educational one (experience interiorization and learning). The more an experience is repeated also at level of fantasy, the more the activated synapses become hypertrophic and the nervous connections stabilized, making memory more alive and lasting. Since mental training (motor education through the promotion of mental images of movement) works as an internal activity of the brain which is able to activate homolateral areas of movement, according to Ghelarducci and Gemignani (2002), it can reasonably be a possible strategy for the recovery of CP, partic-

4

ularly in malformative syndromes and periventricular lesions. Homolateral re-organization always remains incomplete due to the extreme difficulty in the re-configuration of the neuronal network.

Even the simple observation of another person who is performing a certain action can facilitate the learning of its execution (**learning through imitation**), through the activation of specific neurons positioned in area F5 (cortical convexity) and defined as "mirror" to evidence the double "execution/observation" value of their reaction (Rizzolatti et al., 1996). Mirror neurons not only encode the execution of a specific movement of the hand, foot or mouth, but they are also stimulated during the observation of a mirror analogous action accomplished by another individual. *"Each time we observe a person performing an action, as well as activating visual areas, there is a simultaneous activation of motor cortical circuits that are usually active during the execution of those actions (activations organized in somatotopic way in specific sectors of our pre-motor cortex). Although we do not reproduce the actions that we are observing, our motor system activates as if we executed the actions that we are observing"* (Rizzolatti et al. 1996). Mirror neurons seem to encode not just the objective of the action, but also the way this objective is achieved. According to the functional interpretation of mirror neurons, these neurons are part of a system allowing us to understand the actions of individuals. This system could work with a visual-motor mechanism involving the action observed and the action accomplished. Since action observation evokes motor representation of the action in the observer, this mechanism could allow us to understand the meaning of the action itself. In other words, neuronal activation evoked by the observed action is the same that would be evoked when a similar action is accomplished (Gallese et al. 1996; Rizzolatti et al. 1996). The visual stimuli involved in evoking the activation of mirror neurons are those actions in which the interaction between the experimenter and the subject of the action is visible, i.e. in which the interaction between the agent of the action and the object of the action is visible. This is certainly one of the most effective tools to teach infants and children with CP how to organize and accomplish a certain motor activity, as it is not influenced by bottom up components of the executing locomotor system (see chapter 12).

Recent experiments (Murata et al. 1997; Fadiga et al. 2000) showed that around 20% of F5 neurons (posterior side of the arcuate sulcus), encoding the target of some specific actions, are activated also by the visual presentation of 3D objects of different shape and dimension, even in the absence of active movements by the investigated animals. These neurons have been called "canonical" neurons. While mirror neurons activate during the observation of actions like grasping, manipulating, holding, or breaking objects, canonical neurons activate during object observation. Very often, a close relation was noticed between the type of prehension encoded by a neuron and the intrinsic characteristics (shape and size) of the object which can evoke a "visual" response in the neuron. These visual responses of pre-motor neurones have been interpreted by saying that the observation of an object, also in a context that does not entail an active interaction with it, determines the activation of the motor program, which is employed in the interaction with that object. Therefore, seeing an object means automatically evoking a potential motor action, the idea of movement towards the observed object (Fadiga et al. 2000).

The idea that the brain is not satisfied with the simply measurement of the physical parameters stimulating senses, dates back to Anokhin (1966) and his model of action acceptor (from Latin *acceptare* which means both accepting and approving), a cortical system specialized in the analysis of complex sensory afferents, which represent the result of the action. This analyzer would evaluate the correspondence between incoming afferents and the action that had previously been prepared on the basis of previous experiences. If the action acceptor detects inconsistency related with his prediction, the CNS will have to perform another analysis by adding new elements to the decision-making process.

The **competence** of an action is not the exclusive product of the need-response, movement-perception equation, etc. It is also influenced by formal rules imposed by the society we live in (**context framing**) due to the fact that some performances, although effective, are inhibited as being considered as inadequate in the executive aspect and/or in the expected standard. Crawling at nursery school can be an adequate way to move, doing it in kindergarten can still be tolerable, but at primary school it is considered as an absolutely unacceptable performance. Eating sitting on the floor is socially incorrect in western societies, while it is not in eastern societies, and so on. Also the image of ability that each of us wants to show to other people (**consonance**) can represent a limit that forces us not to perform activities which instead we would be able to do, although not well enough to be in line with our general standard. Drawing and singing can be two good examples for many of us.

By **self-organization** of CP with regard to the child's development stage, we refer to the logics followed by his CNS for the construction of the most important performances of motor development (posture control, locomotion, manipulation, etc). In spastic syndromes, the recognition of this logic and the main adopted strategies allow us to recognize the existence of different clinical forms within general categories, like tetraplegia, diplegia, and hemiplegia. Within clinical forms, **performance** stages refer to the way in which each child develops his performance over time. For example, gait pattern starts at a certain age and transforms later.

When evaluating a motor performance it is necessary to be able to make a distinction between **defects** and **deficiencies**, both central (top down) and peripheral (bottom up) (see chapter 12), and **internal compensations** (which the CNS applies to reduce the consequences of errors that cannot be avoided) and **substitutions** (solutions adopted to achieve the result by other means or ways). Treatment has to be able to distinguish those elements that can be **directly modified** from those that can be **indirectly modified**, as an effect of changes induced in other components or sites, and, of course, those that **cannot be modified** at all. In gait of diplegic children belonging to the first form (see chapter 15), for example, trunk antepulsion and hip flexion can be considered as the main defects; knee flexion is the internal compensation for hip flexion and talipes equinus is the compensation for trunk antepulsion. The use of the upper limbs to defend and support himself represents a substitution for the CP patient. Obviously, knee flexion and talipes equinus "are" defects, but during performances they also perform tasks of internal compensation related to the main defect, or the defect which is more difficult to correct (hip flexion). In the natural history of this form, with age, when gait becomes too slow and tiring, an electric-powered wheelchair becomes a different and definitive substitution modality to allow the patient locomotion autonomy. In diplegic children of the second form, knee flexion is the main

4

defect, while hip flexion is the internal compensation for it. Foot plantiflexion, although still remaining a defect, is a defense against knee flexion deformity increase, and for this reason it should be respected as much as possible. When the foot gives way and tours into calcaneous, upper limb substitution becomes fundamentally important to maintain a support reaction, which is progressively decreasing (crouch gait). In diplegic children of the third form, the knee compensates hip flexion and talipes equinus compensates trunk antepulsion, while the upper limbs are vital to balance the trunk that swings on the frontal plane. In the fourth form, the defect remains localized on the foot, while knee flexion in foot contact phase and "dynamic" talipes equinus in full stance are the internal compensations. In this form of diplegia there is no need for substitution. Often two opposite defects can mutually compensate: anteversion of the femoral neck, with subsequent intrarotation of the thigh and internal "strabismus" of rotula can be compensated by tibia extratorsion and foot valgus-pronation and vice versa, with unavoidable torsion conflict of the knee. In these cases, it is not possible to correct a defect without accentuating the other.

The knowledge of the natural history of the different forms of CP and the logic of their self-organization must guide possible therapeutic choices not only from a physiotherapy point of view, but also from drug, orthosis and surgical one's. They will be more effective if they manage to become part of the self-organization system, following its internal logic and improving it. As a consequence, motivation, learning ability, and the possibility to modify self-organization of the related clinical form will be the pre-requisites to be able to use the word "therapy" for the activities undertaken to support the child with CP.

References

Anokhin PK (1966) Cybernetics and integrative brain activity. Vop. Psychol., 3, n.°10

Bax M, Goldstein M, Rosenbaum P et al (2005) Proposed definition and classification of cerebral palsy. Dev Med Child Neurol 47:571-6

Bernstein N (1967) The coordination and regulation of movements. Pergamon press, London

Berthoz A (1997) Le sens du mouvement. Odile Jacob Edition, Paris. English edition: Berthoz A (2000) The brain's sense of movement. Harvard University Press, Cambridge, Ma

Berweck S, Heinen F (2003) Treatment of cerebral palsy with botulinum toxin. Principles, clinical practice, Atlas Child & Brain, Bonn, Berlin

Bruner JS (1966) Studies in cognitive growth. John Wiley and Sons, New York

Changeux JP (1983) L'homme neuronal. Fayard, Paris

Damasio AR (1985) The frontal lobes. In: Heilmal KM, Valestein E (eds) Clinical neuropsychology. Oxford University Press, pp 339-403

Eccles JC (1952) The Neurophysiological basis of mind. Oxford University Press, Oxford

Fadiga L, Fogassi L, Gallese V, Rizzolatti G (2000) Visuomotor neurons: ambiguity of the discharge or 'motor' perception? Int J Psychophysiol 35:165-177

Fodor JA (1983) The modularity of mind, an essay on faculty. Psychology, The MIT Press, Cambridge, Mass

Gallese V, Fadiga L, Fogassi L, Rizzolatti G (1996) Action recognition in the premotor cortex. Brain 119:593-609

Gentilucci M, Rizzolatti G (1987) Organizzazione corticale del movimento. In: Leo T, Rizzolatti

G (eds) Bioingegneria della riabilitazione. CNR Gruppo Nazionale di Bioingegneria. Patron editore, Bologna

Gheralducci B, Gemignani A (2002) Cognitive factors and motor learning in normally developing individuals and those with brain damage. Dev Med Child Neurol 44:8

Grenier A (1981) La motricité libérée par fixation manuelle de la nuque au cours des premières semaines de la vie. Arch Franc de Péd 38:557-561

Hennemann E (1984) Organization of the motor systems – a preview. In: Mouncastle (ed) Medical Physiology, XIV Edition. B. Saint Louis The C.V. Mosby Company, pp. 669-673

Keele SW (1968) Movement control in skilled motor performance. Psychological Bulletin vol. 70 n° 6 part 1 387-403

Jasper K (1959) Allgemeine phsycopathologie, 7 ed. Springer, Berlin

Jeannerod M (2006) Motor cognition: what actions tell to the self. Oxford University

Milani Comparetti A (1965) La natura del difetto motorio nella paralisi cerebrale infantile. Infanzia anormale 64:587-628

Milani Comparetti A (1978) Classification des infirmités motrices cérébrales. Médicine et Hygiène 36:2024-2029

Milani Comparetti A, Gidoni EA (1971) Significato della semeiotica reflessologica per la diagnosi neuroevolutiva. Neuropsichiatria infantile 121:252-271

Morasso P, Ruggiero C, Baratto L (1987) Generazione e apprendimento dei movimenti. In: Leo T e Rizzolatti G (ed) Bioingegneria della riabilitazione. Patron editore, Bologna

Mountcastle VB, Lynch JC, Georgopoulos A et al (1975) Posterior parietal association cortex of the monkey: command function for operation within extrapersonal space. J Neurophysiol 38:871-908

Murata A, Fadiga L, Fogassi L et al (1997) Object representation in the ventral premotor cortex (Area F5) of the monkey. J Neurophysiol 78:2226-2230

Piaget J (1936) La naissance de l'intelligence chez l'enfant, Delachaux et Niestlè, Neuchàtel

Rispal-Padel L, Cicirata F, Pons C (1982) Cerebellar nuclear topography of simple and synergistic movements in the alert baboon (Papio Papio). Experimental Brain Research 47:365-380

Rizzolatti G, Fadiga L, Gallese V, Fogassi L (1996) Premotor cortex and the recognition of motor actions. Brain Res Cogn 3:131-41

Rumelhatr DE, Mc Clelland JL (1996) Microstructure of cognition. MIT Press, Cambridge, Mass

Sabbadini G (1995) Manuale di neuropsicologia dell'età evolutiva. Feltrinelli editore, Bologna

Sabbadini G, Bonini P, Pezzarossa B, Pierro MM (1978) Paralisi cerebrale e condizioni affini. Il Pensiero Scientifico editore, Roma

Schmidt RA (1988) Motor control and learning: a behavioural emphasis. 2nd ed Champaign, IL, Human Kinetics

Perceptive Defects

5

A. Ferrari

The currently accepted international definition considers cerebral palsy (CP) predominantly as a posture and movement disorder (Mac Keith et al. 1959; Bax, 1964; Mutch et al. 1992; Behrman et al. 1998; Aicardi and Bax, 1998; Dan and Cheron, 2004; Bax et al. 2005), unacceptably neglecting the influence of perceptive disorders as well as cognitive, communicative and emotional problems on the "nature of the defect" and on the "natural history" of each clinical form (Ferrari, 1990). Although we are aware that it is methodologically incorrect to analyze CP from a single point of view (see chapter 11), on this occasion we would like to deal with this complex problem mainly from the perceptive one.

Perception is a sensory interpretation, an opinion expressed on the information received from the system, and an adjustment of the system to the information itself. The perceptive process is useful to automatically guide the selection of movement patterns for specific activities, and plays a fundamental role in the programming of developmental patterns for specific and personalized goals (Gifoyle, Grady and Moore quoted by Capelovitch, EBTA Conference, Verona, 6-7 September 2000).

To understand the influence of perception on movement, and vice versa, it is sufficient to think about the concept of motor control (Gibson, 1979). An incorrect movement, for whatever reason, provokes the collection, elaboration, and representation of altered perceptive information. The consequence is an inevitable "secondary" incapacity to program, plan, and realize correct movements. Indeed, a correct movement presupposes correct available perceptive information and, on the other hand, the collection of correct perceptive information requires a correct movement (Ferrari, 2000). We will prove why these two postulates are impossible in CP and how, at the prognostic level, they significantly affect the patient's recovery possibilities.

Action Organizes Perception

Put your hand in your pocket: if you are able to distinguish a key from a coin and to further distinguish if it is a house key or a car key this means you are able to produce, through a certain use of your hand, those "specialized" movements that are needed for perceptive recognition (tactile, pressure, thermal, etc) of the characteristics of the object you are exploring (dimension, surface, profile, consistency, temperature, weight, etc), until you find what you are looking for. We could state that the movements of your hand guide your sensory systems (orientation and activation of receptors), and that only by making adequately "selected" movements will you be able to collect, differentiate, and process that meaningful and discriminating sensitive information necessary to recognize the object you are looking for. Henry Poincaré stated almost a century ago "None of the senses is functional without movement" (1905). Therefore, we can easily understand why a CP child can have a sensory functions disorder, which does not necessarily directly derive from the presence of specific CNS lesions but which results from the difficulty in collecting information needed for motor control, due to the incapacity to produce the necessary specialized movements.

Perception Leads Action

Imagine you have to grab an object, after being informed that it could burn, dirty, or sting, or slip from your hand, or be extremely heavy or fragile. The way you grasp it will be influenced by the nature and the degree of the sensory information you will collect as soon as you touch it, and provided that you have previously chosen the most suitable way to execute this task. We could state that your movement is guided by sensory information (modalities to approach the object, type of grasp, speed of execution, strength applied, length of action, etc). Paraphrasing Poincaré we could state that "None of the movements is functional without senses". "*Perception and action are in fact interdependent, in the sense that perception allows us to have an adequate action, and action is necessary to collect adequate perceptive information*" (Gibson, 1979). Indeed, sensations and perceptions are not passive states of consciousness that are awakened when stimuli strike sensory organs, as stated by idealistic philosophy (Meraviglia, 2004). They are "active" processes whose results are widely anticipated in the organism, consciously or unconsciously. In the active perception of intelligent organisms, the distinction between sensory and motor variables tends to disappear: perceptive and motor processes are considered as mechanisms for the development of multimodal sensory patterns that are parallel, arranged, and adaptive (Meraviglia, 2004). "*The brain does not just make sensory-motor transformations: at different levels, motor commands influence treatment of sensory data ... Thanks to anticipatory control, the brain guides and actively tunes perception also through an active process of selection, calibration, suppression, etc, of the information filtered by the most suitable sensory receptors for the task, choosing for every circumstance the most necessary for the task at hand. Action influences perception at the source ... Starting from motor control, action is seen as an essential element for neuronal functioning, making it possible to study how this organizes perception and not just how perception determines action ... It is therefore necessary to abandon the distinction between sensory and motor: this is why I say that the border between sensations and motricity is cancelled*" (Berthoz, 1997).

Ecological approach to perception and action

"The ecological approach to perception and action stresses the mutual relationship between organism and environment, claiming that the processes of perceiving and acting take place in organism-environment systems, not merely in organisms. In traditional information processing theory, perception is thought of as dealing with the incoming sensations and stimuli identification process, while action is thought of as dealing with the response programming processes and sending commands to the muscles. In this way, perception and action are treated as separate and mutually exclusive. However, in the more recent ecological approach, perception and action are necessarily integrated: we not only have to perceive to be able to move, but we also have to move to be able to perceive. Perception and action are thus considered as mutually dependent, where perception subserves action and action influences perception"
(Van der Meer et al. 1999)

It is therefore quite easy to state that movement and perception are two sides of the same coin (Lee et al., 1997), although we must recognize that in case of motor disability these two sides could be differently impaired.

What allows a child with poliomyelitis to achieve outstanding levels of ability in comparison to any other motor disabled individual is certainly due to the preservation of unaltered perceptive capacity. Conversely, what leads a child with leprosy to progressively lose the most exposed motor segments due to mutilation is the severe impairment of thermo-painful sensibility. These are extreme cases. However, no rehabilitation physician would issue a functional recovery prognosis for a child affected by obstetric palsy, sensitive-motor hereditary neuropathy, or myelomeningocele based only on the assessment of the patient's residual motor repertoire. We all know that the central representation of the paretic segment, and consequently its operating potential in time, is proportional more to the quantity and quality of the remaining perceptive information than to muscle tone, residual strength, ROM, etc. Beyond the preserved motor repertoire, the condition of a patient with severe motor impairment but with satisfactory sensory capacity is certainly more favorable in terms of use than the opposite, due to the importance of the perceptive component in guiding the movement execution, with regard to both posture and gesture.

To better understand why this is and what specifically happens in CP, we can ideally analyze the destination of sensitive and sensory information on three different levels of analysis, going from the periphery towards the center:
- first level: sensations
- second level: perceptions
- third level: representations

First Level: Sensations

At the *first level* we find the capacity to collect basic information (sensations). Peripheral receptors (transducers) have the task of providing information (output) on the nature and degree of the incoming stimuli (input), translating signals of completely different natures into a homogeneous language (action potential). "*The five sensory organs are carriers of conscious information, while organs that carry information needed for behavior control and those carrying unconscious information are many more, for example the propriocep-tive organs ... or vestibular ones ...*" (Starita, 1987). The characteristics of the outputs coming from transducers depend on the type of input energy and on transducer layout. The task of transducers is to modify the input format (degree), respecting its content (nature) and making it more accessible to higher levels (perception and representation). The properties of transducers can be understood depending on their corresponding input and output properties (Fodor, 1983).

Peripheral receptors are:

- specific for each domain (nature of information). This means they are highly specialized and can detect only certain types of input (they are "encapsulated" according to the type of information). Differently from the wide range of inputs, outputs from each type of receptor are packed homogeneously as action potentials in order to be accessible to central processing;
- they are made up of a fixed, therefore autonomous, neural architecture;
- they have an obligated functioning (constant and passive). This means that they come necessarily into action every time the specific type of input they are in charge of detecting is present (automatic), however they can be centrally regulated (amount of conveyed information), therefore they can be calibrated (adjustable);
- they have a high functioning speed, that can be centrally regulated to synchronize messages (a higher speed for messages coming from more distal regions from the brain and a slower one for those coming from more proximal ones).

Sensory systems are organized in a serial way: peripheral receptors project to first-level neurons, which then project to second-level ones, which finally project to the highest level. Information on most sensory modes is transmitted by more than one serial channel. The different characteristics of a complex stimulus are processed by different channels, each one transmitting different information to the CNS. The different parts of the peripheral receptive surface, or receptive field, are represented in an orderly fashion in the CNS; therefore the proximity relations existing in the peripheral levels are recognized by the CNS and analyzed according to the action goal.

Given that there is only one form of energy by which information travels and its only variables are frequency, amplitude and the number of fibers activated, at the central level what mechanism allows us to perceive stimuli differently from each other? The nature and the degree of the information received (output) depend on the character of incoming energy (input) and on receptor layout. At the central level, during the first period of life, these two requisites allow the CNS to define specific cerebral areas that acquire specific competences by being stably connected to specific receptors, which are activated only by specific stimuli. The different central regions then interact by gathering the different sensitive and sensory aspects of the explored reality into one consistent perception. *"This perceptive invariance shows that the brain can generalize and abstract some properties that are common to the sensation. Therefore, learning occurs in a trans-modal way, in other words by transferring the acquired experience from a sensory mode to another. The brain perceives very different sensitive stimuli in an identical way, that is to say it generalizes by starting from equivalent receptors and creates what is called perceptive invariance in stimuli constancy"* (Meraviglia, 2004).

We will call each group of receptors "configuration", emphasizing that the brain controls the configuration of the specified receptors at the same time the movement is programmed (Berthoz, 1997).

Sensations

> *Sensitivity* (exteroceptive, proprioceptive and enteroceptive information)
> Touch, temperature, pain, kinesthesia, baresthesia, bathesthesia, pallesthesia ...
> *Sensoriality*
> Sight, hearing, smell, taste, balance ...

For motor control, surface or exteroceptive information is needed, coming from tactile sensibility (in particular from mechanoreceptors that, by measuring pressure and friction on the skin, can provide information at the beginning of a movement or on the presence of an obstacle during movement) and proprioceptive information, obtained from kinesthetic sensitivity (sense of movement or arthresthesia), baresthesia (sense of pressure), bathesthesia (sense of position), and pallesthesia (sense of vibration). All the above-mentioned sensitivities, together with statognosia (space position of a segment in relation to the body) and vestibular information, which assess the movement of the head in space, provide information about proximity. Instead, information on distance is provided by hearing, smell and above all by sight, which measures the flow of the external world image on the retina and the positions of the objects in the space. Other sensitive modalities, like hylognosia (nature of the matter), stereognosia, or morphosynthesis (surface, shape, and size of the object), topognosia (position in the body and its segments), graphoesthesia (localization and recognition of signs, symbols, numbers, or letters) and the capacity to distinguish between two points, are to be considered as integrated and complex sensitive activities, namely, second-level performances (see later).

First-level information is determinant both for posture control (position of segments, load distribution, support stability, etc) and for the production of specialized gestures (exploration, grasping, transport, etc).

"According to traditional neurophysiology, sensations are processed by specific structures like the primary somatosensory, visual and acoustic areas (occipital lobe: visual analyser; temporal lobe: hearing analyzer; parietal lobe: tactile-kinesthetic analyzer); perceptions

are processed in parietal and temporal associative areas, while movements are controlled in motor and pre-motor areas of the frontal lobe. This model establishes a dichotomy between a part of the brain that *knows* things, that consists of postrolandic associative areas, and another part that *does* things, made up of motor and pre-motor areas"
(Umiltà, 2000)

According to Turkewitz and Kenny (1982), the development of the different sensory systems during embryogenesis is sequential in order to determine their mutual independence. While during fetal life both exteroceptive and proprioceptive proximity relations prevail (Gottlieb, 1971), during extrauterine life, after a short competition between smell first and hearing later, sight will definitely prevail (sight is in fact the predominant sense in primates, like smell is for other mammals). Only during a more mature stage of postural control, visual predominance is reduced and children become able to accurately integrate multiple sensory afferences (Forssberg and Nashner, 1982).

Each sensitive or sensorial mode can be measured either quantitatively (from hyper acuity to deficiency) or qualitatively. If we measured the visual capacity of animals (acuity), we would see the hawk competing for first place with the lynx, while the last one would certainly be the mole. Instead the adjectives "epicritical" and "protopatic" qualitatively refer to the "purity" of the signal, that is the "clarity" and specificity of the information that has been collected.

The modern approach to the study of sensations started at the beginning of the 19th century with Weber (1846) and Fechner (1860), who discovered that sensory systems are able to extract four different elements from the analyzed stimuli: modality, intensity, duration and location, which are then fused together.

> *Modality.* In 1826, Müller formulated the law of "specific energies of sensations" according to which modality is a property of sensory nerve fibers. Different stimuli activate different nerve fibers. The stimulus that specifically activates a particular receptor, and therefore a nerve fiber, was called "adequate stimulus" by Sherrington (1906). Actually, the specificity of a nerve fiber response to a certain stimulus is not absolute. If a stimulus is sufficiently intense, it can activate different types of nerve fibers. For example, the retina is very sensitive to light, but in a way it is also sensitive to mechanical stimulation (blind children, for example, rub their eyes to obtain chromatic sensation; this phenomenon is called spintherism).

> *Intensity.* The intensity of sensations depends on the intensity of the stimulus. The lowest stimulus sensitivity an individual can detect is called sensory threshold. It is determined by a statistical process (50% response rate). However, from the earliest studies, it seemed clear that sensory thresholds are not fixed, and that, according to circumstances, they can be higher or lower, since they change with practice, tiredness, emotions, affectivity, context characteristics, etc. We can understand why sensory thresholds can change, if we consider the following aspects:

- the absolute possibility to detect the stimulus, to be interpreted as the capacity of the sensory system to collect information related to the stimulus;
- the criterion that the individual uses to assess the presence of the stimulus; this indicates the individual's attitude or inclination towards the sensory experience.

This aspect leads the individual to experience false positives (like a sprinter at the starting blocks who believes he has heard the shot and therefore starts running), and false negatives (the wounded soldier during a battle who feels the pain only after seeing his blood).

> *Duration.* The sense of duration is determined by the relation between the objective intensity of the stimulus and the intensity subjectively perceived. Usually the longer a stimulus persists, the more the sensation perceived by an individual tends to diminish, due to a phenomenon called "stimulus fatigue".

> *Localization.* The capacity to distinguish the spatial properties of a stimulus can be assessed by determining both the capacity to localize the site of stimulus application, and the ability to recognize two stimuli applied to two nearby points as distinctively different. The minimum distance between two stimuli that are recognized as different is called the threshold between the two points. It varies according to the innervation of the explored body area, and increases in the proximal-distal direction.

Analysis of sensations

> *Quantitative axis*
  Acuity: hyper-…; hypo-…; a-…
> *Qualitative axis*
  Differentiation: epicritical – protopatic

In spastic syndromes we observe the existence of sensitivity alterations which can significantly reduce patient motor performance. Thinking about the affected hand of a hemiplegic child, for example, it is easy to understand how a qualitative and quantitative impairment of basal sensations, including stereognosia (hylognosia and morphosynthesis) and perceptive rivalry (Tizard et al. 1954), can significantly influence the motor prognosis, progressively impoverishing and deteriorating also a part of the repertoire of movements that were initially spared by the palsy. According to the body segment where the patient possesses a sufficiently sensitive discrimination, he can implement different compensation mechanisms to perform grasping activities (coping solutions). In case of a severe impairment of sensitivity along the entire upper limb, he will fix objects between chin and chest, he will place them between his thighs or put them in his mouth. If sensitivity below the shoulder is lost, he will learn to trap things in the armpit; if sensitivity is lost on the forearm, he will use the elbow; if sensitivity loss reaches the wrist, he will use the radial surface of the carpus in order to hold it against the chest. Conversely, if sensitivity loss reaches the fingers, he will use the dorso-lateral surface of the thumb or the lateral surface of the index finger to create a cluster grasp and a digital lateral grasp as the sensitivity

5

preservation extends peripherally (see chapter 16). The only alternative to this destiny is the use of sight, allowing the patient to guide "externally" the activity of a hand that he cannot feel or control "internally". Thus, the plegic hand can become a somewhat reliable tool, often positioned and adapted by the unaffected hand, in order to be used as a functional support. Interdigital grasp is typical of this approach: the object is literally trapped between the thumb and the fingers or between the fingers and the palm, functionally exploiting the existing hypertonia and relying on the unavoidability of pathological flexor synergy. Obviously, this type of compensation is only possible in spastic forms of hemiplegia, in which the magnet reaction prevails over the avoiding one and grasping predominates over the releasing capacity. Conversely, in dyskinetic forms of hemiplegia, the instability of the committed error does not allow the patient to develop any practical compensation. To be functionally useful, synkinesia induced by the unaffected limb must be consistent, meaning that it can always produce the same motor result in the paretic hand. Synergies must be functional in relation to their task and they must be evoked through the movement of a proximal controllable joint station, for example the elbow, without concurrent hyperkinesia, allokinesia, etc. Of course, the extreme difficulty in building a central representation or a global mental image of the manipulated object still exists. This is due to the discordance between the sensory information collected by the two hands (altered perceptive collimation, see later), also considering the hyper-specialization that the unaffected hand has achieved in the meantime.

As well as errors by deficiency, the first level includes errors by excess. The most common ones are: intolerance to load (flight reaction), intolerance to contact (avoiding reaction), and intolerance to stimulus (startle reaction). These defects frequently influence the behavior of dyskinetic syndromes.

The assessments made so far are already sufficient to state that a rehabilitation approach that only focuses on evoking the absent motor patterns and remains indifferent to the perceptive components of motor control is inevitably bound to fail. Similar considerations are also valid for orthopedic surgery (Goldner et al. 1961), for topical, zonal or systemic drugs, and for the use of orthosis, if functional results are to be achieved instead of just aesthetic or analgesic ones. Thus, any improvement in the quality of sensory information leads to significant progress also in patient motor capacities (van der Weel et al. 1991), especially regarding the functional use of residual motor repertoire.

Second Level: Perceptions

At the *second level* there is the capacity to compare, integrate, and interpret sensitive and sensory information collected at the first level (output), trying to recognize any intrinsic coherence. "*Each sense disassembles sensitive reality into components that are then newly composed and connected. Indeed, a real physiology of perception has to give up isolating sensory functions, and instead deal with their multi-sensory character. Therefore, the concept of coherence is the core, since information collected through senses possesses properties that keep its separate, and make its fusion difficult, that to say ambiguous*"

(Berthoz, 1997). A good example of how a child should learn to cope with information ambiguity is offered by lightening and thunder. *"The problem of coherence is not just related to geometry and dynamics. It presupposes central active mechanisms that allow the subject to remove ambiguity, recover or anticipate differential delays between receptors, unify space reference through astute biological mechanisms that are not just changes in coordinates"* (Berthoz, 1997). What we perceive through our senses is a "cognitive product" which derives from a series of elaboration processes performed on the incoming sensations at the CNS level (Smith Churchland 2008). Thus sensitive and sensory information is subject to an associative process and a careful modulation before being incorporated into the cognitive structure (Mesulam, 1998). From now on we will talk more appropriately about *perception*, meant as an active and adaptive integrated and complex process, through which sensory stimulation is transformed into organized experience. *"We should conceive external senses in a new way, as active rather than passive, as systems rather than channels, and as interactive rather than mutually exclusive. If they are used to collect information and not just to evoke sensations, their activity will have to be described differently. We will call them perceptive systems"* (Gibson, 1966).

Perception

> *Complex psychic function that is able to organize sensations produced by stimulating sensitive systems and sensory organs, and to interpret and integrate them into experience, hence allowing the individual to become aware of the environment.*

> *Integrated and complex process that allows us to select a limited number of incoming stimuli, in order to recognize and assess them.*

> *Multisensory convergence process based on the comparison of information encoded by different reference systems aimed at reaching a consistent interpretation of the reality.*

> *"Integrated process through which sensitive and sensory information is transformed into an internal simulation, that is to say into an anticipatory configuration or a collateral copy of the action plan"* (Berthoz, 1997).

> *"The aim of perception is to represent the world in such a way as to make it accessible to thought"* (Fodor, 1983).

The "percept", according to Morasso (2000), is the joint product of stimulation and the comparison of collected information. Berthoz extends this concept to include active exploration, considering perception as a question posed to the world, a challenge, a pre-selection. *"Perception is not just an interpretation of sensory messages, but is closely influenced by the on-going activity. It is action"* (Berthoz, 1997). *"In fact the environment has to be considered as a group of possibilities for action (affordances), that the organism needs to detect through perception"* (van der Meer and van der Weel, 1991). Thus perception is an invitation to act, "readiness to move", as Bernstein stated (1967). *"Acting successfully includes the perception of the environment possibilities as related to us. It is not just the objects that are perceived by the organism, but rather what these objects offer in terms of*

5

action. What each specific object can allow necessarily depends on the perceiver's dimensions and possibilities of action. These possibilities cannot be fixed: they must be continuously updated during life in order to adapt to the changes that occur to the ability to act and the individual's somatic characteristics. This phenomenon is particularly clear during childhood, when new abilities appear, and the body dimensions change" (van der Meer and van der Weel, 1999).

At the center of perception is the fixation of a belief and this phenomenon, according to Fordor, is already a conservation process that is sensitive to what the perceiver already knows. Input analysis can be encapsulated according to the type of information, but perception cannot (Fodor, 1983). In different organisms, the same object, situation or event can evoke completely different behaviors. Just think about what happens between predator and prey.

With regards to systems for the analysis of outputs coming from peripheral receptors, cognitive architecture employs, at least from a perceptive and linguistic point of view, "intermediate" processing structures, "specific interpretation frames" (which Fodor calls modules) able to transform these outputs, deriving from inputs collected and converted from the peripheral receptors, into mental representations. These representations are then offered to the core element of the cognitive system and constitute the primary component of thought structure. The existence of these interpretative frames can be compared to what happens when we get into a simulator, even a simple one in an amusement park. The overlapping of images projected on a semi-circular screen, stereophonic sounds, and chair movements (sensations) make us feel as if we were inside a spacecraft that is moving at a high speed (perception), maybe towards still unknown worlds. According to Fodor, interpretative frames that provide coherence to sensations, being intermediate-analysis systems, have a central access that is limited to the representations they compute; in other words, they are relatively inaccessible to the central states of consciousness. Therefore, perceptions do not depend on the intensity of sensations, but on the concordance between sensations and the hypothesis formulated by the brain, which is strictly related to the characteristics of the interpretative frame that is used. This situation provides perception with objectivity and realism, framing it in space and time, making it constant and passive, keeping it independent from will. However, perceptions themselves are qualitatively different from the physical properties of stimuli, since the CNS first extracts certain information from the stimulus and then interprets it in accordance with previous experience. Although perception is a cerebral construction, it is not arbitrary. For example, although the perception of object size and shape is different from the images that form on the retina, it corresponds to the physical property of the objects and is a reliable prediction of external reality obtained through an inferential operation, since we can measure what we see. Thus perceptions are reliable representations of reality, functional for action, obtained through an accurate reconstruction of the essential properties of objects that also allows us to use them later on. In a few words, perceptions are not a discrete registration of the surrounding world, but they are internal constructions with rules and limits imposed by CNS properties. Kant (1781) called these intrinsic limits (time, space, causality) "innate categories". According to the German philosopher, differently from what empiricism stated, knowledge is not just based on sensory experiences, but also on the existence of innate categories that organize these sensory experiences. Thus, the mind can only see what it is prepared to see.

This vision of perception helps explain the dysperceptive disorder in some children with CP, for example the "falling child" form (see chapter 14): if central access were not linked to the characteristics of the interpretative frame, these patients could easily manage to realize the errors made during information analysis.

At the second level it is possible to imagine the existence of a perceptive *attention/suppression* (hypoprosexia-hyperprosexia) axis, or *awareness/habituation*, and an axis of perceptive *tolerance/intolerance*. In all languages, different words are used to define the attention devoted to a perceptive task from a quantitative point of view: seeing and looking, hearing and listening, tasting and savouring, scenting and smelling, etc. Instead, from a qualitative point of view, we can mention words like observing, scrutinizing, admiring, contemplating, and from a qualitative/quantitative point of view, words like glancing and eavesdropping.

Then, for each type of perception it is possible to identify a measure that is specific for each individual and makes the collected information tolerable or intolerable, with subsequent acceptance-conservation or refusal-removal processes. A person suffering from vertigo stops before climbing a ladder not because of motor incapacity, but because he is aware of not being able to tolerate the perceptions that he would inevitably feel if he decided to execute the action (see chapter 12).

In CP we can recognize the different clinical behaviors of children with perceptive vigilance deficiency towards information necessary for motor control, while others pay too much unjustifiable attention to each new piece of information, and for this reason they are not able to concentrate on anything.

"Stand up" diplegic children (see chapter 14) belong to the first group. These individuals perceive correctly, but they are not able to pay adequate attention to kinesthetic, baresthesic and bathesthesic information, and, only secondarily, to visual information fundamental for posture control. Actually, the "stand up" child is able to correct his posture every time he is externally informed about his wrong posture, otherwise he starts to slouch after a few seconds. Therefore, it is not a movement problem, otherwise he would not be able to adjust his posture autonomously. It is not a problem of muscle strength either, because, as patients with neuromuscular problems do, he would avoid the continuous need to make the effort to lift himself up against gravity. Nor is it a difficulty in collecting basic information needed to guide the requested movement, since postural correction occurs quite adequately (functional use of motor repertoire). It is not even a tone problem, because this would mean confusing causes with consequences. Rather, the "stand up" child shows the inability to keep diachronically stable attention levels towards the information needed for postural control, above all when he has to simultaneously pay attention to other hierarchically higher activities like speaking, reading, listening, etc. Thus, he lacks a "simultaneous control" and he is not able to make the acquired position automatic by correcting it with the necessary gradual adjustments should it risk being altered or compromised. "Stand up" diplegic patients need supplementary information coming from the outside every few seconds, such as the words "stand up", "keep upright", "don't slouch", because the information coming from the inside is not taken into consideration with sufficient attention. Only gaze, if directed at an extra personal target, can inform the individual about what is happening to his posture, starting a spontaneous self-correction process although with difficulties in integrating proprioceptive information.

Differently from "stand up" diplegic patients, among dyskinetic patients, especially athetoid, some individuals are captivated by each new stimulus coming from the internal or external environment, regardless of importance or meaning. Thus, they are able to achieve very high levels of attention, but they are unable to concentrate, interpreting concentration as selectively stabilized attention. Therefore, they do not have a sufficient "sequential control".

Analyzing the perceptive information devoted to postural control (sense of space, body, stability and movement, etc.) along the axis of perceptive tolerance/intolerance, we can understand what happens to the "falling" child (see chapter 14). This type of patient, generally a diplegic child, can receive information (intensity) and be attentive, but he does not have enough perceptive tolerance, up to the point that he thinks he is falling even when he is laying supine on the floor. His "vertigo", as Berthoz would say, is an illusion without solution, determined by a fragmentation of the representation of space and by a difficulty in finding coherence between multiple body references and sensory information (visual-proprioceptive conflict). Any postural variation or external or internal stimulus (acoustic, tactile, proprioceptive, etc.), even if modest, results in an unbearable threat to this child. Dragged by his weight he feels he is losing control over his posture and is continuously falling down; just like in a nightmare, he feels his body is disintegrating and disappearing. The "falling" child expresses his malaise and anguish through successive low-threshold startle reactions, generalized extension spasms, defensive optic reactions and defensive grasping reactions, vasomotor disorders, emotional distress, lucidly verbalizing what he thinks is happening to him: I'm falling, I'm falling! In theory, he would be able to collect information on the depth of the surrounding space, on posture stability, and on the consequences of current movement, but he is not able to tolerate it, because he can not construct a border to his body by separating the intra-personal space from the peri-personal one, the sense perceivable space from the action practicable one.

> *"Intrapersonal space: it is the Self space. It is perceived by our senses and localized within the limits of our body (cenesthesia). It is the real border of the body*
> *Peripersonal space: it is the space through which our gestures operate, the accessible space (near space). It represents the ideal border of the body*
> *Extrapersonal space: it is the space perceived by our remote receptors (far space). It represents the imaginary border of the body"*
> Grüsser and Landis (1991), modified

This is the reason why he decides not to move ("intentional" palsy as a defensive modality, see chapter 9) and creates, if necessary, a protective shield based on a special form of spasticity, a sort of "glue" that gathers all the parts of the body together and which could be consideredes a "second skin", as proposed by Bick (1968, 1986). Unfortunately, this is an exhaustible response (in this form of diplegia there is not enough spasticity!), which most of the time is not sufficient to adequately defend the patient, and, above all, cannot last long enough. It is true, however, that in these diplegic children any intervention aimed at reducing spasticity, especially systemic drugs or functional orthopedic surgery, ends up increasing patient difficulties, and especially malaise. Only in water, where sudden and heavy movements become light and slow, do children take motor initiatives and obtain satisfaction in movement.

Conversely, along the perceptive tolerance/intolerance axis, we find the individual who converts a certain movement into an intransitive repeated and manneristic action, due to a lack of harmony in his relational behavior, which is usually a supplementary component of CP. This child does not use movements to adapt to the environment or to adapt the environment to his needs, but uniquely to feel pleasure. And this is also a form of intentional palsy (see chapter 9)

A more detailed and complete description of the signs of dysperception disorders in CP children, especially concerning the startle reaction, is reported in chapter 14.

Not just in "falling" diplegic children but also in normal individuals, some perceptive conditions beyond a certain intensity become so intolerable as to impair their capacity to move. Indeed, perception is not a "passive" mechanism bound to receive and interpret sensory data, rather it is an "active" process for the anticipation of action sensory consequences. It is therefore a consistent connection between sensory and motor patterns. *"Perception is an internal simulation, judgement, choice, anticipation of action consequences"* (Berthoz, 1997). *"In computational terms, this implies the existence in the brain of some type of "internal model" which acts as a bridge between action and perception"* (Morasso, 2000). Motor programming therefore implies an anticipatory balance of the information that will be collected when doing a certain action (indicated by neurophysiologists as "corollary discharge"). This balance is necessary in order to know if that action can be accomplished and to have same feedback about what we are doing (Figure 5.1). If the balance indicates potential intolerance towards the expected result, the perceptive consensus to the action (conscious or unconscious) will be missing, regardless of the fact that the motor program is more or less feasible. This is why jumping from a diving board is different from jumping from a street curb, and putting a hand in a fire is not just a problem of pointing and reaching the goal. To achieve perceptive consensus for the action, judgement is based on a perceptive recognition process, in which the classification of sensitive and sensory data coming from the perceptual conversion of the motor program requires a comparison with the information that has already been memorized. *"Human beings, establishing mental analogies and models, are able to simulate future actions and immediately eliminate the absurd ones, therefore providing the action with greater safety"* (Meraviglia, 2004). *"This procedure allows our hypotheses to die instead of us"* (Popper, 1996).

The anticipatory balance implies, inside the CNS, a comparison between the outgoing signal ("efference copy" or corollary discharge) and the corresponding "sensory re-afference": the continuous control for coherence between the two representations is the basis for the stability of our perceptive world (Morasso, 2000). To act successfully, it is necessary to anticipate future events on the environment. This requires a perspective control (van der Meer et al. 1991). *"The brain questions receptors by adjusting sensitivity, combining messages, pre-specifying estimated values, in order to carry out an internal*

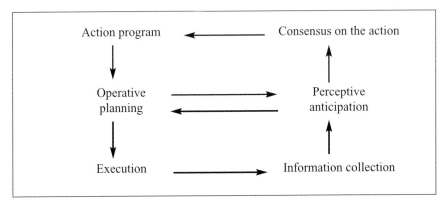

Fig. 5.1 Diagram showing the interpretation of motor control. It is useful to explain movement disorders in children with CP. The action program is the transformation of a thought into a potential action (ideation). An intermediate stage analyzes the program and translates it into executive terms (operative planning). A copy of this executive program is translated into perceptive terms (collateral discharge) in order to have an anticipatory simulation (feed-forward) of what we would perceive if we decided to accomplish the action that has been imagined. This perceptive anticipation is submitted to cognition judgement in order to obtain the perceptive consensus on the action. If the judgement is positive, the action will be carried out and the planned program will pass on to the locomotion system effectors for its execution, otherwise it will have to be re-formulated or abandoned. During program execution, information is collected (sensations) and then compared to the expected perceptive result in order to make, if necessary, some adjustments to the ongoing operative program (feedback)

simulation of action consequence ... In other words, perception is a restrained action, but, above all, it is related to a goal directed action" (Berthoz, 1997).

Information such as "be careful because you are alone", instead of improving patient control over performance and thus the quality of the final result, can on the contrary increase motor difficulties in some diplegic patients with dysperceptive problems, with immediate performance worsening (see chapter 14). The individual who manages to stand with his back a few centimeters from the wall without touching it, while he is not able to do it if he moves one step forward, does not have any motor problems, but rather a perceptive intolerance towards the information that is related to emptiness, distance, and depth of backward space. What should we think, then, of the *motor learning* of these individuals, which Woollacott and Shumway-Cook (1995) defined as adaptative modification, obtained through a complex perceptive-motor-cognitive process, considering that this process cannot be separated from attention and memory? In order to be anticipatory of the future, perception has to be based on the past, on similarities, and on correspondences (Berthoz, 1997). During motor learning, then "*... experience data is organized, or better organizes the learnt structures within which perceptive-motor information is articulated in a chronological order as "action programmes" and in a formal and space synthesis as "knowledge" images*" (Militerni, 1990).

Can we teach not to perceive? Can we teach not to remember? "*The brain is an element comparing and measuring the gap between our predictions based on the past and the information it currently receives from the world according to what it wants to achieve"* (Berthoz, 1997). Is it really possible to provide re-education that does not take into account patient capacity to learn and remember?

Therapeutic stretegies in disperception

The therapist must be able to carefully calibrate the use of attention and distraction according to perceptive errors made by the child. Mistakes due to suppression: increase attention towards information to be collected. Mistakes due to intolerance: reduce attention orienting it in other directions (dual task). Teaching not to pay attention, is actually a contradiction, since attention is the fundamental tool in achieving any form of learning. The learning process in this case can only be indirect and proceeds through imitation, delayed experience processing, subsequently acquired awareness of one's own capacities, and therefore, a subsequent improvement of self-esteem.

Some diplegic children (third form, see chapter 15) know how to walk but cannot stop, and constantly lean forward as if following the projection of their barycenter. Usually, they swing laterally with trunk and upper limbs in the frontal plane; they find it easier to move fast rather than slowly; they always slow down too late, and if they want to stop, they need to find something to hold onto. We can think that their motor behavior is due to a perceptive intolerance of backward space, and that propulsion does not represent a defect but rather a CNS strategy to prevent them from falling backwards. Other children of this form walk "only" if they feel the therapist's hand, even just one finger, on their shoulder. Does that hand have a motor or a perceptive facilitation task, considering that it is sufficient for the patient to think he still has it on the shoulder to keep on walking, while the doubt of not having it blocks him? For these children, the therapist's hand is something more than a motor facilitator: it is an orientation compass, a balance counterweight, a defensive shield, an encouragement to walk.

In the rehabilitation field, in order to respect the concept of perceptive tolerance, before wondering if a CP child can carry out a specific motor action, we should ask if he can bear its consequences from the perceptual point of view. Do movement and perception mature at the same time during development? Can the availability of motor repertoire be developed earlier than motion perceptive tolerance, especially in pre-term children or in CP children? This doubt creates some reservations about the concept of *early re-educational treatment*, which rehabilitation physicians have always agreed on. The recently consolidated presence of physiotherapists in neonatal intensive care units is a counterproof of this. Aren't we trying to reach quietness, tolerance, and autonomic control capacity in the pre-term child, by reducing perceptive conflicts, restricting intensity of disturbing environmental stimuli, limiting the aggressiveness of medical procedures performed on the child and favoring an improved state of well-being through correct postural hygiene (nest, hammock, pouch)?

It cannot be stated that the problem of perceptive intolerance only affects pre-term chil-

5

dren or CP ones. Imagine you are at the foot of a mountain face and you see two young alpinists, climbing above you on a very exposed route. What do you feel? Some feel a mixture of curiosity, interest, and admiration, but would never want to be in their shoes, some others could not even manage to look at them, since the sight of those climbers "holding on to nothing" makes them feel uneasy. Only a few people would feel a bit envious and somehow regretful. Perceptive intolerance can therefore be so intense as to make the sight of other people performing an action unbearable, due to a self-identification process (Ferrari, 2000). Perceptive data ends up overlapping the emotional field, especially for those children with self-integration difficulties (Marzani, 2005).

Illusion	Hallucinations
False interpretation of information. Errors of senses. Wrong data collection. Inaccurate synthesis. Solution found by the brain when facing a lack of coherence between collected information and the deriving anticipatory internal representations. Solution to perception problems that are ambiguous, inconsistent, contradictory between themselves or with the internal hypothesis that the brain has made of the external world, and therefore not compatible with the environmental data (Berthoz, 1997).	Perception without objectivity. Hallucinations are created by the brain itself since they do not originate from sensations that the brain cannot integrate into a consistent perception, but they are produced by endogenous memories about perceptions that suddenly are changing. In a certain sense, hallucinations are dreams made when awake, they are an autonomous functioning of the internal circuits that are usually utilized to simulate the consequences of an action (Berthoz, 1997).

On this subject, it might be useful to differentiate the concept of experience from the concepts of illusion and hallucination. Experience always refers to past events in personal background (positive or negative): we can imagine a child who, after falling many times with negative consequences, is now afraid of falling. Instead, *illusion* is an interpretative error made by the CNS, which considers some actually false perceptive information to be true. It is therefore a distorted perception, an inadequate representation of the object or of the situation, the result of an involuntary processing of real sensations made by the brain. A paradigmatic example of this concept is the Müller-Lyer's illusion (see image below).

In this illusion, even after measuring the lengths of the two lines and verifying that they are absolutely the same, observers cannot help seeing one line longer than the other, due to the orientation of the angled ends.

A hallucination is instead an impression built by the mind, and of which we become

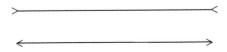

convinced, despite the absence of any real data ("perceptions without *objectivity*", Esquirol, 1838); "*false perceptions that are not distortions of real perceptions, but which appear in association with them and become something completely new*" (Jasper, 1959).

For the individual who perceives them, illusions and hallucinations are not different from normal sensory experience, with which they share some common characteristics such as: practicability, objectivity, spatiality and temporality. Thus the individual is not able to avoid hallucinations. We all have experienced the very strong illusion effect of moving when, sitting on a stopped train at the station, we see the train on the next track start to leave, or when we watch water run under a bridge, we have the impression that the bridge is moving (vection). When traveling by car in the summer, the hot asphalt makes the road look wet although our experience, and the subsequent confirmation we make later, demonstrate the opposite: it is obviously an illusion. Illusions are therefore solutions produced by an endogenous repertoire of motor or perceptive forms, with which sensory inputs are then matched. In this sense, for the brain they are the next best possible hypothesis to solve the problem (Berthoz, 1997).

The phenomenon of illusion is well known and exploited by magicians and ventriloquists.

If the "falling" child's (see chapter 14) fears were the expression of a previous experience, there would have been previous accidents with unpleasant consequences in his past. In any case, it would be materially impossible to fall from a 2 cm thick rug lying in the supine position. What the child reports when he says he is falling is a "prejudice", due to a perceptive illusion, which makes the surrounding emptiness and the depth of the extrapersonal space unbearable for him, and which does not allow him to verify the stability of the support, the real distance that separates him from the ground, the posture arrangement, the danger of the surrounding environment, etc.

A similar process can be found in amputees with the "ghost limb perception". This phenomenon shows us the existence of mental representations in our body, internal models of different segments, independent from their presence. A perceptive decision is needed to attribute a perceived part of our body to the body itself (Berthoz, 1997).

To better understand why CP children's behaviors can be so non-homogeneous, according to the perceptive channel used, and why they can lead to illusory and hallucinatory experiences, we have to consider the possible processes for the regulation of transducers and information manipulation carried out by the CNS (Ferrari, 1995). The brain is able to actively intervene on receptors in an anticipatory way, by selecting, tuning, amplifying, and suppressing information coming from the environment.

> *Calibration*: capacity to set peripheral receptors by pre-determining the quantity of information to be collected.
> *Amplification*: possibility to increase the reception capacity of sensitive and sensory systems by modifying their functional setting.
> *Collimation*: capacity to compare different types of sensory information in order to build a coherent representation of reality.
> *Rivalry*: capacity to distinguish between two stimuli simultaneously proposed in two symmetrical parts of the body.

5

> *Selection*: capacity to be attentive to an interesting stimulus by separating it from others.
> *Competition*: self-generation of information aimed at competing with other information that is considered negative.
> *Suppression*: mental process that helps us identify the problem but not to take it into consideration.
> *Dysgnosia*: mental inability to decode specific sensations by recognizing their meaning, even if sense organs and information transmission channels to the CNS are not impaired.

By *perceptive calibration* we mean the CNS's capacity to pre-determine the quantity of information to be collected and transmitted, by selecting and tuning it at the source so as not to exceed the tolerance threshold. Protecting the nose from very intense smells with a tissue, plugging the ears against a very loud noise, or semi-closing the eyes, peering just between the eyelids when looking at bright images: these all are behaviors showing the above-mentioned properties. In fact, control mechanisms are much finer and they are performed by inhibiting neurons located in the spinal cord that control sensory fiber activity, before they get to the target neurons in the posterior horns. Other mechanisms carry out this filtering on the first neuronal relay of the spinal cord and cerebral trunk. This pre-synaptic inhibition is a mechanism to block sensory input and calibrate its range in order to select messages according to the intentions of a specific moment (Berthoz, 1997). Gamma motoneurons of neuromuscular spindles, for example, modulate the sensory information of the muscles at its origin, regulating it to movement requirements (posture and gesture) or simulating the movement without executing it, in collaboration with Golgi tendon organs. This ability is fundamentally important for the specification of sensory messages that accompany action planning.

Sometimes perceptive calibration towards a stimulus occurs very rapidly: this is the case of a stale odor that we smell when entering a poorly-aired room, which we do not smell anymore if we remain in the room for a few minutes, or the case of tactile receptors that stop firing when the exploring surface is held still for a few seconds on the explored area. Also diplopia is a transient phenomenon: instead of two images that disturb each other, the brain learns to analyze only one, perceptively recalibrating the other one. These solutions allow us not to uselessly overload the CNS with constant signals. Neuronal inhibition is one of the fundamental mechanisms in the production of movement, and its flexibility, without doubt, is the main sensory-motor mechanism (Berthoz, 1997).

But not all information can be easily shielded. From the perceptive point of view, it is easier to climb up rather than climb down a ladder, differently from what we would think if we were guided only by physical tiredness. A person suffering from vertigo who has to cross a space exposed to emptiness cannot avoid closing his eyes, therefore paradoxically exposing himself more to the risk of motor errors, which are worse than those he would make if he looked carefully at what he was doing.

In children with CP, the perceptive tolerance threshold is often exceeded by the sum of several types of information. If the child looks at what he is touching, both an avoiding reaction and an upper limb flight reaction can appear, being typical expressions of perceptive intolerance, which would not occur if he would first look and then touch (temporal dissociation between stimuli). Some diplegics' load intolerance is higher when walking barefoot rather than wearing shoes, and further diminishes if the shoes have an anti-shock sole instead of a stiff sole (see chapter 15). Similarly, the use of parafoveal vision adopted by some dyskinetic children increases when the foveal image generates sensations that are too intense or too difficult to tolerate.

Among the main sensations that the CP child can receive with an intensity which is higher than his tolerance is information about depth, emptiness, and instability. This information is the basis of the "falling" child phenomenon (see chapter 14).

By *perceptive amplification* we mean the CNS's ability to increase the sensory system receptive capacity, by modifying the functional setting. "Keeping your eyes open and your ears peeled" describes this phenomenon, without which it would be more difficult to reach an adequate perceptive attention level. Pribram (1991) described this process in detail, finding that it is often impaired in CP children. Some young patients seem to be able to process visual, proprioceptive, tactile, or vestibular information, but they are totally unable to modulate their perception through anticipatory control. To improve their motor performance, in some cases it can be useful to enrich the environment with some particular sensory information (extraperceptual information, according to van der Weel et al. 1991). This "supplementary" information can be generated by the individual himself, for example clapping his hands at each step or tapping his feet on the ground in order to create an external rhythm, or it could be introduced through adaptative modifications of the environment, like making colourful footprints on the floor, which act as gait facilitating patterns through visual reference. For some diplegic patients, catching a moving object can be more difficult than grabbing a still object, as Lough (quoted by van der Weel et al. 1991) showed, because supplementary information improves timing and reduces the presence of involuntary movements. Some CP treatment methods, for example A. Petô's conductive education (Cotton, 1974), have made great use of the perceptive enrichment produced by the child himself (when during the activity he emphasizes the aim of his actions by singing rhythmic songs) and through a rigorous adaptation of the therapeutic setting and the patient's personal living environment.

By *perceptive collimation* we mean the CNS's capacity to match and compare information coming from different receptor systems. The CNS does not like information incongruence. A clear example is motion sickness (sea sickness, car sickness, air sickness, etc.), a situation in which information provided by orientation receptors does not correspond to the information provided by movement receptors. Visual information, which in absence of a sufficiently mobile horizon suggests environmental stability, does not match with proprioceptive and vestibular information, which instead indicates the instability of posture (sea sickness) or vice versa (car sickness). In CP, errors of different origin are possible, for example sight and proprioception can provide conflicting information to the CNS: sometimes a change in floor color makes the child climb down or up an inexistent step therefore inducing him to make a mistake by deficiency (passage from bright to dark), or by excess (passage from dark to bright). Other times, a step height, calculated at visual level, does not correspond with what had been estimated and transferred at the proprioceptive level during lifting of the lower limb to be moved forward. Therefore the patient often stumbles since he makes a mistake by deficiency, or strikes the floor with the foot thus making a mistake by excess. To improve the quality of movement, the child soon learns to use only one perceptive channel at a time or not to consider conflicting information, for example by not looking at his feet while he is walking.

By *perceptive rivalry* we mean the CNS's incapacity to distinguish between two stimuli proposed on two symmetrical parts of the body that arise at the same time. Usually the patient suppresses the stimulus on the most impaired side, or he is not able to understand which part the stimulus is coming from. For example, a hemiplegic individual is able to recognize the presence of a tactile or painful stimulus. He is also able to recognize the difference between these two stimuli or between two points, and he is able to recognize the presence or absence of an object that is pressed against his body surface and localize it, but he can not do so when the stimulus is bilateral, simultaneous, and symmetrical, and ends up suppressing the stimulus on the plegic side. The same thing occurs when, analyzing the visual perimeter, the visual stimuli are simultaneously present in the two visual fields: the hemiplegic child's eyes invariably turn towards the preserved hemi side (Sabbadini et al. 2000). The principle according to which re-educational treatment is based on the temporary penalization of the preserved hemisomal activity to facilitate plegic hemisomal recovery (constraint induced movement therapy) is widely based on this phenomenon.

Perceptive selection indicates the CNS's capacity to direct attention to the most interesting stimulus, keeping it tuned on a specific signal. This can occur within the same perceptive modality, for example visually separating a specific figure from the background, or the selected sound from the surrounding noise, or between different perceptive modalities, devoting attention to the most interesting information. In its absence, the individual's attention is captured by the most intense or the last stimulus, which is not always the most meaningful. In a few words, by concentrating on everything, the individual is not able to concentrate on anything. Among the possible compensation strategies used by this type of patient is the possibility to voluntarily increase the intensity of the interested stimulus he wants to maintain, for as long as he wants to. For example turning the volume on the TV up, even if he is not hypoacustic, as some dyskinetic children do.

By exploiting *perceptive competition* the individual learns to self-generate specific information to intentionally reduce the intensity of other sensations he does not want to receive, but which he is not able to sufficiently shield. For example, thermal or pressure information can contrast with pain information. This is why we immediately run to put our finger under cold water when we crush it, or we hold it tight, or otherwise we blow on it. Of course, the primitive information we try to reduce has not disappeared but its central representation has a lower intensity. This mechanism can also be exploited in an anticipatory way, by preceding an unpleasant stimulus with a more tolerable one that is able to compete with the following unpleasant stimulus. This is why we close our fists or we bite the pillow while we are waiting for an injection that we expect to be painful, or we spray ethyl chloride to induce a competitive cold sensation.

Perceptive suppression is not a real strategy but rather a mental process that helps us remove what we are not emotionally able to tolerate. According to cognitive theory on adaptation to sensory conflicts, perceptive suppression means keeping elementary signals at a distance. This adaptation process depends on a mental manipulation, which helps to identify the problem but teaches us not to take it into account. This mechanism is the basis of getting used to repeated stimuli. It justifies the indifference to pain shown by children subject to serious psychological disorders and the behavior of the "stand up" diplegic patient (see chapter 14), who, not being able to relate to the peri- and extra-personal space, ends up turning off the proprioceptive information that would inform him about his position and the displacements he is making.

By *dysgnosia* we refer to a mental incapacity to decipher sensations, by recognizing their meaning, although sense organs and transmission channels to the CNS are intact. In the perceptive field, dysgnosia is a cognitive disorder related to the processing and interpreting of information collected by sense organs. It is possible to distinguish between: tactile, visual, hearing, smell, topographic (etc.), dysgnosia.

Third Level: Representations

The *third level* comprises central representations, or mental images, namely, maps representing the final destination for information, after being collected and processed through experience (coding of reality, according to Bruner, 1968; re-descriptions of reality according to Karmiloff-Smith, 1992). These maps are part of the procedural memory heritage on which anticipatory mechanisms are based and are dynamically updated during movement itself. The re-description of representations is a process through which information, implicit in the mind, becomes explicit for the mind, initially related to a particular domain (group of representations that support a specific knowledge area) and then extended to other domains (Karmiloff-Smith, 1992). In any case, word representation has to be interpreted as something inside the child's mind and not as a depiction, meant as an exteriorized form of representation, such as in drawings or sculptures. The representative level is distinguished from the perceptive one: representations, differently from perceptions, can be evoked even in the absence of a promoting stimulus. "*The brain contains a library of prototypes of shapes, faces, objects, movements, synergies and there are as many sensory-motor spaces as body segments*" (Berthoz, 1997).

"*Twenty years of study have shown that children come into life with predispositions that guide the way they process specific domain inputs ... Predispositions can be specified as the architecture of the various parts of the brain, in terms of computational mechanisms the brain is equipped with and in terms of space-time limitations on cerebral development*" (Karmiloff-Smith, 1992).

"*The process of space representation is activated through active movement experience in the environment. This facilitates the emerging of spatial maps, through which sensory coordinates are transformed into spatial coordinates, which are relatively a-modal and lead and modulate movements and postural compensations. The different maps of space coordinates, based on neural perceptive-motor maps, interact to produce a spatial coherent reference system made up of invariant relations between perceptions*

and movements, namely topological aspects. These spatial references, by acting in parallel, produce spatial representations. Spatial maps are based on the coexistence of parallel representations that are initially topological (related to reciprocal spatial relations – of proximity and distance, etc – between objects and between objects and the body), then Euclidean (tied to internal relations inside each spatial configuration with regard to reference coordinates)"
(Camerini and De Panfilis, 2003).

According to Mandler (2000), topological reactions would be initially more accessible to the child than Euclidean ones. In other words, the innate mechanisms for the control of movement in space are "tested" by matching the environment, in order to generate new spatial maps, as a result of learning and trial/error strategies.

During development, different forms of space consciousness (knowledge) emerge, and the individual becomes more or less aware of them. Therefore, they can be explicit or implicit. Implicit, or procedural, knowledge, includes a series of interactive innate motor actions that are evoked and modulated by the first perceptive experiences. Explicit, or declarative, knowledge instead, evolves through learning acquired from experimentation with new motor actions (Camerini and De Panfilis, 2003).

Many recent studies, carried out with special brain CT scan techniques, have shown that, when an accidental loss or prolonged immobilization of a finger occurs, cortical projections of tactile receptors of the different hand segments are very rapidly re-organized, modifying the topographic setting of the sensory cortex. This re-organization also depends on the degree of use of that finger in grasping and manipulation tasks. However, information coming from the external world does not lead to a unique description of the stimuli, the "percept": events, objects and their spatial position are described again and again and for different aims. Together with the "visual" description of stimuli, which is necessary to compare objects and interiorize them, in parietal-frontal circuits multiple descriptions are usable for the different motor responses that the same stimulus can determine (Murata et al. 1997; Umiltà, 2000). According to this new motor system concept, the main constitutive element is represented by a series of circuits connecting in both directions a frontal area with a parietal area. The primary goal of these cortical circuits is not to provide a "perception" of stimuli, but to organize suitable responses to stimuli. Perception is a phenomenon produced by the integration of multiple sensory-motor circuits. Therefore, we can conclude that the spatial perceptive localization of the objective to be reached is determinant for the generation and active modulation of movement (Pierro, 1995).

"The brain uses several systems of reference for perception, in relation to the task to be accomplished, and to the available and more useful sensory indexes. Body pattern represents the sum of these reference systems"
(Berthoz, 1997).

Also at the level of mental representations it is possible to observe the presence of errors, among which the most typical is neglect, in its different forms. We talk about

perceptive neglect when the patient (acquired hemiplegic) does not process basic information, namely, sensations related to the left side of his body. Instead, we talk about personal
neglect if the patient does not pay attention to the situation on the left body side; we talk
about motor neglect when the individual does not use his left limbs, although their motility
is intact. Finally, we talk about extra-personal neglect when the patient does not pay attention to objects that are located on the left side of the environment that surrounds him. In
particular, perceptive and personal neglect can explain the presence of postural control
disorders in hemiplegic patients. Another example confirming the existence of body
mental representations in the brain is the ghost limb phenomenon, which is an error due to
a discrepancy between the internal model, which continues to feel the existence of a certain
body part, and the external reality, according to which that part no longer exists. Other
examples are given by agnosoagnosia (incapacity to recognize one's own illness or paralysis), inter-hemisphere disconnection (split brains), blind ness, etc. But the most impres-
sive mistake that our brain can make in terms of mental representations is give by
autoscopy (Brizzi et al. 1976), a rare event, also called ghost mirror image or visual hallucination of the other self (Lhermitte, 1951), already known in the times of Aristotle, and
probably due to a damage of the girus angularis (Blanke et al. 2002). During such events,
the individual has the sensation of leaving himself and becoming a second self (a double),
alive and thinking, projected into the surrounding space and observing himself as a hollow
wrapper, emptied of his active part.

For a CP child, what can be the destiny of perceptive information at the cognitive level?
Which internal representation of external reality will the child make if he cannot rely on
complete perceptive information, but rather on altered or conflicting information, collected
through a limited and distorted movement repertoire? As Anokhin (1966) stated, representation is not only about an external reality, but also about the construction of the most suitable action to operate on it, on single movements, and the related motor and perceptive
sequential feedback.

If our investments are based on the search for pleasure, how will the CP child invest in
movement if this provokes malaise instead of pleasure, conflict instead of integration, and
if the satisfaction is not worth the effort it produces? How will his self-esteem grow and
how will his personality develop? Learning does not just mean selecting and remembering,
but also suppressing and removing. What makes us successful and gives us pleasure will
be preserved, but failure and negative experiences must be removed. During this process,
perceptive and cognitive aspects have an utmost responsibility and represent the prerequisite for the development of any function.

Is the *containment* we mentioned in relation to pre-term infants a purely physical and
perceptive dimension, or does it include the whole interior world of the child?

Is *stillness* just the lack of movement or the expression of the achievement of autonomic
control? Is it passive or does it imply an interior commitment? Is it total immobility or a
pleasant continuity of a constant and controlled movement, like being cradled? Is it indifference or openness towards the environment? Is it a renouncement or a predisposition of
being, without which any form of action would be hostile?

What happens if during re-educational treatment we induce incorrect, inadequate, or
harmful perceptive experiences in the CP child? It is easy to demonstrate that, most of the

5

time refusal and renouncing are facilitated, therefore that "intentional" palsy, which, together with "motor" and "perceptive" ones, represents the third dimension of cerebral palsy.

References

Aicardi J, Bax M (1998) Cerebral palsy. In: Aicardi J (ed) Diseases of the nervous system in childhood. 2nd Ed. Mac Keith Press, London, pp 210-239

Ayres AJ (1974) The development of sensory integration. Theory and practice. Kendall Hunt Dubuque, Iowa

Anokhin PK (1966) Cybernetics and integrative brain activity. Vop Psykhol, 3, n°10

Bax M (1964) Terminology and classification of cerebral palsy. Dev Med Child Neurol: 6:295-297

Bax M, Goldstein M, Rosenbaum P et al. (2005) Proposed definition and classification of cerebral palsy. Dev Med Child Neurol 47:571-6

Behrman RE, Kliegman RM, Arvin AM (1998) Nelson essentials of Pediatrics, 3rd Ed. WB Saunders, Philadelphia, chap. 1, 50-52

Bernstein NA (1967) The co-ordination and regulation of movement. Pergamon Press, Oxford

Berthoz A (1997) Le sens du mouvement. Odile Jacob Edition, Paris. English edition: Berthoz A (2000) The brain's sense of movement. Harvard University Press, Cambridge, Ma

Bick E (1968) The experience of skin in early object relations. Int J Psychoanal 49:484-486

Bick E (1986) Further consideration on the function of the skin in early object relations: findings from infant observation integrated into child and adult analysis. Brit J Psychother 2:292-299

Blanke O, Ortigue S, Landis T, Seeck M (2002) Stimulating illusory own-body perceptions. Nature 19; 419:269-270

Brizzi RE, Ferrari A, Mainini P, Parma M (1976) In tema di autoscopia. Edizioni AGE, Rivista sperimentale di Freniatria C, IV:876-884

Bruner J, Olver R, Greenfield P (1966) Studies in cognitive growth. John Wiley and Sons, New York

Camerini GB, De Panfilis C (2003) Psicomotricità dello sviluppo. Carocci Faber editore, Roma

Capelovitch S (2000) The perceptual - motor diade. EBTA Conference, Verona 6-7 Sept

Cotton E (1974) Improvement in motor function with the use of conductive education. Dev Med Child Neurol 16:637-643

Dan B, Cheron G (2004) Reconstructing cerebral palsy. J Ped Neurology 2:57-64

Esquirol JE (1838) Des maladies mentales considérées sous les rapports médical, hygiénique et médico-légal. Baillière, Paris

Ferrari A (1990) Interpretative dimension of infantile cerebral paralysis. In: Papini M, Pasquinelli A, Gidoni EA (Eds) Development, handicap, rehabilitation: practice and theory. Elsevier, Amsterdam, Excerpta medica international congress series 902:193-204

Ferrari A (1995) Paralisi cerebrali infantili: appunti di viaggio attorno al problema della classificazione. Giorn Neuropsich Età Evol 15, 3:191-205

Ferrari A (2000) Motor related perceptual problems in cerebral palsy children. EBTA Conference "From perception to movement" Verona 6-9 sett. 2000: 32-37. Atti a cura della ULSS 20 di Verona

Fodor JA (1983) The modularity of mind, an essay on faculty. Psychology, The MIT Press, Cambridge, Mass

Forssberg H, Nashner LM (1982) Ontogenic development of postural control in man: adaptation to altered support and vision. J Neurosc 2:522-545

Gibson JJ (1966) The senses considered as perceptual system. Houghton Mifflin, Boston
Gibson JJ (1979) Principles of perceptual learning and development. Appleton-Century-Crofts, New York
Gibson JJ (1979) The ecological approach to visual perception. Houghton Mifflin, Boston
Goldner JL (1961) Upper extremity reconstructive surgery of the hand in cerebral palsy or similar conditions. AAOS Instructional course lectures, vol. 18 p. 169 Mosby, St Louis CV
Gottlieb G (1971) Ontogenesis of sensory function in birds and mammals. In: Tobach E, Aronson LA, Shaw E (eds) The biopsychology of development. Academic Press, New York, pp 67-128
Gruesser OJ, Landis T (1991) Visual agnosia and related disorders. In: Cronly-Dillon J (eds) Vision and visual dysfunction. MacMillan, Basingstoke (UK)
Jasper K (1959) Allgemeine Psychopathologie, 7 ed. Springer, Berlin
Kant I (1781) Kritik der reinen Vernunft. Laterza, Bari (1966) (Italian edition)
Karmiloff-Smith A (1992) Beyond modularity. A developmental perspective on cognitive science. MIT Press, Cambridge, Mass
Lee DN, von Hofsten C, Cotton E (1997) Perception in action approach to cerebral palsy. In: Connolly KJ, Forssberg H (eds) Neurophysiology and neuropsychology of motor development. Clinics in Dev Med, n° 143/144. Mac Keit Press, Cambridge University Press, Cambridge 257-285
Lhermitte J (1951) Les hallucinations. G. Doin, Paris
Lough S (1984) Visuo-motor control following stroke: a motor skills perspective. PhD thesis, Edinburgh University
Mac Keith RC, Mackenzie ICK, Polani PE (1959) Definition of cerebral palsy. Cerebral palsy Bulletin 5:23
Mandler JM (2000) Perceptual and conceptual processes in infancy. J Cogn Dev 1:3-36
Marzani C (2005) Psicopatologia e clinica dei disturbi mentali nei bambini con paralisi cerebrale infantile. In: Ferrari A, Cioni G (eds) Le forme spastiche della paralisi cerebrale infantile. Guida all'esplorazione delle funzioni adattive. Springer-Verlag Italia, Milan
Meraviglia MV (2004) Complessità del movimento. Franco Angeli editore, Milano
Mesulam MM (1998) From sensation to cognition. Brain, 121:1013-1052
Militerni R (1990) La diagnosi neuroevolutiva. Idelson, Napoli
Morasso PG (2000) Modelli di controllo del movimento: apprendimento ed esecuzione. In: Giannoni P, Zerbino L (ed) Fuori schema. Springer-Verlag Italia, Milan
Murata A, Fadiga L, Fogassi L et al (1997) Object representation in the ventral premotor cortex (area F 5) of the monkey. J Neurophysiol 78:226-230
Mutch L, Alberman E, Hagberg B et al (1992) Cerebral palsy epidemiology: where are we now and where are we going? Dev Med Child Neurol 34:547-551
Pierro MM (1995) Lo spazio e l'attività, il movimento e la coordinazione sensomotoria. Introduzione ai disturbi spaziali nei bambini. In: Sabbadini G (ed) Manuale di neuropsicologia dell'età evolutiva. Zanichelli editore, Bologna
Poincaré H (1932) Le valeur de la science. Flammarion, Paris
Popper K (1996) Knowledge of the body mind problem. Routledge, New York
Pribram K H (1991) Brain and perception: holonomy and structure in figural processing. Erlbaum, New York
Sabbadini G, Bianchi PE, Fazzi E, Sabbadini M (2000) Manuale di neuroftalmologia dell'età evolutiva. Franco Angeli editore, Milano
Schilder P (1935) The image and appearance of human body. Phycol Monographs n°4, Kegan, London
Sherrington CS (1906) The integrative action of the nervous system. Yale University Press, New Haven, CT
Smith Churchland P (2008) Neurofilosofia una nuova scienza. Giornale di neuropsicofarmacologia anno 2008 n° 1 gen-mar 2008 pp 5-9 CIC edizioni internazionali

Starita A (1987) Metodi di intelligenza artificiale in rieducazione motoria. In: Leo T, Rizzolatti G (ed) Bioingegneria della riabilitazione. Patron editore, Bologna

Tizard JPM, Paine RS, Crothers B (1954) Disturbance of sensation in children with hemiplegia. J Am Med Assoc 155:628-632

Turkewitz G, Kenny PA (1982) Limitations on input as a basis for neural organisation and perceptual development: a preliminary theoretical statement. Developmental Psychobiology 15:357-368

Umiltà MA (2000) L'area premotoria F5 ed il riconoscimento delle azioni. Tesi di Dottorato di Ricerca in Neuroscienze. Università degli Studi di Parma

Van der Meer ALH, van der Weel FR (1999) Development of perception in action in healthy and at-risk children. Acta Pediatr Suppl 429:29-36

Van der Weel FR, van der Meer ALH, Lee DN (1991) Effect of task on movement control in cerebral palsy: implication for assessment and therapy. Dev Med Child Neurol 33:419-426

Woollacott MH, Shumway-Cook A (1995) Motor learning and recovery of function. In: Motor control: therapy and practical applications. William & Wilkins, Baltimore, pp 23-43

Praxic Organization Disorders

6

S. Muzzini, F. Posteraro, R. Leonetti

Definition of Developmental Dyspraxia and Pathogenetic Hypotheses

The word "apraxia" was first used in 1781 by Steinthal to indicate an incorrect use of objects provoked by non-recognition. Therefore, at the beginning, the word included the idea of both "agnosia" and "apraxia", as interpreted today.

In 1900, Leipman redefined apraxia as a specific primitive disorder of motor function, consisting of an inability to use movement for intentional actions, with an unquestionable separation of the concept of apraxia from agnosia and emphasizing the intentional character of movement.

For many years, the study of apraxia remained limited to the field of adult neurology and, therefore, acquired disorders. Only during the 1960s did the first references to "developmental dyspraxia" begin to appear. The main reference was to *clumsy or awkward children* for any motor performance, even for the most common activities of daily life, like washing, dressing, using silverware, handling objects and tools, riding a bike, writing or drawing.

In the past, the words "clumsiness" and "awkwardness" were used as synonyms in the literature, and their meaning often coincided with dyspraxia during the developmental age. Children affected by developmental dyspraxia were, therefore, described as "clumsy", and again, in 1992, Smith proposed *"abnormal clumsiness in children otherwise normal"* as the definition.

Since then, many different terms have been applied to this childhood disorder and there is still no agreement, even the most influential diagnostic manuals use different nosological labels: the DSM IV defines it as developmental coordination disorder, the ICD 10 as specific developmental disorder of motor function. We prefer rather to use the term developmental dyspraxia because of its simplicity and its clear reference to the neurological adult disturbance.

No doubt, the miscellanea of terms reflects poor knowledge of the underlying nature of the dysfunction.

Gubbay (1985) refered to children characterized by a *"disorder in the ability of executing correct and intentional movements"*, who show virtually normal motor func-

6

tioning during the neurological examination, normal cognitive levels and normal sensorial functions. In this way he starts to define a clinical framework of a poorly defined pathology, which remains in the uncertain condition between syndrome and symptom even today. All subjects showing disorders in praxic abilities within other major neurological, cognitive or psychological pathologies are automatically excluded; however, this is not enough to clarify the nature of this disorder.

During recent years, the recognition of new developmental disorders concerning non-verbal abilities, such as the attentional deficit and hyperactive disorder (ADHD), has complicated the uncertainty of diagnostic criteria even more. Although the developmental coordination disorder (DCD), according to the DSM, is considered completely separate from the other nosological entities concerning non-verbal skills, such as the developmental receptive language disorder (DRLD) and developmental reading disorder (DRD), the same child frequently shows a combination of these with a prevalence of one, (Henderson and Barnett, 1998).

It is also quite easy to verify that many signs recognizable in dyspraxic children are described in the profile of nonverbal learning disorders (NVLD) (Rourke, 1989; Levi et al. 1999).

Some of the authors who have dealt with clumsiness have tried to identify the possible pathogenesis and analyze the links with probable etiological factors, questioning whether praxic disorder is an independent pathological condition or not, whether it consists of a single disorder or several differentiable conditions. Moreover the questions regularly asked by neuropsychology in relation to a functional disorder: "Is there a correspondence between sign and structure? What is the biological substrate? and In any case, what is the error that provokes its manifestation?" have not yet been answered.

So far several albeit non-exhaustive hypotheses have been formulated. Although developmental dyspraxia is considered a specific disorder, the studies regarding its nature are all but univocal. The concept of "minimal brain damage" proposed by Touwen (Touwen and Sporrel, 1979), reformulated by Jongmans in 1998 and Hadders-Algra in 2003, does not really provide any specific explanation, for it only establishes an etiological continuity between the presence of "minor neurological signs", dyspraxia, and perinatal conditions at risk of causing neurological dysfunction.

Some hypotheses regarding a possible involvement of the left parietal lobe or a cerebellum dysfunction have been formulated without evidence of any specific morphological damage to the CNS in MRI. Tanaka suggested that the basis of dyspraxia is a disconnection of the fibers between the right and left parietal lobes, emphasizing the role played by the corpus callosum (Tanaka et al. 1996).

In the past other authors interpreted dyspraxia with hypotheses focused on functional organization such as an inter- or intra-hemisphere integration disorder, or as an alteration of kinesthetic perception analysis (Bairstow and Lazlo, 1985) or, as a visual-kinesthetic modal transfer disorder and visual-spatial perception defect (Hulme et al. 1982; van der Meulen et al. 1991).

More recently, a group of Italian authors (Bassi et al. 2002) emphasized the recurrence of perception deficits, errors in the estimation of visuospatial parameters, and difficulties in representing movements.

It seems that the disperceptive-disgnosic nature of dyspraxia is finding a greater consensus among those in the clinical field. However, there is no positive connection between deficit or alteration of a single perception modality and praxic disorder. Losse et al. (1991) analyzed single perceptual modalities in a group of dyspraxic children and found no or variable involvement, therefore suggesting the hypothesis of a higher level integration disorder that acts during both the programming and control phase.

Dyspraxia and Infantile Cerebral Palsy

Most authors seem to agree on two principles:

1. Dyspraxia is not simply a movement disorder, but an *action disorder*, that means a disorder of intentional movements, or, more precisely, movement combinations learned to achieve a specific goal;
2. It is only possible to speak of dyspraxia when there are no other major neurological, cognitive or emotional pathologies that may interfere or limit motor learning.

The consequence of the first statement is that dyspraxia must be considered a motor learning disease; therefore, it does not concern the development of genetically programmed primary motor functions, but possibly their use within learned skills. The implication of the second statement is that dyspraxia is a motor learning disorder in an otherwise normal child. This last point seems to contradict those referring to dyspraxia in cerebral palsy (CP). However, as others before us, we believe that not all motor impairments in CP children are due to palsy when interpreted only as a motor disorder. During the 1970s, Sabbadini pointed to the existence of dyspraxia as a hidden phenomenon in CP: *"we realize that the motor disorder of 'Cerebral Palsy' is the result of the interference (or sum) of several factors, which can all be expressed as executive and cognitive disorders at high integration level. They are not only added to spasticity, rigidity, dystonia, ataxia, but mostly influence motor disorder itself in a quite significant way.... Supposing it is possible, even temporarily, to remove spasticity, children affected by cerebral palsy would still show an only-apparently motor (more precisely executive) disorder, which can be expressed as clumsiness or awkwardness. Actually, this 'executive' disorder is nothing more than the result of the sum or interference of various disorders that we may generally define as 'apraxia' and 'agnosia', where these two terms outline a series of 'executive' and 'cognitive' disorders at high integration level"* (Sabbadini, 1978).

At that time, due to the lack of hard scientific evidence, Sabbadini asked his readers to rely on their imagination to support these "intuitions", and to mentally remove spasticity from a spastic child in order to see him "beyond" the palsy.

Recent studies carried out on dyspraxia, which are supported by action control models and highlighted by information coming from neurophysiology studies on motor action, can now provide insights that go beyond intuition and make it possible to start the discussion on an empirical basis.

Motor Control Models

During the second half of the twentieth century, neurosciences tried to provide an explanation of those processes that are the grounds for voluntary movements, or actions. Various theories have been formulated, and various models have been proposed, which are often contradictory. We do not intend to start a discussion on the various theories, which have been described very well by other authors (Zoia, 2004), but we have chosen to illustrate one model among the most significant ones which deal with this subject. The selected model was proposed by Laszlo and Bairstow (1995). We referred to this model in one of our recent clinical studies for the experimental evaluation proposal and data discussion (Muzzini et al. 2002).

This model is built on of four levels or processes (Fig. 6.1):

1. The first level consists of input components, which make it possible to receive the following:
   a) Inputs regarding environmental conditions where movements must be executed, such as intrinsic features of objects and spatial relationships among various objects. For this task, visual information obviously plays an important role.
   b) Inputs regarding body and limb position, supported by visual and sensorial information concerning muscle tone, coming from neuromuscular spindles and tendinous and articular receptors. All information originating from these receptors is integrated to form kinesthetic information.
   c) Any further information regarding the movement to be performed, for example, verbal instructions. However, it seems that the role played by this type of information is not very relevant.
2. The second level consists of central processes, which are divided into standards and motor programming systems (MPS); they do not directly refer to any specific anatomic entity, but they are used to describe two different functional systems.

   In fact, the "standard" is the level where input information, originating from corollary discharge and sensitive/sensorial feedback, is processed, stored (in the form of mnesic traces related to previously carried out attempts), and then used to formulate action programming. After motor programming has been established, the standard "instructs" the MPS, which is responsible for selecting and activating those muscles involved in the execution of a movement. So, while the action plan formulated by the standard defines the overall approach that should be used to achieve a goal, the MPS establishes how this will be reached through the activation of different combinations of muscular motor units. It is interesting to note that, at this level, the goal or the purpose for the execution of a motor action is also considered. For example, in physiological conditions, the way an object is grasped is completely different depending on the destined use. This means that the same movement (grasping) is programmed in a different way only because that object has two different destinations. Based on this characteristic it is possible to evaluate the functioning or non-functioning of the MPS with the following test: the person is asked to grasp a specific object and alternatively throw it into a large container, or introduce it into a correspondingly shaped hole. The two grasping patterns

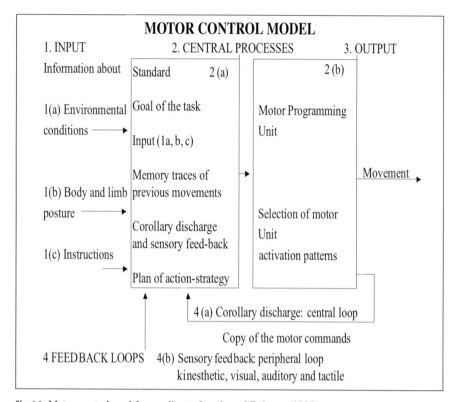

Fig. 6.1 Motor control model according to Laszlo and Baistow (1995)

will be completely different in normal individuals, while they will not appropriately vary in the case of pathological individuals. Unfortunately, this methodology is not very reliable in CP, where the presence of rigid motor patterns may be a prominent feature of the clinical picture and does not necessarily imply a motor programming disorder.

3. The third level is indicated as output and refers to muscular response, which is naturally different depending on whether there are isometric or isotonic contractions.
4. Finally, the fourth level refers to feedback loops, which consist of a central loop (corollary discharge) and peripheral loop (sensory feedbacks).

Due to corollary discharge, the standard receives a copy of the motor command sent to the output level, which contains information regarding the number of activated motor units, their time sequence and, activation frequency. The corollary discharge is only generated if the subject actually performs active movements, but it is not produced if the subject passively performs the same motor action with assistance. This information regarding motor programming is stored in memory and ensures the effectiveness and further improvement of successive motor performances. However, the corollary discharge does not contain any information regarding the purpose of movement, while information regarding performance success or failure is generated by sensory feedbacks.

Within feedback data, kinesthetic and visual information always plays the most important role, while the role of tactile and auditory information can have different relevance according to the motor task.

Neurophysiological Basis of Action

At the basis of any upper limb praxic activity, there are apparently simple motor actions. Relatively recent studies in neurophysiology (Rizzolatti et al. 1996, 2001) have shown the basic mechanisms required for programming and executing any upper limb movements aimed at reaching, grabbing, and handling an object, which is the praxic function.

Approaching the subject, we need to ask ourselves several questions:
1. How are movements planned?
2. How can sensory information give feedback to motor plans?
3. How are these messages translated?
4. How do motor areas give feedback to neurons for performing an action?

In summary, how does our CNS work? In particular, what happens before any motor action, during the so-called anticipatory phase?

According to which code is perceptive information translated into motor sequences? After a previous hypothesis, which considered joint coordinates as crucial – i.e., the rotation angles of every joint segment compared with the previous ones - it is now believed that the translation code is based on spatial coordinates. In this particularly fascinating system, hand positioning and requested movements are specified by a vector whose components are measured by a system of Cartesian axes that has the body of the subject as its center. This system offers a more abstract representation of movement, because it does not consider kinematic restrictions imposed by joints and muscles. Experimental data confirm that the CNS uses this system in determining upper limb movement direction.

Neurophysiological studies carried out during the 1980s on monkeys and subsequently confirmed on humans - to which primate experimental models may be transferred – have assigned an autonomous and differentiated function to area 6 or the pre-motor area, as compared with area 4 or the primary motor area. For this purpose, much experimental evidence has been collected.

In area 6, three zones have been differentiated: the mesial or supplementary zone, and the upper and lower motor areas. Upper area 6, or F2, mostly receives inputs from area 5; therefore, it processes proprioceptive information. Lower area 6 receives impulses (inputs) mostly from the lower parietal lobe; therefore, it processes both somatosensory and visual information. In turn, this area may be divided into two subareas, called F4 and F5, which are functionally different from each other. In F4, we find neurons responding to somatosensory and tactile stimuli; their receptive fields are located mainly on the face, but also around the body. We find neurons responding to visual stimuli coming from the peripersonal space, in particular from a moving object. Processed information differs from

visual sensory cortex information because it is not retinal. These neurons codify the position of an object in peri-personal space, in relation to body position, and may provide
instructions on the point that the hand should reach in order to grab a given object. They
discharge when the arm performs a movement towards that specific position in space or as
a consequence of visual information, which is passively determined by the presence of the
object in that specific area. Therefore, we can identify a relationship between a visual
response and a motor one. It seems that this area is particularly interested in the arm transport component (proximal movements).

The activation moment of neurons in the F4 area depends on the depth of the visual
field, which is the distance between object and body; this decreases in relation to the speed
of the object approaching the body. This fact should indicate that visual transformations
occurring in this area are plastic, in the sense that they show learning abilities, making it
possible to predict the time required for the object to enter the peri-personal space: the
faster the object approaches, the earlier involved neurons are activated in order to ensure
fast programming of upper limb movement.

In the F5 area we find two types of neurons, canonical and mirror, with completely
different features: *canonical neurons* are responsible for a vocabulary of different movements and discharge when the monkey performs hand movements aimed at grabbing and
handling objects (distal movements). These neurons are able to specify the kind of movement requested, that is, they are activated in relation to the kind of grasping movement
needed (accurate grip, finger-palm grip, interdigital grip, etc.) or in relation to object
features (small - a seed, or long - a stick). This activation occurs on the basis of intrinsic
visual stimuli, i.e., regarding object shape and size. Neuron discharges are not related so
much to simple movements (such as finger prehension), but rather mostly to complex
movements which are goal-directed. In certain situations, movements using the same
muscles but for different purposes fail to activate the same neurons, while movements
performed by different effectors (hand, mouth, foot) but having the same purpose
do. Thus, the brain decodes goals not movements. Interestingly, some neurons
also respond when one monkey observes another one performing the same action or a
similar one. These neurons are called *mirror neurons* because the observed action seems
to be reflected as in a mirror. They discharge even if the monkey does not move (anticipatory response) but only watches the action performed by the experimenter. This aspect
may be very important for motor learning processes: watching another individual perform
a given action automatically activates mental representations of the observed action , i.e.
motor programs, independently from whether this action is then performed or not. It
seems that these same neurons allow for the correct interpretation of action meaning,
when performed by others. This has significant effects in terms of social relationships
between one animal and another, and between one person and another, and opens a new
perspective in rehabilitation (Buccino G et al. 2006)

To perform an action, it is not only necessary to activate a motor program, but it is also
necessary to have a specific motivation to do so. Therefore, we should not be surprised by
the fact that the pre-motor area can also be activated without performing movement.

In humans, positron emission tomography (PET scanning) has shown that when an
individual imagines he is performing a specific action, the pre-motor area is activated even

if the imagined movement is not carried out. This gives a new meaning to intentionality, which does not simply refer to motivation, and assigns a specific neurophysiological role to it in the execution of motor programs.

The importance of the parietal lobe in action planning is well documented. In fact, lesions to the parietal lobe can produce apraxia syndromes in humans: individuals no longer know how to perform a praxic movement, or they do not know to use an object. Recent research carried out on the lower parietal lobule, or area 7, which has been shown to convey information to lower area 6, can shed some light on this subject. Numerous subareas have also been identified in area 7, each involved in specific processes; in particular, two areas have been analyzed: the ventral intra-parietal area (VIP) and the anterior inter-parietal area (AIP). In the VIP, there are neurons that respond to tactile stimuli from facial receptive fields, and to visual stimuli from objects situated in determined peripersonal space sectors. These have extremely similar properties when compared with area F4 neurons, and a direct connection between the two has been shown in subsequent studies. Both these areas are involved in processing extrinsic object features when the arm is reaching for an object (reaching phase).

Likewise, in the AIP, neurons are specific for each kind of prehension to be performed, and their properties are quite similar to those of area F5 neurons (grasping and handling phase). Therefore the existence of a circuit involved in hand praxic movements was hypothesized. Accordingly, the lower parietal lobule is connected to the lower pre-motor area, where neurons not only send motor instructions to area 4 for movement performance (for example, prehension) but also send a copy of the same instructions to the parietal area. This area is responsible for checking correct movement performance through visual and motor information, meaning that it plays a feedback role for object grasping and handling. This suggests that the CNS has evolved to achive very complex patterns of connectivity among areas. Such connectivity is the basis of complex neural circuits. They must integrate information from visual, auditory, somatosensory, and limbic sources to support skilled hand motor functions.

Clinical Hypotheses

The above-mentioned neurophysiological studies provide new information on motor action planning processes that occur during the anticipatory phase. It seems that this phase is more crucial in interpreting praxic disorders than the executive phase. This is particularly interesting in CP, considering how difficult it is to differentiate motor palsy from dyspraxia during the executive phase. If the hypothesis that dyspraxia originates from a problem in the anticipatory phase is correct, the presence of a distinct disorder recognized as dyspraxia is not only acceptable, but provides a new interpretation of an important part in the executive disorder of CP. Evidence of the role played by the anticipatory phase in the origin of developmental dyspraxia clearly emerged from the studies by Smith (Smith, 1991). Smith stated that children with developmental dyspraxia show difficulties in programming their movements, and this creates a dependence, which is greater than normal, on action regulation systems during action performance (feedback). It was shown that the time required for the performance of complex motor sequences (not yet learned) is longer for clumsy people than for a control group; this time difference is not dependent on the kind of sensory control used (auditory, visual, or tactile control). This would show that the longer time required and lower fluency of action in dyspraxic people should depend on what precedes the action, i.e., processes supporting intentional movement planning.

Actually, the importance of mechanisms involved in motor control whose activation precedes the beginning of movement has been known for many years. At the beginning of the 20th century, neurophysiologists referred to movement "representation" only in general terms. Then in 1926, Head introduced the concept of motor "scheme", which initially referred only to posture but, later on, also included the existence of an internal model of a still or moving body. Based on these findings, several motor control models were developed such as the "information processing" model by Marr (1982), the "top-down bottom-up control" theory and the "hierarchical organization" by Jeannerod, etc. All these models assumed the existence of a motor programming level consisting of mechanisms which are activated before the primary motor area.

This motor control level may be affected separately, as in developmental dyspraxia or in complex diseases involving different motor control aspects, such as CP, which makes the clinical picture more complicated and interferes with the rehabilitation process.

Therefore, in CP we need to differentiate three types of problem strictly connected which influence motor performance:
1. Action-planning problems:
   - information processing (perceptive inputs)
   - perceptive – motor integration
   - operational strategies formulation
2. Executive problems:
   - selection of single movement and/or movement combinations
   - executive sequence control
3. Skeletal-muscle system problems:
   - deficits and acquired defects of the skeletal-muscle system

It has been widely demonstrated that CP children may be affected by significant disorders in perception and analysis of space, which cause an inability to control peri-personal space. Furthermore, the spatial relationship among various body segments can also be involved: this alters knowledge of them, both for static and to a greater extent dynamic conditions, thus creating a distorted body scheme. If a difficulty in analyzing kinesthetic information, the main feedback control mechanism together with visual information, is present, it is easily understood that CP children may have difficulties in action planning. This can be due to an alteration in perceptive information, which is indispensable for building and generating appropriate motor programs.

Motor difficulties in CP children are not only executive problems, due to symptoms like spasticity, excessive primitive reflexes and involuntary movements, etc, but they quite frequently involve the programming and planning of goal directed motor actions.

Forssberg H (1992) carried out an interesting study concerning motor action compo-

6

nents, during an upper limb motor task, in hemiplegic and diplegic children. Compared with normal subjects, a lack of "modulation" of motor unit anticipatory activation was documented in these children related to an object grasping and lifting task.

During a lifting task requiring a precision grip, a normal adult programs the increase of grip and load force in advance. If force increase modulation depended only on proprioceptive feedback, there would be a long latency period during which an excessive grip force and a fast acceleration of the object should occur. In reality, programmed forces are based on an internal representation of the object's physical features (size, weight, shape). This anticipatory control of forces leads to low initial speed, which ensures good vertical acceleration control. Therefore, for an unknown task, in normal subjects there is a learning period during which an irregular force profile can be registered on a graph for both dynamic (grip and load) and static (object suspension) phases; after several task repetitions this profile acquires a typical bell shape – corresponding to an ability to suitably and anticipatorily dose required forces. This is not the case of CP children, in whom the post-learning change is irrelevant and only related to the static phase. It is as if CP children face the same task every time for the first time. In fact, while the static phase shows a small change based on proprioceptive feedback, the force required for the grip and load dynamic phase remains mostly overestimated, showing the failure of anticipatory planning.

From the clinical viewpoint, the association between CP and disorder in anticipatory action planning provokes a discrepancy between the available motor repertoire and its use in a goal directed sequence. In addition, considering that the motor programming phase is indispensable for learning new motor behaviors, the association between dyspraxia and palsy makes it even more difficult to obtain any further improvement in motor abilities. Therefore, dyspraxia should be considered a disorder of goal directed motor learning which is not related to genetically-programmed motor functions, but to their use in newly learned abilities during development.

The problem of how to identify this disorder in CP children, when associated with executive motor difficulties, still remains to be solved.

Assessment: a Clinical Proposal

The complete use of test material normally proposed for developmental age, such as the protocol recently proposed by Bassi et al. 2002 or Sabbadini L. 2004, may be a problem in CP children due to the typical executive disorder of palsy. The greater the executive disorder, the more difficult it is to separate the executive palsy components from the underlying motor programming disorder. In the most serious cases, such as tetraplegias, the executive deficit is so severe that it is impossible to distinguish dyspraxia. We can reasonably suppose that tetraplegic children can also be dyspraxic, but it is impossible for us to clinically demonstrate it. In any case, this may be irrelevant in relation to prognosis and treatment.

Contrarily, in more favorable clinical conditions, such as diplegia and hemiplegia, if these children fail to perform apparently simple tasks, or tasks for which they have the required executive tools, we may suspect dyspraxia. In these cases, identifying the presence of a dyspraxic disorder, in addition to executive-motor palsy, is crucial for properly choosing the rehabilitation program, thus avoiding extremely frustrating experiences for both the children and their families. The core element for observation is the discrepancy between available motor repertoire and its use for a goal directed action; this justifies a neuropsychological investigation when trying to understand the nature of a motor disorder, especially where palsy alone does not provide sufficient explanations. Since anamnesis is always the first step for an accurate investigation, parents should be extensively interviewed regarding learning periods and modalities for basic praxic abilities involving daily life activities.

Provided that a neurological examination, an observational analysis and a functional assessment have already been carried out, a cognitive assessment is also important. It is well known that a discrepancy between verbal IQ (Intelligence Quotient) and performance IQ of at least 10 points is one of the main diagnostic criteria for developmental dyspraxia. A significant difference between verbal and performance abilities is certainly an extremely important factor, although not sufficient, also in CP children. At this point the use of an Intelligence Scale Test based on child age would be helpful. The use of non-verbal scales, such as those of Leiter and Raven, provides extremely valuable information regarding spatial analysis abilities, crucial in praxic disorder in CP children, although they do not permit any comparison between verbal and non-verbal intelligence.

The assessment of hand praxis with or without objects may be carried out using a standardized battery of tests now available for the developmental age, suitably composed of simple and complex tasks, monomanual and bimanual activities. Verbal, non-verbal, and imitation procedures must be followed. Facilitation by operators, whose importance and effectiveness are useful tools in order to assess individual operating strategies, is permitted.

It is crucial that the tester knows the physiological development of praxic skills corresponding to the age and is always aware of the effort required and the level of assistance provided. In fact, the assessing procedure and type of facilitation considerably influence the response quality, as recently demonstrated by Zoia (2004).

The analysis of constructional praxis must be as accurate as possible, considering how recurrent constructional disorders are in CP children, even when present as an isolated disorder. Block-building tests, Goldstein "sticks" and VMI (Visual Motor Integration) – used as a graphic constructional task - have been shown to be particularly sensitive and easy to administer.

Perceptive and gnosic components are the most difficult to investigate. For the spatial - visual perceptive component, geometrical shape sequences and figure-matching tests, like the VPT, are very significant. To evaluate the perceptive-kinesthetic component, besides the traditional neurological test, which asks for passive finger movement direction, two other possible tests have been proposed by Bairstow and Laszlo (1995): the simpler one measures the ability of discriminating different heights to which hand is raised; the more complex one requires the child to recognize the spatial form of a passive hand movement and match it to a graphic model. Given that the latter also includes a modal transfer, it cannot be considered "pure" when interpreting the results.

The assessment of gnosic abilities involves two main components: stereognosis and visual gnosis. Small-objects matching tasks are particularly indicated to assess stereog-nosis, specific educational "bingo games" made of commonly used wooden objects are available, standardized batteries of familiar objects have also been set up. After a visual acuity deficit has been accurately excluded, visual gnosis may be investigated by using the Gollin test (fragmented figures) or analogous visual closure tasks.

Obviously, this set of tests represents only a minimum reference for the neuropsycho-logical assessment; a deeper investigation may be needed according to the data which emerges during evaluation.

Psychomotor and general motor coordination tests, such as Movement ABC or Oseretsky are not taken into account, since the executive motor component in CP is in any case conditioned by palsy.

Assessment: an Experimental Methodology

The need for identifying any motor programming disorder in CP children has led us to develop a new methodology for assessing movement anticipatory control. This test may be used when a dyspraxic component is associated with the executive disorder, but also makes it possible to study all those clinical situations where a motor programming disorder is isolated or associated with other deficits.

The MRVS (Motor Response to Visual Stimulation) test is based on the neurophysio-logical data mentioned above and uses a reaction time paradigm. This test was developed as follows: on a PC monitor a with blue background a yellow circle or a yellow square of similar size appears. The visual stimulus is preceded by a warning sign (a cross), which appears 1.5 or 2.5 seconds before the test starts. Three wooden cubes, 4 cm per side, are placed at a reachable distance of the child's dominant hand, then the child receives the following instructions: "When you see the yellow square, press the space bar as quickly as possible on the keyboard, and touch one of the three cubes with your finger tip (simple motor task). When the circle appears, press the space bar as quickly as possible, and build a tower with the three cubes (complex motor task)". After a first trial of 10 stimulations, 4 sessions of 20 stimulations each are performed a few seconds apart, for a total of 80 stim-ulations.

This test was used with a sample group of 28 normal children who attended the first year of primary school (average age 6 years and 11 months), 14 boys and 14 girls.

It was possible to observe that reaction time for the complex motor task was signifi-cantly longer than that for the simple motor task ($p < 0.5$). This time difference, due to the need to program a longer and more complex action, was present during the first test session and later disappeared in the following sessions. A good explanation for this can be that the motor sequence, after several repetitions, becomes automatic and no longer requires the role played by the programming level.

To be sure that the difference in reaction time length is dependent on the motor programming component, and its disappearance in the second, third, and fourth test session is due to task automatization, a control test was carried out with some variations. In fact, if the change of reaction time was related to the transition from task learning to automation, when the two motor tasks to be performed in each session are changed, the difference in length of reaction time should remain constant. Therefore, three test sessions were performed and three pairs of different motor tasks were used, always combining a simple task with a complex task. The first session pair consisted again of touching a cube or building a tower with the three cubes; the second pair consisted of grasping a rope or winding it around a rod, and the third pair consisted of grasping a wooden bead or slipping it onto a stiff wire.

This new test was used with a group of 35 normal children, 10 of whom attended the first year of primary school (average age 6 years and 7 months), 15 children the second year (average age 7 years and 3 months), and 10 children the third year (average age 8 years and 4 months). A preliminary interview made it possible to ascertain that none of the children had any neuropsychiatric pathologies and/or sensory deficits, and that all children had normal cognitive, psychomotor and language development. The resulting data analysis confirmed that in all the three sessions, the difference between the simple task and the complex task reaction time was statistically significant.

It seems that this methodology is effective in assessing the role played by the motor programming component in executing simple or complex motor actions. In fact, in the case of a motor programming disorder , we may expect two different results:

a) The difference in reaction time length, depending on the task complexity, after many repetitions remains constant (in this case, the subject is not able to "automate" the motor program).

b) The lengthening of reaction time before a more complex motor action is never obtained (in this case, the motor programming level is inefficient).

In conclusion, MRVS can be useful in assessing the possible dyspraxia in CP, since:

a) It does not require any complex performance at the input level: perceptive information is very simple and does not require high discrimination effort; no specific visual-motor performances are required, such as drawing copying, etc.; in addition, three important conditions are kept constant: environment, body and limb posture, and verbal instructions.

b) The performance relative to standard is elementary (see Laszlo and Bairstow model): the only purpose is to touch the cube (in the simple task) and build the tower (in the complex task) and no other variation is expected.

c) The executive task is very simple and the skeletal-muscle executive component involvement is minimal; therefore, it may be used in both hemiplegic and diplegic children, although the reaction time on average is obviously longer.

d) Data are obtained from the comparison between performance obtained by the same subject in different experimental conditions and not from the comparison with normal subjects.

6

Recommendations

A recurrent neuropsychological profile typical of dyspraxia in cerebral palsy, is emerging from the data of clinical experience and specific studies. Dyspraxia in CP mainly assumes the character of constructional apraxia. However, while in adults this disorder is almost always caused by an error in visual-spatial data analysis or processing (Van der Meulen et al. 1991a, b), in CP children this has yet to be proven. Single perceptive ability investigation in CP children does not always lead to the identification of a specific deficit, but more frequently a variable combination of perception defects is present.

We can therefore suppose that there are several problems simultaneously affecting, to different extents, the various components related to praxic organization disorder (gnosic, visual-spatial, and kinesthetic abilities). Consequently it might be said that the basic issue in the clinical phenomenon is an information processing or a higher-level integration disorder that involves the various perceptive modalities and interferes with motor planning (Muzzini et al. 2006).

Keeping this complexity in mind the rehabilitation approach becomes even more difficult: In what way can we deal with the praxic disorder in a CP child? Is dyspraxia rehabilitation possible in CP, and how? Therapeutic recommendations deriving from the various theoretical models of motor development and interpretations of disorder nature (neuropsychological, psychomotor, and emotional) lead to different rehabilitation practices. Completely different therapeutic procedures have been prescribed to young patients depending on the current school of thought or the determined overriding component (Bassi et al. 2002).

In approaching dyspraxia rehabilitation, firstly, we need to identify the specific characteristics of the disorder in each child and then select and develop cognitive and support strategies. Recognizing the form of dyspraxia and the neuropsychological profile makes it possible to choose the most effective support procedures. For instance, it is clear that recommending the commonly used verbal facilitations in a child who rather shows greater performance improvement through visual-tactile information may be completely inappropriate. We should also consider that efficacy of facilitations varies with age, for example, verbal education is quite ineffective during the first years of primary school, but it may become more and more useful after the age of ten (Zoia, 2004).

Rehabilitation should not consist mainly of or be limited to "exercising" missing skills (Polatajko HJ et al. 2005), but rather in stimulating the child to look for and identify alternative solutions which use his abilities and activate recovery-support-replacement strategies. This is particularly true for some functional defects that cannot be as easily changed as others, for example defects outside the realm of daily routine activities. Therefore, these have to be accepted as they are or handled with substitutive means and tools.

Praxic disorder in CP children, may have important consequences on learning processes, and negatively influence school activities. Therefore, despite the prevalence of the main neuromotor disorder this aspect cannot be ignored or considered as irrelevant .

Recognizing, analyzing, and managing the praxic disorder is an important part of the rehabilitation project in CP children. Although our knowledge about its nature is still incomplete, it is possible to define rehabilitation strategies according to an objective framework and decide when and how to attempt to modify certain specific functional defects during certain specific developmental phases.

References

Aglioti S, Della Sala S (1990) Fenomenologia, basi neurali e meccanismi dell'aprassia. Europa Medicophisica 26/1,16

Barnett AL, Koistra L, Henderson SE (1998) "Clumsiness" as syndrome and symptom. Human Movement Science 17:435-447

Bassi B, Siravegna D, Rigardetto R (2002) I disturbi minori del movimento: la disprassia evolutiva. Gior Neuropsich Età Evol 22:325-47

Bilancia G (1994) La disprassia evolutiva: contributo neuropsicologico. Saggi, anno XX, vol 1

Bilancia G (1999) Bambini goffi: i disturbi dello sviluppo prassico. Prospettive in pediatria 29:91-99

Buccino G, Solodkin A, Small SL (2006) Functions of the mirror neuron system: implications for neurorehabilitation. Cog Behav Neurol vol 19, n. 1

Crawford SG, Wilson BN, Dewey D (2001) Identifying developmental coordination disorder: consistency between tests. Phys Occup Ther Pediatr 20(2-3):29-50

Crenna P (1998) Variabilità contesto-dipendente dei meccanismi neurali che controllano il movimento. Gior Neuropsich Età Evol, vol 18, supplemento 2/1998

Davis NM, Ford GW, Anderson PJ, Doyle LW (2007) Developmental coordination disorder at 8 years of age in a cohort of extremely-low-birth weight or very preterm infants. Dev Med Child Neurol 49:325-330

De Renzi E (1990) L'aprassia costruttiva in neuropsicologia clinica. Ricerche di psicologia. Franco Angeli editore, Milano

Eliasson A, Gordon A, Fossberg H (1991) Basic co-ordination of manipulative forces of children with cerebral palsy. Dev Med Child Neurol 33:661-670

Eliasson A, Gordon A, Fossberg H (1992) Impaired anticipatory control of isometric forces during grasping by children with cerebral palsy. Dev Med Child Neurol 34:216-25

Elliot JM, Connolly KJ, Dovlea JR (1988) Development of kinaesthetic sensitivity and motor performance in children. Dev Med Child Neurol 30:80-92

Ferrari A, Cioni G (1993) Paralisi cerebrali infantili: storia naturale e orientamenti riabilitativi. Edizioni Del Cerro, Pisa

Gordon AM, Forssberg H, Johansson RS, Westling G (1991) Visual size cues in the programming of manipulative forces during precision grip. Exp Brain Res 83:447-482

Hadders-Algra M, Huisiyes HJ, Towen BCL (1988) Preterm or small for gestational age infants; neurological and behavioural development at the age of six years. European Journal of Pediatrics 147:460-467

Henderson SE, Barnett AL (1998) The classification of specific motor coordination disorders in children: some problems to be solved. Human Movement Science 17:449-469

Hulme C, Brigger Staff A, Moran G, Mc Kinlay I (1982) Visual kinestetic and cross modal judgement of length by normal and clumsy children. Dev Med Child Neurol 24:466-471

Laszlo JI, Bairstow PJ (1995) Perceptual-motor behaviour: developmental assessment and therapy. Praeger scientific, New York

Levi G, Diomede L, Mazzoncini B (1989) Disprassie evolutive e rappresentazione del movimento. I care 2:41-43

6

Missiuna C, Polatajko H (1994) Developmental dyspraxia by any other name: are they all just clumsy children? Am J Occup Ther 49:619-27

Muzzini S, Leonetti R, Maoret A (2006) Praxic organization disorders in diplegic children. Dev Med Child Neurol suppl n. 107, Oct, vol.48, 16

Pieck JP, Coleman Carman R (1995) Kinaestetic sensitivity and motor performance of children with development co-ordination disorder. Dev Med Child Neurol 37:976-984

Polatajko HJ, Cantin N (2005) Development coordination disorder (dyspraxia): an overview of the state of the art. Semin Pediatr Neurol 12(4):250-8

Rigardetto R, Siravegna D (2000) I disturbi minori del movimento in età evolutiva. In: Il bambino che non parla. Edizioni Omega, Torino

Rizzolatti G (2006) So quel che fai. Raffaello Cortina Ed, Milano

Rizzolatti G, Craighero L (2004) The mirror neuron system. Annual Rev Neurosci 27:169-192

Rizzolatti G, Fadiga L, Gallese V, Fogassi L (1996) Premotor cortex and the recognition of motor actions. Brain Res Cogn Brain Res 3:131-141

Rizzolatti G, Gentilucci M, Camarda RM et al (1990) Neurons related to reaching-grasping arm moments in the rostral part of area 6. Exp Brain Res 82:337-350

Sabbadini G, Bonini P, Pezzarossa B, Pierro M (1978) Paralisi cerebrale e condizioni affini. Il pensiero scientifico editore, Roma

Sabbadini G, Sabbadini L (1995) La disprassia in età evolutiva. In: Manuale di neuropsicologia dell'età evolutiva. Zanichelli editore, Bologna

Sabbadini L (2005) La disprassia in età evolutiva. Metodologie Riabilitative in Logopedia, vol 12. Springer-Verlag Italia, Milano

Sims K, Henderson SE, Hulme C, Morton J (1996) The remediation of clumsiness: an evaluation of Laszlo's kinaesthetic approach. Dev Med Child Neurol 38:976-987

Smyth MM, Handerson HI, Churchill AC (2001) Visual information and the control of reaching in children: a comparison between children with and without developmental coordination disorder. J Mot Behav 33:306-20

Smyth TR (1991) Abnormal clumsiness in children: a deficit in motor programming? Child Care Health Dev 17:283-294

Smyth TR (1994) Clumsiness in children: a defect of kinaesthetic perception? Child Care Health Dev 20:27-36

Tanaka T, Yoshida A, Kawahata N et al (1996) Diagonistic dyspraxia. Clinical characteristics, responsible lesion and possible underlying mechanism. Brain 119:859-873

van der Meulen JH, Denier van der Gon JJ, Gielen CC et al (1991) Visuomotor performance of normal and clumsy children I: fast goal-directed arm movements with and without visual feedback. Dev Med Child Neurol 33:40-54

van der Meulen JH, Denier van der Gon JJ, Gielen CC et al (1991) Visuomotor performance of normal and clumsy children II: arm tracking with and without visual feedback. Dev Med Child Neurol 33:118-129

Wilson PH, Mackanzie BE (1998) Information processing deficits associated with developmental coordination disorder: a meta-analysis of research findings. J Child Psychal Psychyatry 39:829-840

Zoia S (2004) Lo sviluppo motorio del bambino. Le bussole. Carocci Ed, Roma

Visual and Oculomotor Disorders

A. Guzzetta, F. Tinelli, A. Bancale, G. Cioni

Introduction

Consensus has been reached on the concept that infantile cerebral palsy (CP) is a complex disorder which is limited neither to motor disability nor to the simple association between motor disability and possible disorders of other functions. Conversely, as extensively shown in this book, CP is currently considered as the result of the interaction between the different residual motor, sensorial, perceptive, or cognitive abilities or functions and their adaptative transformation grounded on evolution, that is to say a "continuously evolving disability of an individual who is continuously evolving". The issue of visual-perceptive development (and of its disorders) in CP must be viewed within this frame-work, also considering the central role it plays in the child's neuromotor, cognitive, and affective development, becoming the first tool for the interaction with the surrounding world.

Oculomotor function holds a prominent position, being essential in allowing the use of visual function. It allows us to focus the fovea on a visual target, shifting it on different parts of the localized object or on different places of the same space and maintaining foveal contact with the target during its movement or the object's movement, and to beneficially use the anatomical connections of the eyes to the head, both to compensate perturbations coming from the moving object and to facilitate the above mentioned tasks. An oculomotor dysfunction distorting three dimensional perception may, therefore, impair many of the basic adaptative functions, such as grasping, posture balancing, and locomotion, which are all functions requiring an unitary multisensorial perception in a stable environment (Pierro, 2000).

As a consequence, the clinician needs to perform early detection of visual and oculomotor disorders, to continuously monitor their evolution, and to carefully analyze their role with respect to any other development area, which is essential for a proper planning of the rehabilitation program.

The first part of this chapter will provide an overview on the state-of-the art knowledge about the available instruments for early detection of visual disorders in children of development age, with special focus on the most up-to-date technologies providing higher prognostic value. The second part will describe our experience, together with a literature review, on the incidence and on the type of visual damage in children with specific patterns of cerebral lesion, and in children with CP. The third part will be devoted to the more complex visual perceptive disorders and to the correlation between visual abnormalities and other elements related with development.

Diagnostic Tools

Until some years ago, most studies concerning vision in children presenting with cerebral lesions and/or CP were exclusively based on standard ophthalmologic evaluations, due to the lack of appropriate investigation methods to be applied on children and non-cooperative individuals. However, in the last years, new evaluation methods have been developed requiring neither active cooperation from the patient nor special ability from the clinician allowing their routine application already from the first months after birth, or even in children with severe mental retardation or with behavioral disorders.

The main innovation derived from the possibility to measure visual acuity in the infant, by using "acuity cards". Currently, other aspects of vision can also be examined, such as visual field, visual attention, optokinetic nystagmus and color vision. Longitudinal studies performed on samples of normal individuals, have allowed the collection of data on the maturation of the different aspects of visual function in the first year after birth, allowing also the application of such methods to the evaluation of individuals with CP and the comparison of results with other clinical and neuroradiological studies.

Some of the most reliable techniques for the evaluation of visual function disorders of central origin in children with CP are hereby presented.

Visual Acuity

Visual acuity, or *visus*, is the capacity to discriminate a detail. It corresponds to the highest spatial frequencies we are able to perceive. It depends on the position of the image on the retina and it is higher in the foveal region where only cones are located. A possible way to investigate visual acuity is to discriminate the single elements of a repetitive pattern (resolution acuity) in a grid representing a simplification of the visual stimuli perceived in the environment by our visual system. Visual acuity can be expressed as the number of cycles (a lighter stripe followed by a darker stripe) that are clearly perceivable in a degree of visual angle. The highest spatial frequency that a normal adult is able to perceive corresponds to a visual acuity of 45-50 cycles/degree.

In the estimation of visual acuity both behavioral and electrophysiological techniques are applied (Sutte et al. 2000). Behavioral techniques are based on the spontaneous visual response of the child to a specific stimulation. Indeed, infants, as opposed to adults, can neither be easily instructed nor are they able to provide understandable verbal responses. For this reason, behavioral methods must be based on the child's spontaneous repertoire, i.e. eye movements, head rotation towards the stimulus and fixation.

One of the first behavioral techniques to be applied was optokinetic nystagmus (OKN), introduced by Fantz in 1962 to assess the development of visual acuity in the first 6 months after birth (the technique was then abandoned, since OKN anatomical substrates proved to be so complicated as to question their reliability in evaluating visual acuity). Currently, the most popular techniques are based on preferential looking (PL) and its variant, forced-choice PL (FPL).

All these tests originate from Fantz's first observations, dating back to the 1960s, in which children and even infants, if facing two different stimuli, of which one is "config-ured", i.e. non-homogeneous with marked contrasts such as a grid, and the other one is more uniform, clearly prefer the first as evidenced by a longer fixation activity or by eye movements towards it. In PL, the investigator presents to the child a preset number of grids with growing spatial frequency. The direction of the first fixation activity as well as the number of subsequent looking activities and the total time of fixation activities are meas-ured. If, for a pattern, a higher number and/or longer fixation activities are observed, it is possible to conclude that the child can discriminate the grid. A variant of PL is FPL, which differs from PL in that in FPL the observer, placed behind a screen, does not know if the stimulus will come from the right or from the left and needs to assess on which side of the grid it is located on the basis of the child's eye behavior (Dobson and Teller, 1978; Mc Donald et al. 1985).

To formulate his assessment, the observer can use any type of behavioral index, visual or non-visual, that he deems to be providing enough information about discrimination ability. Every spatial sequence is presented to the child a certain number of times, and the percentage of correct answers is calculated. The visual threshold is considered as the value of spatial frequency of the grid for which the observer has provided from 70 to 75% correct answers. These techniques have been applied in many studies on the development of visual acuity in children and infants. However, they could not be applied on a wider clinical scale due to the long time required for test performance.

More than 15 years ago, the "acuity cards" technique was conceived (Teller et al. 1986, 1990), allowing fast data collection on visual acuity. The foundation of this technique is the same as that of PL and FPL. What is exploited is the preference for a non-homoge-neous and high contrast stimulus (the grid), rather than for a homogeneous and uniform stimulus. Cards containing the grid are presented to the child through a rectangular opening located on the side of a uniformly gray screen, aimed at preventing the child from being distracted by the surrounding environment (Figure 7.1).

The test starts when the observer, who is placed behind the screen, is able to attract the child's attention to the center of the opening in the screen. First, a very low spatial frequency card is presented so that the observer can have an idea of the type of reaction the child presents when facing the stimulus (eye deviation, features of looking, face expres-sions, etc.). Subsequently, the child is rapidly presented with cards displaying increas-ingly higher spatial frequency. As in FPL, the observer ignores the grid side and observes the child's behavior through a peep hole located in the center of the screen. If the first grids presented are easily discriminated by the child (as observed in his behavior), it is possible to show the cards just once or to skip intermediate spatial frequencies to directly present grids that are more difficult to discriminate, until reaching the card that does not elicit any

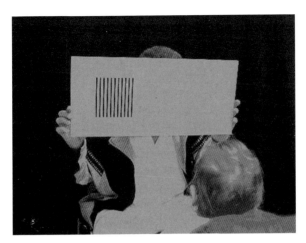

Fig. 7.1 Visual acuity assessment through acuity cards. The child is faced with a stimulus of white and black stripes with increasing spatial frequency. The observer looks at the child from a peep-hole located in the center of the cardboard and is unaware of the position of the configured stimulus. Visual acuity is measured depending on the maximum spatial frequency that the child can discriminate

more reactions in the child. The visual threshold corresponds to the highest spatial frequency the child can discriminate. The duration of this test differs depending on the child's cooperation. In a quiet and awake child, 5 minutes are usually sufficient. Instead, if the child is not paying enough attention, or if he is restless, the duration increases, since between one presentation and the next new systems to attract the child's attention to the center of the screen need to be invented (Hall et al. 2000; Mash and Dobson, 1998; Hertz et al. 1988). Curves for the evaluation of normal development are available (Van Hof-van Duin, 1989).

With older and more collaborative children, optotype tables such as the Rotterdam C-Chart are used. This table is composed by the letters "C" with different directions (rightwards/leftwards, upwards/downwards) and placed on horizontal lines which reduce in dimension by 1/8 per line. Visual acuity is measured in monocular and binocular vision at 40 cm and at 4 m. The child's task is to recognize the direction of the letter. The line with the smallest optotype on which the child provides 4 correct answers of 5 is considered as the threshold of visual acuity. Also for this method, comparable data are available.

Visual Field

The visual field is that part of space in which objects are visible at the same moment when the gaze is kept in a direction, or, as stated by Glaser "an island of vision surrounded by a sea of blindness". Instrumental techniques for visual field examination even at infant age are available, mainly based on a kinetic perimetry, by the old-fashioned Foerster's perimetry, or by the more modern Goldman-type perimetry.

A kinetic perimeter is a device composed of two 4-cm-thick metal sheets, which are fixed perpendicularly and curbed to form two arches, each with a 40 cm radius. The perimeter is positioned facing a black screen, hiding the observer, who can look at the child's head movements through a hole. The child remains sitting at the center of the perimeter staring at a 6-cm-diameter white ball placed in the center of the perimeter. The observer then attracts the child's attention towards an identical ball which, from the side, is moved to the looking point through one of the arches in the perimeter at a speed of about 3 degrees per second. The point in which the child moves the eyes towards the side stimulus is used to assess the limit of the visual field. To assess the visual field in all its range, the ball is sent in from different directions in random mode at least three times (from above, below, left or right). For every direction, the median of the obtained values is then calculated. This method allows one to assess the side preference in the visual field, simultaneously presenting two opposite side stimuli, while the child is looking at the central stimulus (Figure 7.2).

This strategy is extremely useful, for instance, in individuals with congenital hemiplegia who often present with a homonimus hemianopia. In such cases, the deficiency may not clearly be seen from the examination performed on each field, but it may be better evidenced through simultaneous bilateral stimulation. This is probably due to "perceptive antagonism" between the two sides (see chapter 16), which is unmasked only when the two homologous cortex sides are simultaneously stimulated. With this technique, the incidence of hemianopia may be considerably higher.

In patients with severe congenital encephalopathy, it is often necessary to employ less refined evaluation methods, defined as "comparison" methods. The observer places himself in front of the child with his two hands placed at the sides, and while the child looks at his face, the observer slowly approaches his hands to the sides of the visual field. In case of a suspected narrowing in just one field, the width of the visual field in the preserved side may offer the possibility to perform this comparison. Instead of his hands, the observer can decide to use smaller and more colorful objects. This method provides a more reliable feedback if stimulations are repeated more than once. Apart from simultaneous bilateral stimulation, the stimulation of one eye at a time is also useful.

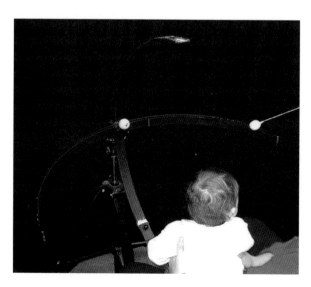

Fig. 7.2 Visual field evaluation through a kinetic perimeter. The child is sitting in the center of a hemisphere with a 40 cm radius, composed of two orthogonal gradual arches. A small white sphere is slowly moved from the side of the visual field towards the center, starting from randomly selected different directions (above, below, left, right). The point in which the child moves his eyes towards the stimulus is considered as the limit of the visual field in that specific direction

Fixation

Fixation can be considered the primary and prerequisite sub-function of every visual function related with vision and object recognition. It indicates the capacity to position and keep the fovea fixed on an object or a light source (macular or foveal fixation). The fixation of the fovea on the target is the main objective of oculomotor function, which must be achieved in a broad range of dynamic conditions. Three systems of eye movements keep the fovea on the selected target, namely, saccadic eye movement, pursuit movement, and vergence movement (Pierro, 2000).

The dynamic stabilization of the two eyes on the target, while the child moves or is carried, allows the perception of a stable 3D environment within which the body moves in three directions. Such perception of environmental stability allows one to:
1. interpret the current space orientation with respect to the environment;
2. discriminate the spatial direction from the perturbating environmental forces of body balance;
3. discriminate the spatial direction of muscular forces compensating for the perturbation;
4. guide the emerging postural changes towards a more adequate configuration to the intentional objective.

In some individuals, fixation can be exaggeratedly persistent, being therefore defined as hyperfixation. In such cases, what is lacking is the capacity to inhibit fixation and therefore to shift the gaze (fixation shift) towards a different stimulus (Cannao, 1999). Conversely, in other cases, fixation cannot be kept or only for fractions of a second, and the eyes orient in every direction, with and without conjugated movements. This is called chaotic gaze. It must be taken into account that, in the very first days of life, the infant may present with eye movements which are still lacking fluency, expressing an immaturity in fixation mechanisms.

Pursuit

Pursuit or follow movement is intended as the capacity to keep fixation on a slowly moving target. To examine the pursuit capacity, a target is placed in front of the child's eyes and it is moved very slowly. In infants it is advisable to use objects presenting contrasts, such as black-and-white stripes, or Fantz's faces (Fantz, 1965), or a target appearing like a checkerboard. In babies or infants, the most effective stimulus can be the observer's face moving in a horizontal direction.

In infants, pursuit may lack fluency and may require frequent subsequent re-fixations. This phenomenon gradually decreases in the first days after birth. In individuals with CP, the number of subsequent fixations may still remain very high.

Evaluation of Saccadic Movements

Gaze saccadic movements are ballistic, jerky movements, with minimum latency, good acceleration, and they are fast and conjugated. Being so rapid, saccadic movement does not allow corrections in its course. If it falls too short or too long, missing the target, another saccadic movement is required to correct the mistake. Its minimum latency indicates that the time lapse between action planning and action itself is very short, around 200-250 ms.

Gaze saccadic movements can be subdivided in attraction movements and localization movements. The first may be evoked by a stimulus suddenly appearing at the side of the visual field, while the second are more or less intentional movements, performed with the aim of locating the position of an object.

Orizontal saccadic eye movements are present at birth, while the vertical ones appear later, and are often immature until the first or second year of age.

Response to Tactile and Visual Threats

This test consists of eliciting an avoidance reaction from the child to a tactile or visual stimulus which is suddenly introduced. The response is usually defined by the simultaneous closing of the eyes and by movements of the head and upper limbs. The visual component of the threat reflex is assessed by using a transparent screen which is located between the child's eye and the rapidly approaching observer's hand. The response to tactile threat is present at birth and it is based on a subcortically mediated tactile sensory input, while the response to the visual threat appears at the age of 4 months and is controlled by the cortex.

Reaction and Pupillary Reflexes

Pupillary constriction, or myosis, and pupillary dilatation, or mydriasis, are either reflexes or associated reactions (the pupillary response to light stimulation is a reflex, with a specific reflexogen area; pupillary restriction during accommodation and vergence instead is an association). Pupillary constriction is a parasympathetic response and the stimulation to one eye determines myosis of both pupils: direct reflex and consensual reflex. Pupillary dilatation instead is governed by the sympathetic vegetative system.

Focusing

When facing a child, it is always very important to try and understand what is the distance at which objects should be placed in front of him, so that he can see them clearly. The infant is unable to focus, due to different reasons, among which is the fact that crystalline at birth is still immature, fixed precisely at the calculated distance of around 19-20 cm. In dyspraxic children, focusing on far objects is often impossible, probably due to "central" reasons.

Vergence

Vergence consists of the capacity of the eyes to move one towards the other. To assess vergence, an object is placed between the eyes and then it is gradually approximated, while asking the individual to fix on it. The control consists both in the observation of the approximation of the two eyes between them and in the appearance of pupillary constriction: accommodation, vergence, and pupillary reaction are associated and synchronous events. A vergence disorder is very rare or totally absent in the outcomes of a congenital or infant encephalopathy, but it is assessed anyway to exclude the (relatively frequent) possibility of internuclear palsies associated with infantile cerebral palsy, especially in the presence of damage to the encephalic trunk.

Optokinetic Nystagmus

Optokinetic nystagmus, OKN, is a physiologic event that is part of reflex movements, in that it cannot be voluntarily performed or inhibited. It is characterized by a two-phase oculomotor response consisting of a regular shift of a slow pursuit component and a rapid return component with saccadic movement characteristics. If optokinetic nystagmus is present, it can be implied that both the fixation-pursuit system (posterior-occipital) and the saccadic system (anterior-frontal) are intact. In cases of lesion to the posterior segment, optokinetic nystagmus is absent, while in cases of lesion to the saccadic system the gaze has a slow pursuit component but remains laterally fixed.

Optokinetic nystagmus can be elicited from a random pattern generated by a computer or simply through a Hemholtz or Barany drum, made of a rotating cylinder on which many vertical (black and white) stripes are drawn with variable spatial frequency. When the observer's gaze is on the rotating drum, the eyes fixing the stripe pursue it slowly until it is visible. Immediately afterwards, the gaze spontaneously moves fast to shift fixation on a different stripe, and so on. The drum can be substituted by a series of stripes horizontally placed in front of the individual, performing a slow movement to the side until the individual lets himself be carried and return seizures appear. This mode is often applied in the examination of infants or babies who cannot cooperate.

Usually, optokinetic nystagmus assessed in binocular vision is symmetrical starting from birth onwards, while optokinetic nystagmus assessed in monocular vision shows a better response to stimulation in the temporal-nasal direction starting from 3-6 months of corrected age (Atkinson and Braddick, 1981).

Stereopsis

Stereopsis is a binocular function in which depth perception is extracted by a nasal and temporal split in the projection of similar retinal images, one from each eye, to the brain. Even though stereopsis implies a normal visual acuity in each eye, a deficiency in stereopsis can also be present in patients with excellent monocular visual acuity. Stereopsis can be evaluated through different tests, easy to perform, which require the patient's collaboration, such as the Titmus test and the Lang test (Donzis et al. 1983)

Color Vision and Recognition

The most frequently applied test in color vision is Ishihara's test, which allows one to recognize only a deficiency in red and green. Other tests also include the recognition of yellow and blue.

Contrast Sensitivity

The test to evaluate contrast sensitivity is done in patients with a minimum visual loss, especially in conditions such as optic neuritis, glaucoma, and glioma. This test may be abnormal when other standard tests, such as visual acuity, color vision and visual field, are normal. Sensitivity to contrast seems to rapidly develop during the first years of life.

Visual Evoked Potentials (VEP)

Visual evoked potentials (VEP) are electrophysiological techniques employed in the examination of visual functions development. VEP are the electrophysiological responses recorded at the scalp, reflecting neuronal processing of visual inputs starting from photoreceptors to the visual cortex.

In clinical applications, visual stimuli are of two different types:
– flash luminance changes (flash VEP)
– spatial contrast changes, with constant lumination (pattern VEP)

Pattern is a repetitive stimulus, usually a checkerboard, or dark and light stripes which can be vertical or horizontal and of different size. In reversal mode pattern, dark elements are alternated with light elements, and vice versa. In the onset/offset pattern or appearance/disappearance pattern, the pattern alternatively appears (onset) and disappears (offset).

Depending on stimulus frequency, VEP (both flash and pattern) are subdivided into transient and steady-state. In transient VEP, a low stimulation frequency (e.g. 1-2 Hz) allows a period of recovery from the visual cortex before the next stimulus is displayed. In steady-state VEP, the higher stimulation frequency does not allow inter-stimulus recovery.

Longitudinal studies on transient VEP demonstrated that latency decreases with postnatal age, and that this is correlated with the development and rapid myelinization of the central nervous system in the first months after birth (Hrbeck et al. 1973; Mercuri et al. 1994; Mushin et al. 1984; Taylor et al. 1984).

Flash VEP

Flash VEP trigger internal retinal activation, and, subsequently, the activation of large portions of visual cortex. Even though the lack of stimulus specificity prevents a precise location of the potential generators registered by the scalp, it is assumed that most deflexions derive from striate and extrastriate cortical areas.

In the clinical field, flash VEP can be considered an important tool for the overall evaluation of visual pathway integrity, especially in infants and in all children presenting with fixation or accommodation deficiencies. Moreover, since flash VEP undergo relevant modifications during maturation processes, they are a valid index of the development of visual pathways.

Pattern-Reversal VEP

These are elicited by a repetitive stimulus, usually checkerboard or stripes, which alternates dark and light elements and vice versa. In the mature response, to every stimulus reversal corresponds a typical negative-positive-negative complex wave. This method has achieved rapid diffusion for three reasons:
1. the waveshape can be easily recognized and remains practically unvaried at all ages;
2. the pattern stimulation can be easily generated by special stimulators, which are largely available on the market;
3. the broad diffusion of this technique has allowed the collection of reliable data.

The disadvantages in the application of pattern reversal VEP are the sensitivity to oculomotor instability, and the need of accurate screen fixation, without which the response is not reliable. Therefore, its application is not possible in pathological conditions, such as nystagmus, and in general, in all situations characterized by scarce collaboration by the patient, which are typical in children.

Onset-Offset Pattern VEP

Onset-offset pattern VEP stimulation is repetitive and consists of stripes or squares appearing and disappearing (on-off), while the average luminance of the whole screen surface remains constant to avoid flash responses.

Onset response is three-phase. The first component, called CI, is positive and of extrastriatal origin. The second component, called CII, is negative and derives from the striate cortex. The origin of CIII, also positive, is controversial; it is probably extra-striatal.

Offset response is represented by a single positive peak whose profile is similar to that of reversal pattern response.

Usually, onset/offset patterns VEP are to be preferred to reversal patterns for the following reasons:
– the response to onset pattern, and especially the CII component, essentially reflects the response to spatial contrast, while reversal pattern responses introduce a component as

a response to reversal, that is the moment of the stimulation. This seems to explain the reason why onset patterns responses are more closely related to behavioral assessments of visual acuity (e.g., acuity cards), than reversal pattern responses;

– moreover, the onset pattern stimulus is especially suggested during development, in case of strabismus, in eye motility disorders (e.g. nystagmus), and in non-collaborative individuals, in that it does not require such accurate fixation and such long attention times as instead required by pattern-reversal stimulation;

– finally, differently from pattern-reversal VEP, onset-offset patterns provide an excellent measurement of the maturation processes of the spatial resolution capacity of the visual stimulus. Indeed, the wave shape recorded with this method develops its typical adult profile only at puberty.

Steady-State VEP

Electrophysiological techniques can also be used to collect more precise information about the onset and the evolution of specific mechanisms of the cortex visual function, such as orientation discrimination. Recent studies have reported the development of a steady-state VEP technique, allowing isolation of the response of selecting mechanisms for orientation and providing information regarding visual cortex capacity to discriminate the different orientation reversals.

Due to the fact that only neurons located in the visual cortex are sensitive to orientation reversals while neurons in subcortical pathways are not, a specific positive response for orientation reversals may be useful to indicate cortex functioning. The application of this electrophysiological technique in a population of normal infants has demonstrated that some orientation mechanisms are extremely immature at birth and produce no significant response to VEP in the very first weeks after birth (Braddick et al. 1986a, b; Wattam Bell, 1983). The response to orientation reversal VEP (OR VEP) may be elicited starting from the 6th week after birth through a low temporal frequency stimulation (3-4 reversals per second), while VEP recorded at a higher frequency (8 reversals/second) can provide a response even at 10-12 weeks, and certainly at 16 weeks.

The simple shifting of phase (pattern reversal, PR) without orientation reversal may instead be observed starting from the first weeks after birth, both at 4 and at 8 reversals per second. Recent studies have also demonstrated the use of VEP as a prognostic marker: while normal OR VEP are associated with a normal visual and motor development, abnormal responses at 5 months to OR VEP at 4 reversals per second, or to PR VEP at 8 reversals per second are associated with abnormal visual and motor development (Atkinson et al. 1991).

Fixation Shift

Fixation shift is a visual attention test assessing the direction and the latency of eye saccadic movements as a response to a peripheral target (stimulus) in the lateral visual field. A central target is used as a fixation stimulus before the peripheral target appears.

While in some tests the central stimulus disappears simultaneous to the appearance of a peripheral stimulus (non-competition), in others the central stimulus remains visible, generating a competition between the two stimuli.

Studies conducted on infants show that they can easily shift their attention in a non-competition setting during the first weeks after birth, while rapid fixations in a non competition setting only appear at 6-8 weeks after birth, and they are easily detected at 12-18 weeks. A re-fixation which is absent or delayed (with a latency over 1.2 seconds) at 5 months is considered as normal (Atkinson et al. 1992). This indicates that while the localization of a single target can be supported by the subcortical mechanism, more complex processes, such as that of shifting attention from an object to another, require the executive control of striate and extrastriate cortex. The same problem was also detected in older children with neurological problems (Hood and Atkinson, 1990).

Visual Disorders of Central Origin in Individuals with Brain Lesions and CP

In visual disorders in CP, reference is made to visual function deficiency secondary to involvement of central visual pathways, i.e., the set of disorders defined by the international literature as cerebral visual impairment (CVI). The development of advanced and reliable clinical tools for the early assessment of vision , described in the first part of the chapter, has in the last years shown the important role played by the disorder in visual perceptive development in individuals with cerebral lesions. Especially, literature on this subject is split in two main areas: on the one hand works dealing with visual disorders in children with CP, and, on the other hand, more recent studies on the development of visual functions in children presenting with neonatal cerebral lesions, irrespective of their neuromotor outcome.

This distinction is respected in this chapter, since it helps to evidence the features and the relevance of the visual disorder in the different types of CP, and it also allows us to understand the early significant markers of visual prognosis in infants with cerebral lesions, providing ground for the neurobiological development models of these functions.

Incidence and Types of Visual Disorder in Children with CP

Available population studies report that the prevalence of visual defects in children with CP is around 50%. However, this value needs to be considered as an underrating of the actual values, since in these studies clinical data are usually obtained from a review of clinical records rather than a systematic and prospective evaluation. A more reliable assessment was made on severe visual deficiencies, which account for 7 to 9% of individuals with CP (Pharoah et al. 1998).

Even less definitive appear to be the epidemiological characteristics of the different sub- types of visual impairment, starting from the distinction between central and peripheral disorders. It is proved that eye diseases present with higher incidence in individuals with CP than in normal controls, and this is not surprising considering that peripheral disorders may share part of their etiopathogenetic dynamics with cerebral disorders. A recent study on a sample population of premature infants below 32 weeks (Asproudis et al. 2002) evidenced a clear difference in the incidence of both retinopathy of prematurity (ROP) and strabismus in individuals with CP versus controls with normal development, with a 9 to 1 and 6 to 1 ratio, respectively. The same study showed that pure refractive defects are more frequent in CP, even if not in an equally significant way.

The main vision defects present in CP will be described, devoting the first part of the description to pure eye diseases and the second to defects of cerebral origin secondary to damage of the retrochiasmatic visual pathways or to other cerebral areas involved in visual stimuli perception and processing.

Ophthalmological Abnormalities

As previously mentioned, an exhaustive eye examination including refractometry, ocular motility, and fundus oculi, should be performed as soon as CP is diagnosed. This appears to be necessary both considering the high incidence of such diseases in individuals with CP and for a correct differential diagnosis with disorders of central origin. A possible example is the relevance of a visual acuity deficiency with or without a refraction defect. Moreover, early ophthalmology assessment in children with CP is essential to establish a correct therapy plan, accounting for all the possible problems arising in the development of the rehabilitation strategy. In a study of 1980, Black reported that a high number of individuals with CP, enrolled in a special school, were never referred to an ophthalmologist but presented with a high frequency of untreated amblyopia.

Pure refraction defects were reported in around 16% of CP cases, with a higher percentage of myopia, in line with the normal population. Ocular defects secondary to ROP affect 15% of the infants with gestational age below 32 weeks who develop CP. Congenital cataract and coloboma, conversely, affect a limited percentage of individuals, which overall is lower than 5%.

Optic atrophy deserves a different perspective, detected in around 10% of individuals with CP but not always considered the main cause of visual deficiency. This is due to the fact that optical atrophy is often associated to extremely severe CP conditions with marked lesions of the occipital cortex and the optic radiations, the main cause of blindness.

Visual Defect of Central Origin

Some authors (Schenk-Rootlieb et al. 1992, 1994; Ipata et al. 1994) carried out an assessment of visual functions in two large populations of individuals with CP, detecting in about 70% of them a reduction of visual acuity which could not be explained by any ophthalmological disease. In both studies, defect distribution was related to the type of CP. Acuity deficiency had a higher incidence in tetraplegia and in dyskinetic palsy, followed by diplegia. Children with hemiplegia usually presented with normal acuity levels, as suggested by previous articles (Guzzetta et al. 2001).

Defects of visual acuity are often associated with other visual disorders, such as strabismus, other oculomotion defects, visual field reduction, and asymmetry of optokinetic nystagmus. These associated disorders, in particular oculomotion disorders, may have a negative influence on the reliability of certain behavioral tests, and especially evaluation with acuity cards.

The reliability of this technique seems to improve in parallel with the age of the tested subjects, due to their higher compliance. In the sample by Schenk-Rootlieb and co-workers (1994), a significant number of individuals presenting with an initial reduction in visual acuity demonstrated an improvement in the second evaluation repeated after an interval of some months. Moreover, a limited number of children who were considered as to be normal at a first evaluation presented an acuity level lower than the tenth percentile at a subsequent examination. In agreement with such data, Van Hof-van Duin and co-workers (1998) reported that results of early visual evaluations performed in the first two years in children with cerebral lesions statistically correlate with visual outcome at 5 years, even if in some individual cases incoherent results and even a visual deterioration may be observed.

Another marker of visual defect of central origin is visual field reduction, detected in more than half of the children with hemiplegia. The defect can be unilateral, in the form defined as hemianopia, or involve both fields with different severity. A recent study (Mercuri et al. 1996) performed on a sample group of individuals with congenital hemiplegia with variable etiology detected a clear association between unilateral lesions (mainly venous and arterial infarctions) and hemianopia contralateral to the lesion. Conversely, in the same sample group of hemiplegic patients, individuals with bilateral lesions (mainly periventricular leukomalacia) often presented with bilateral visual field restrictions. Even though the cause of this field defect is usually attributed to damage of the post-geniculate visual structures, such as optic radiations and occipital cortex, it is not always possible to detect a clear correlation between the involvement of such structures on MRI and field restriction. As a general rule, field defects can be consequent to lesions at different levels of the visual pathway. In optic nerve lesions (e.g., retrobulbar neuritis), a central scotoma can be detected, due to the major involvement of the fibers deriving from macular cones and selectively from foveal cones. In optic chiasm lesions, multiple deficiencies are detected, differing depending on whether lesion involvement is in the chiasm or in the lateral areas, leading to bitemporal hemianopia, central area defects, or irregular defects.

An important type of disorder which is often related to CP, as clearly evidenced by the studies performed by Giorgio Sabbadini and co-workers (2000), is that of visual exploration. Even though such disorders can be differentiated by perception disorders, they clearly influence visual recognition, which is closely related to a correct and fluent visual exploration.

The main defect of visual exploration is congenital ocular dyspraxia. In Cogan's original definition, formulated in 1952, it is conceived as a form of gaze intentional palsy, with preservation of spontaneous erratic movements, mainly involving the horizontal direction. They are associated with the presence of compensatory movements of gaze "mobilization", such as blinking and head jerks, which are necessary to start the saccadic movement.

Moreover, fixation spasms are also present, expressing the inability to inhibit fixation.

Cases of pure Cogan type dyspraxia are extremely rare in the literature, and its etiopathogenesis is still unknown. Conversely, a form of ocular dyspraxia with similar features, defined by Sabbadini as "Cogan like dyspraxia", can be commonly detected in individuals with CP, but with some important differences. Firstly, palsy involves all directions of gaze, both horizontal and vertical. Secondly, other dyspraxic symptoms are almost invariably associated, such as verbal, gesture, gait, writing dyspraxia, etc. (see chapter 16). Apart from that, the symptoms are very similar, with hyperfixation and compensatory strategies of gaze mobilization.

Another relevant compensatory strategy of visual origin is macular "translocation", by which gaze displaces from one object to another along a sequence of objects placed at very small distance. Indeed, when objects are located at a distance that is lower than 15°, a tangible displacement of the macula on adjacent objects is produced, but without a loss of fixation.

In dyspraxic individuals, saccadic movements are generated with difficulty and can also be inaccurate. These individuals often present with saccadic movements which are dysmetric, hypometric, and hypermetric, i.e., characterized by a measurement error corrected by subsequent swinging movements, until the target is reached.

The role played by visual exploration disorders in object recognition will be described later in the text.

Central Visual Disorder in Individuals with Congenital Cerebral Lesions

As a consequence of the progress achieved in the techniques for the management of neonatal neurological diseases, it is currently possible from the first days of life, even in pre-term and/or extremely low birth weight infants, to detect the presence and the characteristics of lesions to the CNS. This is possible through neuroimaging techniques, especially ultrasound (US) and magnetic resonance (MR). This scenario has led the clinician to face the difficult task of predicting the consequences of brain damage, even in the earliest stages of life, when clinical signs and symptoms lack specificity. In the following section, some of the main profiles of the perinatal cerebral lesions frequently associated with evolution towards CP will be described, and the possible associations with visual function disorders will be analyzed. Some general remarks on the correlation between lesion and function will follow.

Periventricular Leukomalacia (PVL)

Different studies have assessed visual acuity in subjects with PVL, detecting in this pediatric population an incidence of the deficiency of over 60%. Although acuity is usually normal in individuals with prolonged flare, or with type 1 and 2 leukomalacia (according to the classification by de Vries et al. 1990), it is generally reduced in individuals with PVL stage 3 or 4. Visual abnormalities are usually severe in individuals with subcortical cystic leukomalacia, while they are less frequent and less severe in individuals with cystic PVL leukomalacia. Eken and co-workers (1996), reported that in individuals with cystic PVL leukomalacia, visual abnormalities are more frequent in those with 35-37 weeks of gestational age compared to those with gestational age lower than 32 weeks. This difference can be explained depending on the different location of the lesions, since in more mature infants cystic lesions involve subcortical white matter and consequently increase the risk of involvement of the visual pathway.

Different studies demonstrated that the severity of visual impairment in children with PVL is significantly associated with the degree of involvement of the peritrigonal white matter and with the involvement of optic radiations and occipital cortex. Other studies showed that, apart from visual acuity, other aspects of visual functions, such as visual fields and eye movements, are frequently impaired in these subjects.

Recently, our group studied 29 subjects with PVL with a mean gestational age at birth of 32 weeks (range 25–40). At least one of the aspects of visual function assessed was abnormal in all subjects but one. Strabismus was present in 24 children (21 esotropia and 3 exotropia), oculomotor disorders in 21, visual field reduction in 15 and visual acuity redcution in 18. About visual field defects, Jacobson et al (2006) studied six subjects with white matter damage of immaturity of pre- or perinatal origin, born at a gestational age of 28-34 weeks, by means of manual and computerized quantitative perimetry. They found that all the subjects had a visual field defect involving particularly the lower portion of the same.

Intraventricular Hemorrhage (IVH)

Small hemorrhages, both intraventricular and of the germinal matrix (stage I and II, according to Levene et al. 1981), are often associated with normal visual acuity. Individuals presenting with larger hemorrhages may present with a visual deficiency at term age, but tend to improve after a few months. These transient alterations might be explained by the effect of the intraventricular hemorrhage on the thalamus and inferior colliculi, or the bleeding of the germinal matrix in the posterior nuclei of the thalamus and the optic radiations.

Permanent effects on the visual system caused by these lesions do not occur frequently, even in cases of parenchymal damage (stage IV IVH), because the lesions more often involve the intermediate or anterior part of the parietal lobes, sparing central visual pathways.

Hypoxic-Ischemic Encephalopathy (HIE)

Visual abnormalities are extremely common in individuals presenting with HIE. However, the presence of a visual deficiency does not always correlate with the level of HIE at birth. While individuals with stage I HIE, according to the classification by Sarnat and Sarnat (1976), usually show normal development of visual functions, and patients with stage III

HIE always have a severe visual deficiency, the visual outcome of individuals with stage II HIE is extremely variable.

In HIE, the presence and the extent of deficiencies is significantly related to the extent of the cerebral lesion on MRI, especially in case of lesions to the basal ganglia and thalamus. It is also important to remark that not all the lesions involving the occipital lobes are associated with a deficiency of visual functions. According to our experience, individuals with lesions simultaneously involving the basal ganglia and a cerebral hemisphere invariably present with severe and persistent abnormalities of one or more aspects of visual function. Visual abnormalities can also be detected in the first months after birth in patients with isolated lesions of the basal ganglia, even if such lesions tend to resolve within the end of the first year (Mercuri et al. 1997a).

Cerebral Infarction

Although visual acuity is usually normal in individuals with focal lesions, other aspects of visual function, such as visual field or fixation shift, can be altered. However, the presence and the severity of the damage cannot always be predicted depending on the lesion location or its extent on MRI. Unlike adult patients presenting with similar lesions, showing a consistent association between occipital cortex involvement and contralateral visual field deficiency, around half the children with occipital lobe infarction may present with a visual field within the normal range.

Correlation between Lesion and Function

In our experience and in a literature review on the development of visual functions in individuals with cerebral lesions of pre- or peri-natal origin, it becomes clear to what extent visual abnormalities are frequent in these patients, but also how the association between visual pathway lesion and visual deficiency does not always follow the same pattern as shown in adults presenting with similar lesions. Early neonatal MRI has provided a considerable set of data on the existing correlation between vision and cerebral lesion characteristics. A broad consensus has been raised on the following aspects:

a) visual abnormalities tend to be more frequent in pre-term children with HIE, than in term ones. This is probably due to the low incidence of visual abnormalities in pre-term infants with mild leukomalacia or with hemorrhages. However, while in pre-term infants the lesions in the occipital cortex are usually associated with visual function impairment, in term children both unilateral and bilateral occipital lesions may be associated with a fully normal vision. This can be explained by the difference in lesion type and location. In severe PVL, lesions are usually extensive and bilateral. Moreover, severe prematurity is usually associated with many other problems (reduced stimulations, feeding difficulties, reduced oxygenation, infections, etc.), globally involving cerebral activity so to negatively impact on functional reorganization processes after the lesion has occurred.

b) In term infants, the severity of the visual deficit seems to be mainly related to the simultaneous involvement of the basal ganglia and thalamus. The role played by the basal ganglia and the thalamus in visual maturation has not been fully clarified. Neuroanatomical aspects of such a correlation may reside in the existence of many mutual connections between the visual cortex and basal ganglia. Any interruption of such connections may reduce information transfer to other parts of the brain, therefore reducing the possibility for other cortical areas to perform the functions of the damaged occipital regions. In other words, the subcortical structures lesion might, through an inhibition of neural trasmission, prevent the possibility of functional reorganization of the damaged cortex.

c) Visual functions may be abnormal in individuals with a completely normal ophthalmologic examination, and with spared optic radiations and visual cortex. This can be explained by the involvement of parts of the brain other than the geniculostriate pathways, such as the frontal or temporal lobes, which are associated with visual attention or other aspects of visual function. In some cases, visual attention, and in general visual functions, may be disturbed by other clinical problems which are frequent in individuals with cerebral lesions, such as oculomotion impairment or epilepsy.

d) A certain number of individuals may present with transient visual deficits, with gradual recovery occurring in some cases in the first months after birth. Such cases can be described as delayed visual maturation (DVM) (Mercuri et al. 1997b). This term is used to describe individuals with poor vision at birt which subsequently improves, with a complete recovery within the end of the first year. The delay in visual maturation may be an isolated element or it can be associated with ocular and development abnormalities. Different mechanisms have been presented to provide an explanation of these cases, such as the use of extra-geniculostriate pathways, the recovery of a normal excitability of the neurons spared by the lesion, or of the neurons adjacent to it. Although many subjects with DVM present with associated neurodevelopmental abnormalities, correlation with neuroimaging has been poorly investigated. In our sample of term infants with neonatal cerebral lesions, the delay in visual maturation was mainly found in individuals presenting with isolated lesions of the basal ganglia. A possible explanation for this is that the isolated involvement of these subcortical structures may cause a delay in visual maturation in the first months after birth, when visual functions are mainly governed by subcortical structures, and that vision improves in parallel with the maturation of the cortical visual areas taking their places. Further anatomofunctional correlation studies need to be performed on individuals without apparent perinatal problems to rule out the possibility that minor and unknown lesions might cause the delay in visual maturation in such infants.

Complex Visuoperceptive Disorders and Correlation between Visual Abnormalities and Other Aspects of Development

The definition of complex visuoperceptive disorders, as opposed to that of more "simple" disorders, certainly appears to be arbitrary and shows no consistent neurophysiological basis. This is even more evident considering modern theories on visual processing as part of different "systems" largely working in parallel, with complex and multilevel mutual integrations.

Even so, to provide a necessary explanation, we will deal in this chapter with several complex visuoperceptive disorders, meaning visual recognition disorders together with spatial localization and movement perception disorders. This definition makes clear reference to the concept of two visual systems: the first, occipito-temporal, also known as "ventral", involved in object vision, i.e., shape recognition, and the second, occipito-parietal or "dorsal", involved in spatial elements of vision, such as movement and spatial localization of stimuli. Due to their different characteristics, these two systems have also been defined as "what" and "where", and more recently as "who" and "how". In other words, one system is aimed at recognizing what or who we see, and the other is aimed at recognizing where the object is located and therefore how we can act on it (Figure 7.3).

Studies leading to the formulation of these theories were mostly performed on animals used for experimental purposes, and especially on primates, or individuals with focal lesions acquired at adult age (Tanne-Gariepy et al. 2002; Creem and Proffitt, 2001). Conversely, young children with early acquired lesions, and therefore in individuals with CP, the possible presence of disorders similar to those described in adults is extremely controversial (Gunn et al. 2002).

The main studies on complex visuoperceptive disorders during development are described, followed by a brief overview of neuropsychological studies that can be useful for a better classification of such disorders, and finally an analysis of the relation between visuoperceptive disorder and neuropsychic development.

Object Recognition Disorder (Who and What)

Object recognition disorder, manifested as visual agnosia, appears during development and is difficult to differentiate from cortical blindness. If a very young child does not perceive,

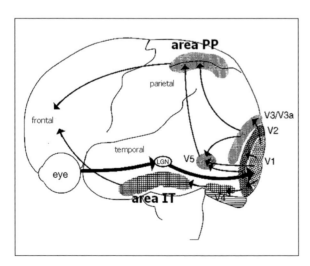

Fig. 7.3 Graphic representation of the visual system. Through the eye, the visual stimulus reaches the lateral geniculate nucleus (*LGN*) and the striate cortex (areas *V1* and *V2*). From the striate cortex, two main pathways originate: the main pathway, which, through area *V4* reaches the inferotemporal complex (*IT*), and the dorsal pathway, which through the areas *V3* and *V5* reaches the posterior parietal complex (*PP*). For the specific functions of these pathways, see text

or perceives in an abnormal way, his recognition possibilities (i.e. his possibility of perceptive and semantic categorization) are impaired. Such cases, even the in presence of a visual
residual capacity, are not considered true visual agnosia but possibly pseudo-agnosia or a
non-primitive defect, which is in some way associated or consequent to acuity deficiency.
In this perspective, Sabbadini states that the terms cortical blindness and agnosia, applied
to development age, may be intended as synonyms "if, by blindness, we intend an
outcome, not a missed acquisition or a severe failure of the vision of the object, but a
preservation of spatial vision".

The possible nature of a visual recognition deficiency was recently investigated by
Stiers and co-workers (2002) in children with CVI and, in most cases, motor disabilities
due to pre- or perinatal lesions. These children were tested at the age of 5 by means of an
object recognition test composed of different tasks, such as the recognition of damaged or
concealed objects, or of objects placed in an unconventional viewpoint (see chapter 10).
To rule out possible effects of the test on a more global delay of nonverbal intelligence,
the results of each subject were evaluated considering the individual's mental age. Even
with this correction, a high percentage of cases (more than 70%), showed a specific
visuoperceptive deficiency which did not turn out to be significantly related to the degree
of the visual acuity defect. The existence of a visuoperceptive disorder as a specific
condition in children with cerebral lesions was recently confirmed by van den Hout and
co-workers (2004).

As mentioned in the previous paragraph, visual exploration disorders may have a
negative impact on visual recognition. In particular, the visual recognition disorder
that seems to be more associated with ocular dyspraxia is simultagnosia. This term
defines the inability to recognize the meaning of an entire object or of an entire scene,
even though details are well perceived and recognized. The individual recognizes every
part in the scene, but cannot perform a simultaneous synthesis of what he is seeing, i.e.,
to give it a meaning. The association with ocular dyspraxia appears to be understandable
if visual exploration is conceived as a crucial active process for the understanding of
the surrounding reality. To be effective, the sequence of saccadic movements for
the exploration must be programmed and continuously re-programmed. It may deal with
a truly present or sometimes imaginary target, and it has to be sequentially organized. The
impairment of these balances may significantly alter the overall recognition of reality.

Fedrizzi and co-workers (1998) previously investigated eye movements and visuoperceptive deficiencies in individuals with CP. Different features of eye motility were
analyzed through video tape recordings while children were performing a visuoperceptive
test consisting of an adapted version of the Animal House, a subtest of WPSSI. In this test,
children with spastic diplegia achieved significantly worse results than controls. In particular, they needed more time to complete the task; they had a higher number of omissions
and more mistakes in sequence and exploration. Moreover, they presented with a reduction
of anticipatory saccadic movements.

The visuoperceptive disorder in children with CP may also be partly due to a deficiency in selective visual attention. Hood and Atkinson (1990) suggested that children
presenting with neurological diseases may show a visual performance disorder subsequent
to a difficulty in shifting fixation from a central target to a peripheral one. Fixation shift

alterations are often not associated with pursuit problems or reduction of visual acuity, but they can be evidenced in individuals with parietal lobe lesions.

Spatial Localization and Movement Disorder (Where and How)

Only recently the investigation of disorders of the occipitoparietal visual system in pediatric age has raised interest, through the implementation of new tools, still in their experimental application, for the behavioral evaluation of these functions (psychophysical techniques) and for the localization of the functionally involved cortical areas (PET, fMRI). This has provided evidence of neural networks which account for the perception of complex movement stimuli in healthy children, and documented their malfunctioning in some cases of cerebral lesions and CP.

Although an exhaustive explanation of the incidence of this type of disorders in children with CP is not available, some preliminary studies seem to indicate that some degree of deficiency in the perception of motion stimuli is not infrequent in individuals with an early cerebral lesion but this was found also in patients with complex genetic malformative syndromes (Down syndrome, Williams syndrome) (Atkinson et al. 2003). In other words, the vulnerability of this system seems not to have characteristics of specificity towards one or another neurodevelopmental disease, but to be sensitive to non-specific perturbations of the CNS. Specific types of motion perception seem to be altered in subjects with periventricular leukomalacia. In particular, recently, we measured coherence sensitivity for global motion along a translational or circular trajectory and found that sensitivity both to translational and rotational motion is on average significantly reduced compared with age-matched controls. Deficits of motion processing were not related to the number of other visual abnormalities. Of particular note, our group (Morrone et al. 2008) found that two children with PVL perceived translational motion of a random dot display to move in the opposite direction, consistently and with high sensitivity. The apparent inversion was specific for translation motion. In this field, scientific investigation is only at the beginning but it has also raised interest, considering the relevant role that such disorders might play in the understanding of other motor difficulties (walking) or of visuoperceptive difficulties of patients with CP.

Main Neuropsychological Tests for the Support of Visuoperceptive Disorders

The evaluation of complex visuoperceptive disorders is based on a number of neuropsychological tests which are commonly employed in development age. Some of the most significant and popular tests are hereby described.

Test for the Evaluation of Visuoperceptive Abilities

L94 Visuoperceptive Test

L94 comprises eight visuoperceptive tests (some are described later in the text) conceived to assess the visuoperceptive abilities of children of pre-school age with multiple disabilities (Stiers et al. 2001). Such tests were selected to investigate three of the main aspects of visuoperceptive dysfunction described in adults with cerebral damage (Figure 7.4).

Visual matching (VISM): ten items are displayed on a computer screen in which a drawn target is shown for a second. The individual has to recognize, among the four alternatives that are presented, the drawn object represented in a different way. This test evaluates the semantic categorization of prototype presentations of common objects, which is delayed in individuals with visual agnosia.

Overlapping line drawings (OVERL): this test is used in the analysis of perceptive categorization disorders. Individuals presenting with this disorder show reduced ability in the visual identification of objects presented in suboptimal conditions. In this test, the patient is faced with an image with many overlapping objects that need to be identified. If the individual is unable to recognize them, then the objects are only partially overlapped, and the task is more and more simplified until objects are presented only as touching, and finally as separated.

Unconventional object views (VIEW): the test consists of asking for the names of the drawn objects, presenting them from an unconventional viewpoint. The object is presented in a sequence of four images that become increasingly similar to the real object.

Occluded by noise (NOISE): the individual is asked to recognize an object which is occluded by a masking pattern made of small squares. Each item starts with a 60% occlusion, and noise can be gradually reduced to 0% in 7 subsequent steps.

De vos (DE VOS) (Stiers et al. 1998, 1999): the individual is asked to recognize an object which is presented or inserted within a context, or with some missing parts, or just with contour, or with omission of one of its typical features, or from an unconventional viewpoint.

Visual Object Recognition Battery

This battery (Bova et al. 2007) allows the study of the visual object recognition abilities in children aged 6 to 11. It consists of neuropsychological tests based on Marr's model (Efron test, Warrington's Figure-Ground Test, Street Completion Test, Poppelreuter-Ghent Test, a selection of stimuli from the BirminghamObject Recognition Battery, a series of color photographs of objects presented from unusual perspectives or illuminated in unusual ways).

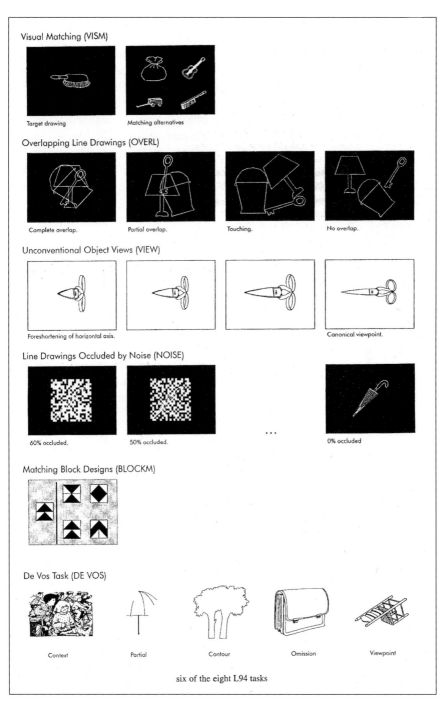

Fig. 7.4 L94 visuoperceptive test. Details on each item are described in the text (from Stiers et al. 1998, modified)

Frosting Developmental Test of Visual Perception

This test (Abercombie, 1964; Ward, 1970) allows the identification of a visual perception deficiency and the measurement of its severity. It is structured on five tasks: visuomotor coordination (drawing straight, curved, or angled lines without guidelines); occluded items (occluded geometrical shapes on a complex background); shape consistency (recognition of geometrical shapes); position in space, discriminating between shape reversal and rotation; spatial relations (copying shapes from simple models).

Benton Neuropsychological Battery

This is ideally subdivided into two parts: 1) tests of orientation detection and of learning, and 2) other tests for the measurement of perception and motricity (Qualls et al. 2000; Benton and Tranel, 1993). The following are among the tests performed: temporal orientation, right-left orientation, serial digit learning, facial recognition, judgment of line orientation, visual form discrimination, pantomime recognition, motor impersistence.

Among the most popular in the recognition of visuoperceptive problems is the judgment of line orientation, measuring perception characteristics and abnormalities in relation to the right and the left hemispheres. It comprises two forms, H and V, consisting each of 30 stimuli, presented in different order but always in increasing difficulty. The individual is simultaneously faced with a multiple choice stimulus (a number of lines with different orientation) and a simple stimulus (a pair of lines, each oriented as a corresponding line in the multiple choice stimulus) that the patient has to detect in the multiple stimulus.

Test for the Evaluation of Visuo-Constructive Abilities

Developmental Test of Visual Motor Integration (VMI): this test (Beery, 1997) consists of evaluating the capacity to copy geometric figures in a preset space per every example.

Matching Block Designs (BLOCKM): this is a discrimination test formula in which the same drawing has to be recognized among four different alternatives.

Constructing Block Designs Task (BLOCKC): a printed drawing must be constructed in a preset space with two or four square blocks diagonally divided in a black half and a white half.

Cerebral Visual Impairment and Mental/Motor Development

Different studies have shown how vision plays a crucial role in motor, cognitive, and functional development. The new approaches on the factors involved in motor development evidence the central role of the different sensor inputs, especially visuoperceptive stimuli, in posture and motor control. The main sensory pathway of development in normal infants is vision, playing a relevant role especially in the early stages of motor development. When head and trunk control are achieved for upright sitting or standing, the child mainly relies on visual information, while in the subsequent phase of complete acquisition of posture control visual dominance disappears and the child is able to automatically integrate multiple sensory inputs. In children with CP, it has been suggested that the inability to acquire normal posture control is strongly related to the need to maintain dependence on sensory inputs, and especially vision, as observed in normal individuals in the stages of learning of new motor and posture competences. The difficulties displayed by children with CP in the integration of multiple perceptive stimuli were described by Lee and co-workers, focusing on individuals with hemiplegia. Collected data suggest that improvement in the quality of visual function, together with other perceptive pieces of information, may produce a significant improvement in the motor performance of children with CP.

Recently, many researchers have investigated the relation between visual and neurological development. Eken and co-workers (1996) found a consistent correlation between neurological development and visual acuity in individuals presenting with perinatal cerebral lesions. Mercuri and co-workers (1999), analyzing a group of term infants with HIE, some with CP, found a strong correlation between the results of visual evaluation in the first months after birth and the development ratio at 2 years of age.

Cioni and co-workers (2000) reported a significant statistical correlation between visual functions at 1 year and motor development at 1 and 3 years of age in 29 pre-term infants with periventricular leukomalacia, most of whom developed CP. Results of a multiple regression analysis indicated that vision defect was the variable with the highest correlation with cognitive level, compared with motor deficiency and with the lesion score of the MRI, suggesting a fundamental role of visual disorders in the early cognitive development of these individuals.

This correlation between cognitive level and central visual disorder was also confirmed in 5-years-old children with pre- or perinatal cerebral lesions, irrespective of the degree of motor deficiency. The impact of central vision disorder on the different functional aspects (communication, emotional contact, cognitive level) in a group of children with CP was investigated by Schenk-Rootlieb and co-workers (1992). These authors demonstrated that the functional level of all these aspects of development was significantly lower in individuals with central vision deficiency, irrespective of the severity of the motor disorder.

The incidence and the relevance of these disorders requires early diagnosis and early treatment with the most advanced and suitable techniques (Sabbadini, 2000).

References

Abercrombie ML (1964) Visual, perceptual and visuomotor impairment in physically handicapped children: VI. Marianne Frostig Developmental test of visual perception. Percept Mot Skills 18:583-94

Asproudis IC, Andronikou SK, Hotoura EA et al (2002) Retinopathy of prematurity and other ocular problems in premature infants weighing less than 1500 g at birth. Eur J Ophthalmol 12:506-11

Atkinson J, Braddick OJ (1981) Development of optokinetic nystagmus in infants: an indicator of cortical bunicularity. In: Fisher DF, Monthy RA, Sender JW (eds) Eye movements: cognition and visual perception. Hillsdale NJ: Lawrence Erlbaum Associates 53-64

Atkinson J, Braddick O, Anker S et al (1991) Visual development in the VLBW infant. In: Transactions of the 3rd Meeting of the Child Vision Research Society. Rotterdam

Atkinson J, Braddick O, Anker S et al (2003) Neurobiological models of visuospatial cognition in children with Williams syndrome: measures of dorsal-stream and frontal function. Dev Neuropsychol 23:139-72

Atkinson J, Hood B, Wattam-Bell J, Braddick O (1992) Changes in infants' ability to switch visual attention in the first three months of life. Perception 21:643-653

Benton A, Tranel D (1993) Visuoperceptual, visuospatial and visuoconstructive disorders. In: Heilman KM, Valenstein E (eds) Clinical neuropsychology 3rd edn. Oxford University Press, New York, pp 165-213

Beery KE (1997) The Beery-buktenica developmental test of visual-motor integration. Administration scoring and teaching manual. 4th edn. Modern Curriculum Press, Parsippany

Black PD (1980) Ocular defects in children with cerebral palsy. Br Med J 16; 281:487-8

Bova SM, Fazzi E, Giovenzana A et al (2007) The development of visual object recognition in school age children. Developmental Neuropsychology 31:79-102

Braddick O, Atkinson J, Wattam-Bell J (1986) Orientation- specific cortical responses develop in early infancy. Nature 320:617-619

Braddick O, Atkinson J, Wattam-Bell J (1986) VEP testing of cortical binocularity and pattern detection in infancy. Documental Ophthalmologica Proceedings Series 45:107-115

Cannao M (1999) La mente con gli occhiali. FrancoAngeli Editore

Cioni G, Bertuccelli B, Boldrini A et al (2000) Correlation between visual function, neurodevelopmental outcome, and magnetic resonance imaging findings in infants with periventricular leucomalacia. Arch Dis Child Fetal Neonatal Ed 82:F134-40

Cogan DG (1952) A type of congenital ocular motor apraxia presenting jerky head movements. Trans Am Acad Ophthalmol Otolaryngol 56:853-62

Creem SH, Proffitt DR (2001) Defining the cortical visual systems: "what", "where", and "how". Acta Psychol 107(1-3):43-68

De Vries LS, Dubowitz LMS, Pennoclùk J, Dubowitz V (1990) Brain Disorder in the Newborn. Wolfe Medical Publications, London

Dobson V, Teller DY (1978) Visual acuity in human infants: a review and comparison of behavioural and electrophysiological studies. Vision Res 18: 1469-1483

Donzis P, Rapazzo J, Burde R, Gordon M (1983) Effect of binocular variations of Snellen's acuity on Titmus stereoacuity. Arch Ophthalmol 101:930-2

Eken P, de Vries LS, van Nieuwenhuizen O et al (1996) Early predictors of cerebral visual impairment in infants with cystic leukomalacia. Neuropediatrics 27:16-25

Fantz RL (1965) Visual perception from birth as shown by pattern selectivity. Annals N.Y. Academic Science 118:793-814

Fedrizzi E, Anderloni A, Bono R et al (1998) Eye-movement disorders and visual-perceptual impairment in diplegic children born preterm: a clinical evaluation. Dev Med Child Neurol 40:682-8

Gunn A, Cory E, Atkinson J et al (2002) Dorsal and ventral stream sensitivity in normal development and hemiplegia. Neuroreport 7;13:843-847

Guzzetta A, Fazzi B, Mercuri E et al (2001) Visual function in children with hemiplegia in the first years of life. Dev Med Child Neur 43:321-9

Hall HL, Courage ML, Adams RJ (2000) The predictive utility of the Teler acuity cards for assessing visual aoutcome in children with preterm birth and associated perinatal risks. Vision Research 40:2067-2076

Hertz BG, Ropsenberg J, Sjo O, Warburg M (1988) Acuity card testing of patients with cerebral visual impairment. Dev Med Child Neur 30: 632-637

Hood B, Atkinson J (1990) Sensory visual loss and cognitive deficits in the selective attentional system of normal infants and neurologically impaired children. Dev Med Child Neurol 32:1067-77

Hrbek A, Kalberg P, Ollson T (1973) Development of visual and somatosensory evoked potentials in preterm newborn infants. EEG in Clin. Neurophysiol 34:225-232

Ipata AE, Cioni G, Bottai P et al (1994) Acuity card testing in children with cerebral palsy related to magnetic resonance images, mental levels and motor abilities. Brain Dev 16:195-203

Jacobson L, Flodmark O, Martin L (2006) Visual field defects in prematurely born patients with white matter damage of immaturity: a multiple-case study. Acta Ophthalmol Scand 84:357-362

Levene MI, Wigglesworth JS, Dubowitz V (1981) Cerebral structure and intraventricular haemorrhage in the neonate: a real time ultrasound study. Archives of Disease in Childhood 56:416-424

Mash C, Dobson V (1998) Long-term reliability and predective validity of the teller acuity card procedure. Vision Research 38: 619-626

McDonald MA, Dobson V, Sebris SL et al (1985) The acuity cards precedure: a rapid test of infants acuity. Investigative Ophthalmology Visual Science 26:1158-1162

Mercuri E, Atkinson J, Braddick O et al (1997a) Basal ganglia damage and impaired visual function in the newborn infant. Arch Dis Child Fetal Neonatal 77:F111-4

Mercuri E, Atkinson J, Braddick O et al (1997b) The aetiology of delayed visual maturation: short review and personal findings in relation to magnetic resonance imaging. Eur J Paediatr Neurol 1:31-4

Mercuri E, Haataja L, Guzzetta A et al (1999) Visual function in term infants with hypoxicischaemic insults: correlation with eurodevelopment at 2 years of age. Arch Dis Child Fetal Neonatal Ed 80:F99-104

Mercuri E, Siebenthal K, von Daniels H et al (1994) Multimodality evoked responses in the neurological assessment of the newborn. Eur J Pediatr 153:622-631

Mercuri E, Spano M, Bruccini G et al (1996) Visual outcome in children with congenital hemiplegia: correlation with MRI findings. Neuropediatrics 27:184-8

Morrone MC, Guzzetta A, Tinelli F et al (2008) Inversion of perceived direction of motion caused by spatial undersampling in two children with periventricular leukomalacia. J Cogn Neurosci 20:1094-106

Mushin J, Hogg CR, Dubowitz LM et al (1984) Visual evoked potentials to light emitting diode (LED) photostimulation in newborn infants. EEG Clin Neurophysiol 68

Pharoah PO, Cooke T, Johnson MA et al (1998) Epidemiology of cerebral palsy in England and Scotland 1984-9. Arch Dis Child Fetal Neonatal Ed 79:F21-5

Pierro MM (2000) La valutazione del rapporto oculomozione/visione. In: La valutazione delle funzioni adattive nel bambino con paralisi cerebrale. FrancoAngeli Editore

Qualls CE, Bliwise NG, Stringer AY (2000) Short forms of the benton judgement of line orientation test: development and psychometric properties. Arch of Clinical Neuropsychology 15:159-64

Sarnat HB, Sarnat MS (1976) Neonatal encephalopathy following fetal distress. Archives of Neurology 33:696-705

Schenk-Rootlieb AJ, van Nieuwenhuizen O, van Waes PF et al (1992) The prevalence of cerebral visual disturbance in children with cerebral palsy. Dev Med Child Neurol 34:473-80

Schenk-Rootlieb AJ, van Nieuwenhuizen O, van Waes PF, van der Graaf Y (1994) Cerebral visual impairment in cerebral palsy: relation to structural abnormalities of the cerebrum. Neuropediatrics 25:68-7

Stiers P, De Cock P, Vandenbussche E (1998) Impaired visual perceptual performance on an object recognition task in children with cerebral visual impairment. Neuropediatrics 29:80-8

Stiers P, De Cock, Vandenbussche E (1999) Separating visual perception and non-verbal intelligence in children with early brain injury. Brain Dev 21:397-406

Stiers P, van den Hout BM, Haers M et al (2001) The variety of visual perceptual impairments in pre-school children with perinatal brain damage. Brain Dev 23:333-348

Stiers P, Vanderkelen R, Vanneste G et al (2002) Visual-perceptual impairment in a random sample of children with cerebral palsy. Dev Med Child Neurol 44:370-82

Sutte CM, Banks MS, Candy TR (2000) Does a front-end nonlinearity confound VEP acuity measures in human infants? Vision Res 40:3665-3675

Tanne-Gariepy J, Rouiller EM, Boussaoud D (2002) Parietal inputs to dorsal versus ventral premotor areas in the macaque monkey: evidence for largely segregated visuomotor pathways. Exp Brain Res 145:91-103

Taylor MJ, Menzies R, MacMillan LJ, White HE (1984) VEPs in normal full-term and premature neonates: longitudinal versus cross sectional data. EEG Clin Neurophysiol 68:20-27

Teller DY, McDonald MA, Preston K et al (1986) Assessment of visual acuity in infants and children: the acuity cards procedure. Dev Med Child Neurol 28:779-789

Teller Acuity Cards (1990) Stereo Optical Co Inc. Vistech Consultants Inc

Tinelli F, Pei F, Guzzetta A et al (2008) The assessment of visual acuity in children with periventricular leukomalacia: a comparison of behavioural and electrophysiological techniques. Vision Research 48:1233-41

van den Hout BM, de Vries LS, Meiners LC et al (2004) Visual perceptual impairment in children at 5 years of age with perinatal haemorrhagic or ischaemic brain damage in relation to cerebral magnetic resonance imaging. Brain Dev 26:251-61

Van Hof-van Duin J (1989) The development and study of visual acuity. Dev Med Child Neurol 31:547-552

Van Hof-van Duin J, Cioni G, Bertuccelli B et al (1998) Visual outcome at 5 years of newborn infants at risk of cerebral visual impairment. Dev Med Child Neurol 40:302-9

Ward J (1970) The factor structure of the frostig developmental test of visual perception. Br J Educ Psychol 40:65-7

Wattam Bell J (1983) Analysis of infant visual evoked potentials (VEPs) by phase sensitive statistics. Perception 14 A33

Neuropsychological Evaluation

8

D. Brizzolara, P. Brovedani, G. Ferretti

Introduction

The study of cognitive and neuropsychological functions in children with cerebral palsy (CP) is relevant both from a theoretical and a practical point of view. From the theoretical standpoint, an analytical documentation of cognitive development and of the neuropsychological patterns associated with the different clinical forms of CP is important for advancing our knowledge on the relations between neurobiological substrate and function. From the practical point of view, a comprehensive cognitive and neuropsychological evaluation represents the starting point for defining the rehabilitation program.

This chapter, starting from a literature review on the factors influencing psychological outcome, will investigate the specific aspects of cognitive evaluation in children in the first two years of life, and, subsequently, will analyze the neuropsychological profiles associated with diplegic and hemiplegic forms. Recent epidemiological studies (for example, European Cerebral Palsy Study, reported in Bax et al. 2006) have contributed to advancing our knowledge on the impact of different factors, such as lesion characteristics and timing, pre-mature vs at term birth, severity of motor and visual deficits, on the cognitive and neuropsychological outcome in the different forms of CP. Finally, short reference will be devoted to the methods for evaluating cognitive, verbal, and non-verbal abilities in children with severe motor disorders (tetraplegia and dyskinesia) in preschool and school age.

Disorders and Factors Associated with CP Influencing Psychological Outcome

Mental Retardation

The incidence of mental retardation in CP is higher than that observed in the normal population. Epidemiological data report a frequency of cognitive disorders ranging from 30 to 60% (Hagberg et al. 1975; Evans et al. 1985; Pharoah et al. 1998; Beckung et al. 2002;

The Spastic Forms of Cerebral Palsy. Adriano Ferrari, Giovanni Cioni
© Springer-Verlag Italia 2010

8

Surman et al. 2003; Sigurdardottir et al. 2008; Andersen et al. 2008). The incidence of mental retardation differs depending on the form of CP. Cognitive function, evaluated through the classical psychometric instruments, is more preserved in dyskinetic, diplegic, and hemiplegic forms than in tetraparetic and ataxic forms.

Epilepsy

The presence of epilepsy, more frequent in cases of tetraparesis and hemiplegia than in cases of diplegia and dyskinesia, is a risk factor for psychological outcome when mental retardation is associated to CP. Carlsson and co-workers (2003) reported that only 15% of the children with CP and normal cognitive development presented with epilepsy, while epilepsy was present in 61% of children with mental retardation. A study by Uverbrand (1988) reports that hemiplegic children with mental retardation present with a frequency of epilepsy 5 times higher than that of children with intelligence within normal range.

The incidence of epilepsy varies in the different studies (from 12 to 90%), probably due to the different clinical features of the patients in the samples. A retrospective study on 85 children with CP by Kwong and co-workers (1998) reports an incidence of epilepsy of 71% in tetraparesis, 32% in hemiplegia, and 21% in diplegia. Moreover, while all cases of diplegia presented a satisfactory control of seizures with single anti epileptic drug, the same result was not achieved in tetraplegic patients. Hadjipanayis and co-workers (1997) report, in a sample of 300 children, an incidence of 50% in tetraparesis, 47% in hemiplegia, and 27% in diplegia. A more recent study (Carlsson et al. 2003) confirms a high incidence of epilepsy in hemiplegic forms (66%) and in tetraparesis (about 43%) and a much lower incidence for diplegic forms (about 16%). Comparable values have been reported by Bax and co-workers (2006). Generally, in the case of diplegia, epilepsy is less frequent in pre-term birth than at term. In particular, periventricular leukomalacia, the most frequent neuroradiological finding in diplegia, is associated with a low risk for epilepsy with respect to the other forms of CP (26%) and the presence of neonatal seizures are strongly associated with later occurring epilepsy (Humphreys et al. 2007). In congenital hemiplegia, epilepsy is mainly associated with cortico-subcortical lesions rather than with periventricular lesions (Cioni et al. 1999; Brizzolara et al. 2002). The impact of factors related with epilepsy on psychological outcome, such as age of onset, frequency and duration of seizures, type of anti-epileptic drugs, has not been systematically analyzed in patients with CP.

Factors Related to the Characteristics of the Lesion

The lesion factor (timing, etiology, location, size, unilateral/bilateral) also plays a relevant role in determining the psychological outcome in children with CP. Even when of the same size, hemorrhagic or hypoxic-ischemic lesions acquired in the last trimester of gestation, usually localized at the level of the periventricular white matter, are mainly associated with milder cognitive disorders than those resulting from hypoxic-ischemic lesions or cerebral infarctions occurring at term, often involving a vast array of cortical areas. More-over, bilateral lesions tend to further reduce the potential for plasticity than unilateral lesions (e.g., more preserved cognitive function in hemiplegia than in tetraparesis). Few studies have attempted at correlating lesion characteristics with neuropsychological outcome (e.g., Brizzolara et al. 2002; Chilosi et al. 2005); however recent advances in fMRI research offer a promising means for understanding the mechanisms subserving re-organization of function in the face of different lesion characteristics (Staudt et al. 2001, 2002; Lidzba et al. 2006a and b; Guzzetta et al. 2008).

Pre-term birth in itself is an important risk factor for psychological outcome, especially in the case of children born very prematurely, and for visuo-cognitive disorders and visuo-motor difficulties. There is a vast literature in this area of research which should be consid-ered when interpreting neuropsychological profiles of children with CP (Roth et al. 1994, 2001; Fawer et al. 1995; Goyen et al. 1998; Foreman et al. 1997; Jongmans et al. 1996; Isaacs et al. 2003; Atkinson and Braddick, 2007; Larroque et al. 2008; Van Braeckel et al. 2008).

Visual Function Disorders

The incidence of severe visual function disorders, defined as retrochiasmatic and visual recognition disorders, is estimated to be around 7-9% of the children with CP (Pharoah et al. 1998). Such disorders, referred to as cerebral visual impairment (CVI) comprise a reduced visual acuity, visual field deficits, oculomotion disorders, strabismus, and difficul-ties in visual recognition. Disorders of visual function are, however, very frequent in chil-dren with CP (more than in 50%) and are described in detail in chapter 7 of this book.

In normal children, visual function plays a predominant role in the initial phases of posture and motion control. In children with CP, the presence of a congenital visuo-perceptual disorder does not only have a negative impact on motion control, but also seems to be a predisposing factor to an unfavorable psychological outcome (cognitive, emotional, adaptative). Cioni and co-workers (2000) reported that in pre-term children with periven-tricular leukomalacia (PVL), the level of visual function impairment at 12 months was correlated with the cognitive level at the same age and at 36 months, being the variable which mainly accounted for cognitive development as compared with the clinical form of CP and with cerebral lesion size and severity. In children born at term with hypoxic-ischemic encephalopathy, many of whom had CP, Mercuri and co-workers (1999) report that the level of visual function in the first year of life correlated with the developmental quotients of the Griffiths scales (1984). Shenk-Rootlieb and co-workers (1992) report a significantly lower level of psychological function (emotional, cognitive, relational) in children with CP presenting with visual function disorders, irrespective of motor disorder severity. As a whole, studies that have related the degree of severity of visual disorders with different variables (such as the severity of the lesion and of the motor deficit) suggest that a severe visual function disorder may in itself impair later cognitive development.

Some forms of CP, especially diplegia and tetraplegia, are more frequently associated with visual function and visual recognition disorders (see section on neuropsychological

8

approach to diplegia), depending on lesion location and size (for a review on the relation between type of lesion and visual disorder, see Guzzetta et al. 2001 a, b and chapter 7). Recent studies have attempted correlating visual function disorders with specific neuronal substrates which could have been damaged by the lesion causing CP, as for example dorsal or ventral pathways of the visual system (Gunn et al. 2002; Fazzi et al. 2004).

Psychiatric Disorders

Psychiatric disorders are factors which can also influence the psychological outcome of children with CP and co-morbidity should be investigated and treated. Mental retardation is associated with a three- to four-fold risk of developing psychiatric disorders with respect to the normal population (American Psychiatric Association, 2000); thus forms of CP with mental retardation have a higher co-morbity with mental health problems (McDermott et al. 1996). Psychiatric co-morbidity could have a biological underpinning (including lesion characteristics, associated mental retardation and prematurity) as well as psychosocial determinants (Goodman and Yude, 2000). The incidence of psychiatric disorders varies from about 25% to 60% (Parkes et al. 2008; Carlsson et al. 2008). The variability of the figures probably depends on the methodology used to assess psychiatric disorders (direct clinical assessment of the child according to DSM criteria vs rating scales or questionnaires filled out by parents and patients). For a comprehensive analysis of the characteristics of psychiatric co-morbidity in children with CP, see chapter 9 of this book.

Factors influencing psychological outcome in CP

> Mental retardation
> Epilepsy
> Factors related to lesion characteristics: etiology, localization, size
> Visual function disorders
> Psychiatric disorders

Cognitive Evaluation in the First Years of Life

Psychometric Approach

In the evaluation of the cognitive development of children with CP in the first two years after birth, the selection of the instruments to be applied differs depending on the degree of motor autonomy achieved by the child. In diplegic and hemiplegic forms, difficulties presented by the child in his relation patterns with objects and in transitive praxies are usually not such as to hinder, as reported in the literature (Fedrizzi et al. 1993; Pagliano et al. 2007; Enkelaar et al. 2008), the use of the most popular psychometric tests such as Griffiths and Bayley scales. The main advantage of these scales derives from their sensitivity, that is their capacity to finely differentiate different degrees of psychomotor development and therefore to detect how much the child's abilities differ from those of the reference sample.

What Are the Limitations of Baby Tests?

The first limitation is their poor validity, detected in normal populations, in predicting IQ of subsequent preschool and school age children (McCall and Carriger, 1993; Slater, 1995). This was interpreted as an effect of the changes involved in development, since psychometric tests on infants mainly measure perceptive-motor abilities, which are later followed by more evolved mental functions, implying the manipulation of symbols, such as language. In contrast with reported data on normal child populations, a study on children at risk due to severe prematurity, with or without association with motor disorder, detected an agreement between development markers at one year after birth and IQ of the same individuals at the age of 8 (Roth et al. 1994). This apparently surprising result can be explained by the fact that in the investigated sample were present, with much higher frequency than in the normal population, extreme IQ values, representing conditions that tend to be maintained in subsequent development stages. More recently, Barnett et al. (2004), in a sample of children with perinatal encephalopathy found that the Griffiths scores had a predictive value on the subsequent development at school age but also a high incidence of "false negatives", i.e. children with cognitive disabilities at later developmental stages but in the normal range in their first two years of life. A second limitation of baby-tests, which is more substantial for the characteristics of children with CP, is that such scales imply normal manipulation abilities, therefore evaluating what the child is truly able to perform. Correlations found by Cioni and co-workers (1997) between brain structural alterations (white matter lesions, cysts, ventricle dilatation) and performance at Griffiths scales were explained by the authors in that many items of such scales require fine motor abilities, which are often impaired as a consequence of white matter lesions. Since executive difficulties alone do not necessarily reflect cognitive development alterations (see dystonic forms), the use of diagnostic tools emphasizing the role of manipulation may sometimes lead to underestimations of the child's actual abilities. The third limitation of baby tests is substantial in the evaluation of children with development disorders: psychometric tests, due to their nature, provide quantitative markers, which do not help in acquiring information about the degree of thought organization or the child's adaptive abilities, which are necessary for the planning of the rehabilitation treatment. Being based on a development model that assumes progressive ability improvement, these scales simply group the child's acquisitions on their temporal concurrent onset, without investigating interdependence elements among the different areas of knowledge or among the acquisition of a certain development level and the next one. A very large number of studies have used the Griffiths scales and the Bayley scales in populations of children with high prematurity or low birth weight, showing that only a minority will develop a motor disability; by contrast, a very limited number of studies have been performed with psychometric instruments on the cognitive development of children with CP in their first years after birth.

Cioni and co-workers (1997) studied a group of 48 children presenting with bilateral spastic forms at the average age of 17 months. The emerging condition is that of a widespread cognitive disability: more than one quarter of the children proved not to be good candidates for testing, and in the remaining 34 the general quotient (GQ) in Griffiths scales was lower than 70. A second element deserving special note in this population is the high variability of IQ compared with the normal population. In another study, Cioni and co-workers (2000) also demonstrated that already at the age of one in cases of tetraplegia and spastic diplegia, cognitive retardation presented an incidence and a severity comparable to that reported in other studies on older children: while all tetraplegic individuals, except one, presented with severe mental retardation, the average scores of diplegic patients were instead within the range. Also in this case, the predictive capacity of a score seems to exhibit a two-fold distribution.

Ordinal Approach

The cognitive evaluation of children with difficulties in expressing even elementary forms of motor activity, especially related to manipulation, is extremely difficult. In these dyskinetic and tetraplegic forms, the issue is how a child can develop an idea of the surrounding environment or think about the possible solution to problems without any direct action. Fortunately, the evolution of thought and the presence of mental representations are not necessarily the lengthening of the sensorimotor activity, as stated by Piaget, and the normal evolution of the notion of object, demonstrated by Decarie (1969) in phocomelic individuals, shows that it can derive from inferences made by the child on perceptive information. Children with neuromotor lesions, as stated by Stella and Biolcati (2003), integrate the lack of motor experiences through perceptive-gnosic reconstruction processes. What remains is the difficulty in highlighting, when patients' actions are reduced or absent, valid indicators of the underlying levels of thought organization. It is therefore necessary to differentiate the development of abilities from the behaviors from which they are usually inferred.

The consequence of these remarks is that the cognitive evaluation of children with CP must be directed not so much at finding the contents of behavior, but to defining the developmental level of the organization structures of thought.

In the cognitive evaluation of a child with motor impairment, it is necessary to:

> Require performances in which execution accuracy is not essential
> Be flexible in the types of material and in stimulus-situations, to adapt them to the different motor characteristics of every single child
> Rule out execution speed as one of the concurring factors for the success of every single test

For infants, a positive response to the above-mentioned needs is provided by the ordinal psychological development scales by Uzgiris and Hunt (1975), representing an application projection of Piaget's theories. It is useful to note that, for these authors, development is conceived as the transformation of intellectual structures through subsequent ontogenetic stages, in which changes are qualitative. Stages are characterized by invariance of their sequence, and by the fact that they progressively include typical structures of the previous stages with the emergence of the most evolved ones.

Uzgiris-Hunt ordinal scale

> I   -   Ability to follow with the gaze moving objects and permanent objects
> II   -   Development of the means to achieve desired environmental events
> IIIa   -   Vocal imitation
> IIIb   -   Gesture imitation
> IV   -   Development of operational causality
> V   -   Development of spatial relationships among objects
> VI   -   Development of relationship schemes with objects

Different from what happens in psychometric tests, the application of an ordinal scale does not imply the strict application of standardization rules, so that it is not necessary to strictly control the features of the employed material, the way it is presented, and the type of response. In the study related to the permanence of the object, to give an example, it is absolutely irrelevant if the child actively searches for the toy hidden by the examiner under a screen: simply focusing gaze in that direction and maintaining it until the discovery action is performed by the adult is enough to indicate that the child has developed the notion of object, and that it is more evolved if the concealing procedures made by the adult were more complicated. Even the simple attempt to act on the activating mechanism of a mechanical toy, even if it fails due to lack of movement precision, clearly indicates that the child has established a cause-effect relationship.

As already mentioned, a development test to be performed on children with CP must also be adapted to make it compatible with the motor abilities of every single child. This can be achieved in two ways: modifying the material or the initial situation, so that the task can be performed by the child, or "become the child's hand", putting the child's intentions into practice. As observed by Robinson and Rosenberg (1987), the two strategies are not fully interchangeable in the different developmental stages. Instead, each can be more or less appropriate depending on the child's evolution level. It has been demonstrated (Bates et al. 1975; Harding and Golinkoff, 1979) that the ability to intentionally direct the adult's action, intended as the awareness of playing an active role, may appear only in sensorimotor stage V, so that before that stage any attempt to act instead of the child, to be "his arm", cannot be successful, since the child is not able to establish a relationship between his attention towards an object and the action the adult makes on his behalf.

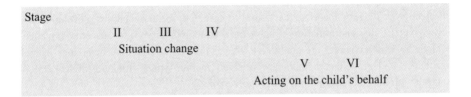

In the identification of the different stages of children's sensorimotor intelligence, Ina Uzgiris (1983) proposed a classification in four stages, which follows, in a simplified way, that by Piaget. This classification does not involve neonatal stage, corresponding to Piaget's first stage, in which objective and subjective levels of reality are still undifferentiated. We report the main features of each of the four levels and the general criteria for the approach to the child, providing some practical examples which could allow the evaluation even in children with more or less severe motor disabilities.

- *First stage* (including Piaget's stages II and III): characterized by the systematic repetition of simple patterns, which are auto- and hetero-directed (looking, bringing objects to the mouth, moving and beating objects). The observer must enable the child to grasp the correlation between his actions and environmental events; therefore special attention will have to be devoted to posture facilitations and to the selection of materials allowing the child to perform actions. Motor activity or direct visual fixation towards the object (it is expected that the child searches for partially concealed objects) is sufficient to indicate active research. To verify the presence of the so-called "procedures", indicating the emergence of the cause-effect relation, parents can help in suggesting the movement games or the vocal games the child considers as more familiar and that activate the child.

- *Second stage* (stage IV): characterized by the intentional coordination of two patterns in a whole, in which one acts as instrument and the other as objective (removing obstacles, use of intermediaries to achieve objectives, etc.). As in the previous level, also in this level it is essential to act on the material and on the environmental conditions, even though it is possible to start teaching the child that he can guide our behavior.
The easiest domain to investigate is that of object permanence (which is now sought after one of the two patterns with visible displacement). The research effort, based on manual attempts and with visual fixations, needs to be verbally requested and essen-

tially rewarded with tangible results, so that the adult must be ready to free the concealed object as soon as the child touches the screen or fixates it with his gaze. In the means-ends domain, this stage involves the typical appearance of the "support conduct", so that it is necessary to make the object to be attracted as one with the place-mat, to allow the action performed on it to always produce a correspondent movement of the object. The adult should second the motor attempts made by the child to make them effective in their results.

• *Third stage* (stage V): characterized by adaptations to the action on the basis of results, with progressive adjustments depending on the correspondence between the result itself and the objective pursued. Having achieved a differentiation between means and ends, it is then possible to become "the child's hand", directly acting on objects on the basis of the child's indications, or assisting and helping the child in motor activity, co-acting with him, to allow him to experience the action. In this level, the child understands the adult's instructions about "showing" where the object was concealed; or, in the means-ends domain, by means of sequential fixations, the child may show awareness of the fact that the objective can be pursued through intermediaries (for example, looking at the string or at the stick that can be used to approximate remote objects).

• *Fourth stage* (stage VI): the transition from practical intelligence to representation intelligence, with anticipation of the results of a motor activity through mental combinations. Adaptations of materials and of environmental conditions are secondary to the importance acquired by gestures, glances, or words (even simple assertions or negations) spontaneously produced also outside the observation session. Much more than in previous stages, the specific behaviors of this stage can be verified: the child, apart from the motor attempts and the use of gaze as indicator, can also direct the adult's attention through continuous confirmations and denials, both in words or in mimic.

From these concepts it is possible to infer that, depending on the child's motor disability, it is not always possible to perform a complete evaluation of the development of all seven domains examined in the Uzgiris-Hunt scales. Even so, the information obtained in only one domain (for example, object permanence) retains its validity, since the marked interdependence among the different domains allows inferences about the child's general level of thought structuring.

On this basis, it is essential to remember that the development pattern detected in children with motor disability, even if characterized by general retardation, reproduces the same stages followed by normal individuals. Indeed, data collected by Cioni and co-workers (1993) on children with CP confirmed the sequentiality of ordinal scales also in these atypical populations.

Evaluation and Rehabilitation

The evaluation of the young child presenting with CP is a process directly involving the family and all the rehabilitation caregivers. Interaction with them reveals information on a broad range of reactions and behaviors regarding the child's life and daily social relationships, which would probably be missed in the observation session. On the other hand,

8

family and caregivers should then receive all the information on the child's level of development and mental organization, essential for the rehabilitation program.

The ordinal approach in the investigation of the child's mental functioning allows the examiner to match data deriving from observation to Piaget's theory, therefore enabling anticipation of which thought organization level will follow.

Each education and rehabilitation approach can be influential only if complying with the principle of "minimum discrepancy" between stimuli and the child's actual development. Messages and proposals deriving from the environment play a propulsive role if they create a positive tension towards growth, remaining compatible and ready to be integrated with the child's degree of thought organization. It is a challenge aimed at recognizing, at every single moment, all the stimulations and experiences which, by questioning the attained structural balance, prompt a cognitive reorganization at higher levels, without inducing in the child reactions of frustration or defense to external intrusions.

Piaget's developmental model, a useful theoretical reference in the process of cognitive development evaluation, must also represent for the family and the caregivers, a reference framework, within which behaviors related to the child's life need to be inserted. It drives to overcome superficial aspects that are easier to observe, to reach an awareness of the existence of a central mental organization aimed at integrating all the ideas that the child himself has built upon himself and his surrounding environment.

Experimental Approach (Human Information Processing)

Recent methods for the evaluation of intellectual development in infants overcome the problem of the reduced predictivity of psychometric tests. The performance within the first year after birth, on the basis of human information processing abilities (HIP), has demonstrated good correlation with IQ levels of subsequent ages (Mc Call and Carriger, 1993). This was attributed to the fact that, while performance required by psychometric testing is age-specific, attention and memory, directly investigated through HIP methods, are instead mental functions which can be supposed to be transversal in development. Usually, they are paradigms based on visual recognition memory processes, which imply longer fixation by the child on the new stimulus than on the familiar one (the so-called "novelty effect"). This method was applied both for the investigation of children with severe motor disorders (Drotar et al. 1989) and on sample populations of children at risk due to severe prematurity, who displayed longer familiarization time spans and a reduced "novelty effect" compared with controls (Rose et al. 1988; Rose, 1983). By means of the Fagan Test of Infant Intelligence (FTII) (Fagan and Shepherd, 1991), Cioni and co-workers (1998) investigated the ability of visual information processing in children presenting with congenital hemiplegia. This test consists of ten tasks in which, after a stage of familiarization with single or pairs of identical stimuli representing human faces, the presentation of a new face follows, associated with one to which the child has already become familiar. The longer time span the child employs to stare at the new stimulus as compared with the familiar ones demonstrates recognition of the second stimulus as differentiated from the first, and the effective processing of the stimuli he was exposed to. The interesting result of this study is that, while all children except one attained scores that were normal or within the range in Griffiths scales, the performance of four of them at FTII fell into suspect or high-risk areas. Such data however must be further confirmed by studies conducted on larger populations of children presenting with different forms of CP. More recently, Guzzetta et al (2006) demonstrated a significant correlation between the performance at the FTII at 9 months and cognitive development at two years of age. The limitation of this type of test, however, is that quite a high percentage of children with CP have a reduced binocular visual acuity, often associated with strabismus, reduction of visual field, and asymmetries in optokinetic horizontal nystagmus (OKN) (Ipata et al. 1994), i.e., conditions which can more or less interfere in the visual analysis of stimuli and represent an obstacle in the application of this method.

Neuropsychological Approach to Spastic Diplegia

Studies on the Development of Intelligence

Global intellectual functioning, measured with psychometric scales largely adopted in clinical practice, is generally preserved in the diplegic forms of CP although IQ scores usually fall below the mean in the majority of children. Data from the literature converge in reporting an asymmetry in the cognitive profile, with higher verbal than performance scores (Fedrizzi et al. 1993; Inverno et al. 1994; Ito et al. 1996; Cioni et al. 2000; Yokochi et al. 2000; Pirila et al. 2004)

Studies analysing early cognitive development in infants are rare. In the study conducted by Cioni and co-workers (2000), 29 pre-term children with periventricular leukomalacia at MRI were evaluated with the Griffiths scales first at one year and subsequently at three years. The aim of the study was to analyze the relationship between visual functions (acuity, visual field, fixation, nystagmus) and neurological and cognitive outcome. Looking at the developmental quotients of the 15 diplegic children at one year of age, the scores on the language scale were higher than the values for the eye-hand coordination and performance scales (Table 8.1). This discrepancy between verbal and non-verbal performance was present in most children, and in some cases it was marked. Since 13 out of 15 children presented with one or more visual function disorder, it was suggested that these disorders significantly contributed to the decrease of non-verbal quotients. A study by Fedrizzi and co-workers (1993) analyzed early cognitive development in 3-year-old pre-term children with spastic diplegia, comparing performance on the Griffiths scale of the premature children with periventricular leukomalacia at CT scan with that of a group of pre-term children considered "at low risk". Again, the cognitive profile of diplegic children revealed better performance in the verbal scale with respect to the eye-hand coordination and performance scales, with differences of 20 to 25 points. As in the study conducted by Cioni, these data suggest that the delay in the acquisition of visuoperceptual and visuoconstructional abilities has early onset, already at pre-school age. The same children in the Fedrizzi et al study, evaluated at six years of age with the WPPSI, showed a VIQ of 96

8

Table 8.1 Non-verbal intelligence disorders in diplegia

Authors	Subjects	Neuroimaging	Visual functions	Results
Studies in the first year of life				
Cioni 2000	n= 29 Premature 15/29 diplegia CA at 1 and 3 (longitudinal	PVL Classification of severity of abnormalities and of lesions to optic radiations and O cortex at MRI	13/15 diplegic with 1 or more disorders of acuity, field, nystagmus, fixation, strabismus	(Griffiths) Verbal DQ = 84 E-H coord. DQ = 76 Perf. DQ = 75 Correlation between visual disorder and MRI abnormalities; between optic radiation damage and non-verbal DQ
Studies in the second year and at school age				
Fedrizzi 1993	n = 20 CA = at 3 and 6 (longitudinal) GA = 27-36 N = 10 premature controls without lesions	PVL of different severity in F, trygonal and O regions CT	4 strabismus 4 refraction disorders 9 strabismus + refraction disorders	3 years (Griffiths) Verbal DQ = 98 E-H coord. DQ = 74 Perf. DQ = 73 6 years (WPPSI) VIQ = 96 PIQ = 70
Inverno 1994	n = 30 CA = 9;5 GA < 37	PVL Classification abnormalities and lesions for 21/30 at MRI	21 strabismus 18 refraction disorders 14 strabismus +. refraction disorders	VIQ = 92; PIQ = 66 (WPPSI and WISC-R) Negative correlation between FSIQ and PIQ and degree of ventricular dilation, PV white matter reduction, posterior CC lesions and optic radiations
Ito 1996	n = 34 CA = 6-13 GA= 28-34	Measurement of lateral ventricle surface and ratio between anterior and posterior horns area	visual disorders excluded	VIQ = 94; PIQ = 69 (WISC-R) 22/34 VIQ>PIQ VIQ-PIQ difference correlates with anterior and posterior horns ratio
Yokochi 2000	n = 31 CA = 3-9 GA = 26-36	PVL PV hyperintensity areas white matter reduction	Not evaluated	30/31 non-verbal intelligence lower than verbal (K-form; WPPSI; WISC-R)
Pirila 2004	n = 15 CA= 5-12 GA= 26-38	PVL at cranial US grades I to III 9/15 cystic PVL in P-O or F-P-O areas	10 strabismus	VIQ 97; PIQ 65 WISC-III, WPPSI-R, impaired visuo-motor and visuo-spatial, spared language memory and learning at the NEPSY

CA, Chronological age; *CC*, corpus callosum; *CT*, Computerized tomography; *DQ*, Development quotient; *E-H coord.*, Eye-Hand Coordination scale; *F*, frontal; *GA*, Gestational age in weeks; *NEPSY*, Developmental Neuropsychological assessment; *O*, occipital; *P*, parietal; *Perf.*, Performance scale; *PV*, periventricular; *PVL*, periventricular leukomalacia; *Verbal*, Verbal scale; *US*, Ultrasonography versus a PIQ of 70, confirming the Griffiths profile (Table 8.1). In a larger sample analyzed with MRI, the same group of authors (Inverno et al. 1994) found a negative relationship between PIQ and severity of ventricular dilation, periventricular white matter reduction, and presence of lesions in the posterior portion of the corpus callosum and in the optic radiations. Also more recent studies confirm that the verbal-performance discrepancy is already present in the pre-school years (Pirila et al. 2004).

The verbal-performance discrepancy was also confirmed at school age by Ito and co-workers (1996) in 34 diplegic children between 6 and 13 years of age presenting with a significant difference between VIQ (94) and PIQ (69). This pattern was evident both at the group level, and in the majority of children (18 out of 25). A more recent study by Yokochi (2000) on 31 pre-term diplegic school aged children with periventricular leukomalacia as seen at MRI reported PIQ scores (or comparable parameters of different psychometric tests) to be lower in all cases except one.

Earlier studies and more recent evidence (Pirila et al. 2004; Fazzi et al. 2004; Korkman et al. 2008) confirm a specific cognitive pattern in pre-term diplegic children, characterized by preserved verbal abilities and impaired or borderline visuo-spatial and visuo-constructional skills suggesting that congenital posterior cortical damage selectively and persistently affects performance abilities. There is lower concordance across studies regarding the correlation between severity of damage and later cognitive outcome but this could depend on the degree of resolution of neuroimaging techniques (e.g., MRI vs CT scan and cranial Ultrasonography).

Development of intelligence in diplegia: summary of data from the literature

> Cognitive profile is not homogeneous: the verbal quotient is within the normal range, while the non-verbal quotient is borderline or impaired
> Verbal -non-verbal intelligence discrepancy is evident already in the first years of life
> The degree of impairment of non-verbal intelligence correlates in some cases with the degree of white matter reduction in the posterior areas and in optic radiations

---

What is the Nature of Visuo-Perceptual Disorders in Diplegia?

The hypothesis of a visuo-perceptual disorder associated with diplegia was originally advanced by Abercombie and co-workers (1964), who reported that performance on the Marianne Frostig developmental test of visual perception (DTVP) was lower in diplegic than in normal children. Only more recent studies, with the advancement of neuroradiological techniques (MRI vs CT scan), have paved the way for a more detailed analysis of the neurobiological underpinnings of these difficulties.

Koeda and Takeshita (1992) evaluated 18 diplegic children with gestational age below 36 weeks, intelligence within the normal range or borderline, presenting only with mild upper limbs disorders. The visuo-perceptual quotient at the Frostig was significantly lower than the overall developmental quotient on the Binet scale. Their objective was to correlate the severity of the visuo-perceptual disorder with MRI data. The authors reported that the peritrigonal white matter volume of the parietal and occipital lobes negatively correlated with the degree of the visuo-perceptual disorder (Table 8.2).

Ito and co-workers (1996) also found a lower perceptual quotient (Frostig scale), a significant discrepancy between VIQ and PIQ, and a negative correlation between visuo-perceptual abilities and severity of the lateral ventricles dilation in the posterior horns at MRI. Recent studies confirm that PVL with a reduction in the amount of occipito-parietal and posterior-parietal white matter is strongly associated with impaired visuo-perceptual performance especially when visuo-motor integration is required (Fazzi et al. 2004). While more specific visuo-motor difficulties seem to be a marker of diplegia in pre-term children with PVL, diplegic children born at term are less impaired on all visuo-perceptual tasks and do not exhibit the specific pattern of visuo-motor difficulties (Pagliano et al. 2007).

Table 8.2 Non-verbal intelligence disorders in diplegia

Authors	Subjects	Neuroimaging	Visual disorders	Visuo-perceptual tests	Results
Koeda 1992	n = 18 CA = 5; 4-9;5 GA = 26-33 IQ = 69-122	PV white matter lesions	Acuity reduction and strabismus in some patients	Frostig scales	PQ = 64-118 PQ < IQ Correlation between severity of visuo-perceptual disorder and degree of PV white matter reduction
Ito 1996	n= 34 CA = 6-13 GA=28-34 PIQ = 69 VIQ = 94	Measurement of lateral ventricle surface and ratio between anterior and posterior horns area	Visual disorders excluded	Frostig scales VIQ-PIQ difference	PQ negatively correlates with VIQ-PIQ difference Negative correlation between severity of visuoperceptual disorder and ratio between anterior posterior horns area
Fedrizzi 1998	n = 15 CA = 4;5-6;9 GA = 27-37 IQ>80	PVL 8/15 NMR 7/15 CT scan	4 acuity disorders 6 refraction disorders 7 strabismus	Visuo-motor test adapted from WPPSI	Right-left sequence deficit, visual scanning, saccadic movements. Difficulty in attention shifting to peripheral target
Fazzi 2004	n= 20 CA = 5-8 GA= 25-33 IQ>60 non severe visual impairment	PVL at MRI	11 refractive (corrected with lenses) 5 visual field 4 nystagmus 14 squint	DTVP	17 VMI 7 NMVPQ 13 GVPQ impaired Visual perceptual impairment correlates with severity of parietal white matter damage

CA, Chronological age in years; *DTVP*, developmental test of visual perception; *GA*, Gestational age in weeks; *GVPQ*, General visual-perceptual quotient; *NMVPQ*, Non-motor visual-perception quotient; *PQ*, perceptual quotient; *PV*, periventricular; *PVL*, periventricular leukomalacia; *VMIQ*, visual–motor integration quotient

> **Summary of the literature results on visuo-perceptual disorders in diplegia**
>
> ❯ Perceptual quotient impaired or definitely lower than FSIQ
> ❯ Perceptual quotient strongly correlates with PIQ
> ❯ Severity of visuo-perceptual disorder correlates with the degree of posterior white matter abnormalities in the majority of studies

Few studies have attempted analyzing in more detail the nature of visuo-perceptual disorders. The widely used DTVP may not be sensitive enough to pinpoint which component of visual information processing may be specifically impaired (e.g., figure-ground discrimination, recognition of images from different view-points and lightings, recognizing the image from its component parts). Some authors maintain that periventricular leukomalacia, such as that reported in the diplegic form of pre-mature CP children, determines a specific visuo-perceptual disorder (Stiers et al. 1999; 2001; 2002) and that the severity of the specific disorder positively correlates with the extent of periventricular white matter damage. These authors have devised a set of experimental visual recognition tasks (the L94 battery, already mentioned in chapter 7 of this book) such as recognition of overlapped figures, or objects shown in unconventional view or embedded in noise. The performance on these tasks by children with different forms of CP was found to be lower than their performance IQ, suggesting a specific visuo-perceptual deficit.

Performance on visuo-perceptual tests could be influenced by eye movement difficulties, frequently displayed by diplegic children (Fedrizzi, 1998), which could in turn be associated to an attentional disorder. Attention has rarely been directly assessed in diplegic children. A recent study by Schatz and co-workers (2001) on school aged pre-mature children with periventricular leukomalacia found that 'inhibition of return effect', which implies a faster shift of attention to a novel position in space than to a position to which attention had been previously engaged, was absent in children with anterior damage. This evidence seems in line with older studies by Hood and Atkinson (1990), suggesting that children with neurological disorders have difficulty in shifting their attention from the center to the periphery ("sticky fixation"), and confirmed by more recent evidence by the same group in terms of deficits in selective attention and executive control of pre- mature children with brain abnomralites at MRI (Atkinson and Braddick, 2007).

Neurobiological Underpinnings of Visuo-Perceptual Disorders in Diplegia: Dorsal and Ventral Streams

The debate on the degree of separation and integration of the two principal visual streams, ventral and dorsal, and their functional developmental trajectories and timing in typical development is ongoing and has received renewed interest in recent times (Milner and Goodale, 2008; Grill-Spector et al. 2008). Lesion data from studies on CP have contributed to the issue and have suggested that periventricular white matter damage is associated with a "dorsal stream vulnerability" (Atkinson and Braddick, 2007) and that in pre-term diplegic children the frequent evidence of impaired visuo-motor performance and relatively spared more general visuo-perceptual abilites may in fact be a marker of a dorsal stream deficit subserved by damage to parietal white matter (Fazzi et al. 2004).

Assessing Visuo-Perceptual Disorders in Diplegic Children

A neuropsychological evaluation should focus on an in-depth analysis of the different processes involved in visual recognition. Ideally, elementary abilities, such as recognition of size, orientation, and line length e.g., Benton line recognition, 1990), should be assessed to exclude that a disorder at a 'lower level' of visual recognition might impair more complex object recognition. Such tests, which have a good theoretical framework and which include more higher-level abilities (e.g., Birmingham Object Recognition Battery, Riddoch and Humphreys, 1993; VOPS, visual object and space recognition battery, Warrington and James, 1991) are already available for adults and have been normed for children in some cases (Temple and Coleman, 2000). Recently, a theory- driven experimental battery of visuo-perceptual tests for children was presented for the Italian population (Bova et al. 2007). Other batteries, constructed from older tests (DTVP, TVPS-R) tapping more complex levels of visual discrimination of geometric shapes with different orientation, embedded in noise or fragmented in smaller parts, have already been discussed. Visuo-motor integration, which seems particularly vulnerable in diplegic children, should also be assessed in copying tasks, such as the VMI. Complex stimuli such as faces also deserve special attention although there is paucity of data on children with brain lesions, except for experimental paradigms. These tests derived from the classical neuropsychological literature should ideally be coupled with psychophysical and electrophysiological measures tapping specific circuitries (e.g., ventral and dorsal streams), which offer a promising means for correlating neuroradiological and neuropsychological data especially in infancy and in the early pre-school years, when assessment with traditional tests is precluded (Braddick and Atkinson, 2007; Morrone et al. 2008; Gunn et al. 2002).

The role of attentional mechanisms in visuo-perceptual processing should also be addressed especially in terms of spatial attention e.g., The Everyday Attention for Children test (Tea-ch, Manly et al. 1999; versions of line cancellation tasks are also avalilabe for pre-schoolers, Laurent-Vannier).

Finally, academic achievement should also be evaluated since 'lower level' visuoperceptual difficulties may negatively affect learning of more complex tasks.

The Neuropsychological Approach to Forms of Infant Hemiplegia

Introduction

Forms of congenital infant hemiplegia, originating from mainly unilateral cerebral lesions, and often involving cortical-subcortical areas performing different cognitive functions, are of special interest in neuropsychological approach. More than a century of anatomo-functional correlation studies and of the application of cognitivist models on patients with cerebral lesions acquired in adult age (Dax, 1865; Damasio and Damasio, 1989), recently supported by functional neuroimaging studies (Springer, 1999; Szaflarski et al. 2006), have provided a large database on the functional architecture of the brain. It is known that lesions of a complex neuronal network involving different cortical-subcortical areas of the left hemisphere produce verbal deficiencies of different type, while lesions of neural circuits in the right hemisphere produce deficiencies in different non-verbal activities, as for example the learning of pathways in space.

The application of neuropsychological models of adults to children with congenital hemiplegia may be useful in the interpretation of cognitive deficiencies associated with lesions of different cerebral location and size, and may guide neuropsychological evaluation in a focused way, always considering that infant brain plasticity and the lesion involving a still functionally immature brain, may induce atypical functional organization processes, with effects on cognitive profiles that are different from those of adults. The identification of the functions which are especially spared by the cerebral damage leading to hemiplegia and of the more vulnerable and less restorable functions, is a challenging issue, whose investigation is relevant both from the prognosis and from the rehabilitation perspective.

Overall Intellectual Development in Children

The majority of studies on the cognitive outcome of hemiplegic children have applied measurements of general intelligence. Among the different forms of CP, those of hemiplegia seem to be characterized by a reduced incidence of mental retardation. Case studies lately reported in the literature seem to confirm observations dating back to the past, when infant hemiplegia was thought to be associated with normal or almost normal cognitive development. The incidence of mental retardation, however, varies among the different case studies, ranging from 15% to 50% (Aicardi and Bax, 1998) also depending on the different clinical characteristics of the investigated populations (Cioni et al. 1999). However, it needs to be remarked that, although many hemiplegic children present with normal cognitive development, as a group their performances are often, but slightly, significantly lower than those of normal controls. The definition of the risk factors involved in a deficient development of intelligence in hemiplegic children, and of the conditions favoring a totally normal development still need to be fully clarified and require further investigation.

Factors Influencing Negative Outcome

Epilepsy

Studies which explicitly examined different risk factors on many samples of children (Wiklund and Uvebrant, 1991; Goodman and Yude, 1996) evidenced that, also in hemiplegic individuals, the presence of epilepsy is the main risk factor for mental retardation. The second of the two quoted studies also reported the age of epilepsy onset as a factor which negatively impacts on the overall intellectual development, in the sense that the earlier the onset of epilepsy, the higher the risk of mental retardation will be. A recent study on a sample of 91 hemiplegic children (Cioni et al. 1999) reports a strong association between epilepsy and mental retardation: 57% of children with cognitive deficiency presented with epileptic fits versus 29% of children with normal development. The incidence of convulsive fits is especially high in children with cortical-subcortical lesion, mainly due to medial cerebral artery infarction with perinatal onset, while it is remarkably lower in children with periventricular white matter lesions, with mainly prenatal onset. Cognitive delay could therefore be caused by the interference of epileptic activity, expression of a more widespread neurological dysfunction, with the functional reorganization processes happening in the brain of children subsequent to cerebral lesions. Other studies (Sussova et al. 1990; Vargha-Khadem et al. 1992; Dall'Oglio et al. 1994; Muter et al. 1997), apart from confirming the negative impact of epilepsy on IQ, also report the presence of linguistic and mnesic deficiencies in hemiplegic children with epilepsy.

Lesion Side and Development of Verbal and Non-verbal Intelligence

Differences in verbal and performance IQ were examined in different studies in relation to cerebral lesion side. Studies conducted on adults with unilateral lesions to the left or the right side demonstrated that patients with left side lesions present with a performance IQ higher than verbal IQ, while patients with right side lesions present with the opposite pattern. However, literature reviews on hemiplegic patients at developmental age do not confirm the results reported on adults with unilateral cerebral lesions (Riva and Cazzaniga, 1986; Nass et al. 1989; Vargha-Khadem et al. 1992; Muter et al. 1997; Ballantyne et al. 1994; Brizzolara et al. 2002). Bates and Roe (2001), in a meta-analysis conducted on 12 studies reported in the literature, concluded that most of these studies did not present significant effects related to lesion side on verbal or performance IQ. A reduction of performance IQ as compared with verbal IQ (largely repeated in different case studies and therefore consistent and reliable) instead seems to characterize hemiplegic children regardless of lesion side.

This dissociation could reflect the fact that the administration mode of performance tests is especially penalizing for hemiplegic children, because many subsets of performance intellective scales require manual motor output, performance execution time thresholds and bimanual coordination. Although Muter and co-workers (1997) found that, even excluding execution time for the "block design" test of the WISC scale, scores of hemiplegic individuals were lower than scores of controls, more recently impaired hand motor function, influencing speed in manual tasks, has been found to be correlated with lesion size and performance IQ in patients with early left-hemisphere lesions (Lidzba et al. 2006a).

"Crowding" Effect

The drop in performance IQ might reflect the so-called "crowding" effect (Lansdell, 1969; Teuber, 1975), by which the right hemisphere should also perform the functions of the impaired left hemisphere. The subsequent competition for the neuronal space of specialized functional circuits would produce a disadvantage for non-verbal right side abilities. Conversely, in congenital left side hemiplegia, a "crowding" effect, i.e., the reduction of verbal ability with full development of visuospatial abilities, would not be observed. The asymmetry in the "crowding" effect is attributed to asynchrony in the development of functional maturation from less specialized areas. Behavior data suggest that the posterior areas of the right hemisphere are functionally more immature than the homologous areas in the left hemisphere, but this hypothesis has not obtained adequate experimental confirmation through neurophysiologic and neuroimaging techniques (Chiron et al. 1997). The "crowding" hypothesis cannot be validly demonstrated through data related to lowering of performance IQ. Indeed, intellectual performance scales are not specific neuropsychological instruments to measure functions of the right hemisphere, such as space perception and knowledge, memorization of non-verbal stimuli, recognition of emotional conditions, faces, etc.

Specific impairments have seldom been reported after congenital left hemisphere lesions: Brizzolara and co-workers (1984) evidenced difficulties in performing visuospatial tasks, such as reading the time on a watch, discriminating the orientation of lines both in visual and tactile modality, as opposed to a normal development of verbal abilities in a child with congenital right hemiplegia.

Carlsson (1997), in patients with right congenital hemiplegia, found a difficulty in reproducing by heart abstract drawings with the left hand, a difficulty not found in patients with left hemiplegia. The authors attribute this result to the "crowding" effect, a specific short-term visual-spatial memory deficiency, and expression of a dysfunction of the supporting right hemisphere. Korkman and von Wendt (1995) instead tried to demonstrate the hypothesis of "crowding" by using hemisphere specialization tests, both for language and for non-verbal functions (discrimination of face expressions). Although cerebral lateralization patterns emerged as a result of the focal lesion, these authors reported a significant individual variability in the inter- and intra-hemisphere reorganization deriving from an early cerebral damage.

Even though the occurrence of specific visuospatial deficiencies deriving from left side lesions proves a lack of functional development from the right hemisphere, it does not provide a direct demonstration of the abnormal specialization of the right hemisphere for language.

The lateralization of language was recently investigated with the application of dichotic listening paradigms in children presenting with congenital hemiplegia. Such studies demonstrated that language is reorganized in the right hemisphere following congenital lesions in the left hemisphere (Nass et al. 1992; Hughdal and Carlsson, 1994; Isaacs et al. 1996). Brizzolara and co-workers (2002) have demonstrated that the factors inducing inter-hemisphere reorganization of language are lesion location in temporal areas of the left hemisphere and perinatal timing of the lesion.

New, non-invasive techniques of functional exploration of the CNS, such as functional MRI (fMRI), have been mainly applied to epileptic patients (Hertz-Pannier et al. 1997; Liegeois et al. 2004) to localize language representation in the brain. More recently, a few fMRI studies have directly measured language lateralization in non-epileptic patients with early left hemisphere lesions.

Right hemisphere organization for language has been demonstrated in patients with unilateral white matter lesions of the early third trimester of gestation (Staudt et al. 2001, Staudt et al. 2002). An interhemispheric language organization has also been found after perinatal left arterial stroke, both in group and in single case studies (Tillema et al. 2008; Guzzetta et al. 2008; Booth et al. 1999; Heller et al. 2005).

Crucial data supporting the "crowding" hypothesis have been obtained only recently with fMRI experiments conducted on patients with pre- or perinatal focal left hemisphere lesions. Adolescents and young adults with right hemisphere language production at fMRI had visuospatial deficits in short-term memory and in mental rotation tasks compared not only to control subjects but also to patients without right hemispheric language preference (Lidzba et al. 2006a); the deficits were related to the degree of right hemisphere involve-ment in language. Moreover, in another study, the same authors showed that verbal and non verbal tasks activated a common right-hemisphere network (Lidzba et al. 2006b).

The identification of mechanisms and factors underlying functional re-organization of the nervous background following early unilateral lesions is still an open issue whose neuropsychological approach, integrated with CNS functional investigation techniques, would provide an essential contribution for the future.

Mechanisms Underlying Language Re-organization

One of the factors that seem to be influencing cognitive outcome is lesion timing. Language re-organization and development may largely differ depending on the moment in which the cerebral lesion occurs, reflecting different levels of anatomo-functional organization and maturation.

Many neuropsychological studies on hemiplegia in children are focused on differenti-ating the effects deriving from prenatal lesions, or from lesions occurring in the first 6 months after birth, and those deriving from a subsequently acquired lesion. The idea that plasticity decreases with an increase in cortical specialization is largely accepted (Stiles, 2001 for a review). Increasing lateralization of language during childhood has been reported both with fMRI (Szaflarski et al. 2006) and with magnetoencephalography (Ressel et al. 2008). An initially more bilateral organization of language may facilitate compensatory processes by the right hemisphere after early damage to the left hemisphere.

Currently available clinical data demonstrate how children with congenital focal lesions of the left hemisphere adequately learn language within the first 5 years after birth (Vicari et al. 2000; Chilosi et al. 2001, 2002), while in children with later lesion onset language deficiencies may occur which are not totally recovered over time (Chilosi et al. 2008). However, it is difficult to assess the relevance of lesion-onset timing as a separate aspect from other factors, such as etiology, location, and size. Within the different types of congenital hemiplegia we can differentiate between prenatal lesions, occurring at different stages of gestational life (encephaloclastic prenatal cysts, white matter lesions due to parenchymal hemorrhage or periventricular leukomalacia), and those occurring at perinatal age (cortical-subcortical lesions deriving from cerebral infarctions), which differ in etiopathogenetic mechanisms from post-natal gliotic lesions due to cranial trauma, infections, etc. (Cioni et al. 1997). Also, cerebral reorganization patterns following early lesions could change depending on lesion timing, as demonstrated in a study on language lateralization in hemiplegic patients with perinatal or prenatal lesions (Brizzolara et al. 2002). The application of dichotic listening tests evidenced that in children with left side cortical lesions that occurred at perinatal age language was lateralized in the right hemisphere, while children who suffered from prenatal periventricular lesions to the left hemisphere, presented with a lateralization for language in the same damaged hemisphere.

The role of lesion site in language re-organization has been recently supported with the use of fMRI in a study by our group on young patients with left perinatal arterial stroke (Guzzetta et al. 2008). Lesion proximity to anterior language regions was associated with atypical right hemisphere specialization. In the same study, the degree of impairment of hand motor function was associated to right hemisphere language organization, giving support to the relationship between gestures and language, well established in typical language development.

Time Elapsed between Lesion Onset and Age of Neuropsychological Evaluation

This factor was considered in two interesting studies (Levine et al. 1987; Banich et al. 1990), which reported how in congenital lesions IQ worsens over time, while this trend is not evidenced in acquired hemiplegia. A longitudinal study by Muter and co-workers (1997) on 38 patients with congenital hemiplegia demonstrated, however, a significant decline only in performance IQ in the age range 3 to 5 years.

Bates and co-workers (1999), in a transversal study on 76 patients with congenital hemiplegia between 3 and 14 years of age, did not confirm the results reported by Banich and co-workers (1990) on a significant correlation between age and IQ, even though IQ tended to decrease with the passing of time. These authors have proposed the hypothesis that IQ worsening might be due to methodology bias in patient sample selection in transversal studies, since older patient groups would report a higher number of children with cognitive disorders, due to the fact that precisely for this reason these children are referred to rehabilitation care centers.

The debate is still open on the possible constant relation between cognitive outcome and lesion onset timing, as well as on the limitations related to plasticity and recovery potential (Bates and Roe, 2001). It could be maintained that in different development stages, when learning new and complex tasks (e.g., written language or calculations), children's brains which suffered from functionally compensated lesions, might face new reorganization processes, with consequent periods of transient difficulty followed by compensations.

Only longitudinal studies on large populations evaluated with a long-term follow-up will provide conclusive information on the existing relation between lesion onset timing and cognitive development pathways.

Specific Neuropsychological Deficits

The neuropsychological approach seems especially useful in identifying the specific deficits and their possible correlation with the characteristics of the lesion underlying the hemiplegic condition. Such an approach is aimed at studying single cognitive functions which could be subdivided into a series of processes on the basis of cognitivist theoretical models.

Neuropsychological studies of the last decades (Bates et al. 1997; Vicari et al. 1998; Chilosi et al. 2001, 2008) yielded remarkable progress from the methodological point of view, compared to the studies that appeared in the 1980s, which included in case studies patients with both congenital and acquired hemiplegia, and which often did not provide, due to the reduced diffusion of neuroimaging techniques, neuroradiological documentation of the lesions. Consistent progress has been achieved also in the methodology of neuropsychological observation, with the introduction of new evaluation instruments to monitor the development of cognitive functions at extremely early development stages (e.g., language in the first three years of life). Synergy among the best instrumental methodologies for the documentation of lesion characteristics, and more refined measurements of behavioral functions applied to large and adequately selected patient populations, have provided reliable data for a better understanding of the development of certain cognitive functions in children with congenital hemiplegia.

Visuospatial and Visuopraxic Abilities

Specific disorders in visuo-constructive activities, such as reproducing spatial configurations with square blocks, drawing from a model, or spontaneous drawing, have been demonstrated in patients with right-side and left-side hemiplegia (Stiles and Nass, 1991; Stiles et al. 1996; Vicari et al. 1998; Akshoomoff et al. 2002). The nature of the deficiency however, changed depending on the lesion side: in the drawing on copy and by heart, children with right-side lesion showed a deficiency in the global organization of the figure, while those with left-side lesions produced less details, but the spatial pattern was preserved.

The difficulty maintained by the authors is that the deficiency subsequent to a lesion of the right hemisphere consists in the difficulty of spatial integration of the local elements.

Hemiplegic patients with left side lesions would instead have difficulties in reproducing details, maintaining, however, a spatially integrated organization, even if simplified.

Evolution Pathways of Visuospatial Abilities

In a longitudinal study, Akshoomoff and co-workers (2002) tried to define the typical characteristics of spatial and visuoconstructive abilities in children presenting with unilateral cerebral lesions, and to highlight the evolution pathway of those abilities. These authors investigated the productions of copied drawings and drawings made by heart with a largely applied test (complex figure by Rey-Osterrieth) to evaluate constructive, visuospatial, and planning and memory abilities at different development stages (at 6, 8, 10 and 12 years of age). Products (Stern et al. 1994) as well as processes and strategies employed in the copy and drawing by heart test were evaluated.

Products were quantified on the basis of the presence, reproduction accuracy and spatial positioning of the configural elements, groups, and details that the drawing was made of. Processes (task planning and organization approach) were instead evaluated according to categories describing the procedures applied in normal development between 6 and 12 years of age (Akshoomoff and Stiles, 1996). In normal development, an analytical and destructured approach, develops into an approach in which global configuration is integrated by detail collocation.

Hemiplegic patients enrolled in this study presented lower scores in products in the lower age group, but subsequently improved their performance which it will never achieve fully normal levels in terms of drawing completeness and spatial positioning of elements, but will become quite accurate.

In terms of strategy, the systematic improvement of normal development was not observed, with persistence of more immature strategies. Especially, no child with right side lesion applied the integrated global/analytical approach, while some children presenting with left side lesions showed a more evolved process.

Differences between hemiplegic children and controls, and between children with right side lesions and left side lesions, are amplified in drawing from memory. Indeed, in this condition, children must use an internal representation of the model, and, at this level, differences among the groups emerge, more of qualitative than of quantitative type. Children with right side lesions produce drawings which are poorly integrated at the global level and more fragmented than those of children with left side lesions, whose production of drawings by heart reflects representations in which global aspects prevail.

Stiles and co-workers' fMRI study (2003) of two children with early focal lesions of the left or right hemisphere has shown that both global- and local-level pattern information is lateralized to the contralesional hemisphere, demonstrating that the developing brain can recruit alternative patterns of brain organization.

Qualitative performance differences discussed in the study by Akshoomoff and co-workers (2002) are also compatible with the neuropsychological models employed in adult patients, with right and left side lesions subsequent to cerebral infarctions (Kirk and Kertesz, 1989). For patients with right side lesions, these authors found visuospatial cognition deficiency and analytical processing. The poor performance of patients with left side lesions was instead attributed to a conceptualization deficiency of the object to be graphically represented, maybe due to the aphasic disorder present in many of them. A study by Carlesimo and co-workers (1993) considered the hypothesis that the role of the right hemisphere in visual-constructive activities is especially important in the manipulation of objects for visual information guidance (manipulative-spatial abilities), offering interesting hints on the possibility to separately study the contribution of motor, visuoperceptive, and manipulative-spatial deficiencies in visuoconstructive performances. Movement speed tests (finger tapping) and tests for the discrimination of spatial orientation which imply no executive responses (discrimination of direction of transverse lines) were performed to that aim. Spatial manipulation abilities have been investigated both with drawings copy tasks requiring analysis of complex spatial stimulations, and with visual tracking tasks, such as drawing a line within preset margins. The authors concluded that patients with left side hemiplegia also find difficulties in visuoperceptive tasks, differently from patients with right side hemiplegia. The examined studies in children and adults with cerebral lesions provide relevant indication on the potential strength of the neuropsychological approach to build neurocognitive models aimed at identifying the elements constituting complex cognitive processes and evidencing possible specific deficiencies and individual differences. This type of cognitivist approach, which so far has not adequately been applied in neuropsychological studies on forms of infant hemiplegia, apart from allowing a more precise diagnosis of the cognitive disorder, might also represent the reference model in the construction of a neuropsychological evaluation protocol and a rehabilitation programme.

Language Abilities

The left hemisphere is involved in language processing. This specialization involves between 95 and 98% of right-handed adults. A full understanding on how this special ability is developed, its nature, and what happens in case a cerebral lesion damages the left hemisphere in early developmental stages has not been fully achieved.

The analysis of language development in children with unilateral congenital cerebral lesions is therefore relevant to understand if the specialization of the left hemisphere is irreversibly determined. In such a case, we would expect an impaired language development in children with left side lesions (Woods, 1983), or perhaps both hemispheres are equivalent at birth and therefore the lesion side is not relevant (Lenneberg, 1967). Overcoming both extreme positions was possible through the investigation performed in the last decades with studies on populations of children with right and left side unilateral congenital lesions, whose language development was monitored at early stages and with adequate evaluation instruments (Thal et al. 1991; Bates et al. 1997; Vicari et al. 2000).

The study by Thal and co-workers (1991) on children with right and left side congenital lesions, evaluated between the first and third year of life, shows that both groups present with a delay in language production, while lexical understanding is more delayed in children with right side lesions. The subsequent study by Bates and co-workers (1997) extended these results to a larger sample and found that, in the first two years of life, children with left side lesions present a selective delay in lexical production, while children with right side lesions present a delay in the production of communicative and symbolic gestures. In the third year, however, the delay is maintained especially in lexicon and grammar in children with left side lesions involving the temporal lobe, and in children with left and right lesions involving the frontal lobe. Data of these initial studies (mainly transversal) evidence a complex developmental framework which cannot be derived from a hypothesis of delay or normal development based on the lesion side, but from reorganization processes which change over time.

Language Evolution Pathways Subsequent to Right and Left Side Lesions

With a longitudinal study on hemiplegic children of Italian language with right or left pre- or perinatal unilateral damage, evaluated in the age range between 13 and 46 months, Chilosi and co-workers (2001) confirmed the initial delay in linguistic development (in production but not in understanding), but also better defined the evolution pathways of language acquisition on the basis of the lesion side.

In children with left side lesions, delay was initially more marked in lexicon than in grammar. At four years, even with a significant progress in linguistic abilities, development could not keep the pace with normal development. These children consistently maintained the initial delay. In patients with right side lesions, who seemed to have a less severe delay, the discrepancy with normal developmental pace progressively increased. The authors underlined that, while left hemisphere plays a predominant role in the initial phases of language acquisition, the shift from simple to more complex forms of linguistic organization may involve a broader neural network and more cooperation between the two brain hemispheres.

In a later, longitudinal study, Chilosi et al (2005) focused on the relationship between neural language (re)organization and developmental language trajectories in two groups of 12 children each with congenital left or right hemisphere lesions. In the area of language, left side specificity was revealed by the presence of a delay both in vocabulary and receptive-expressive grammar that was present from the earliest stages of development. The disadvantage of children with a left hemisphere lesion was even more evident at the end of the follow-up as 10 children showed a persistent delay of expressive language development compared to 4 children with right hemisphere lesions.

The results of the dichotic listening test documenting right hemisphere language lateralization in children with early left lesions supported the power of plasticity in inducing neurofunctional reorganization after left congenital brain lesions. The early delay of language development in most of these children also suggests that reallocation of language functions in alternative regions of the brain has a cost in terms of the slow rate of language acquisition.

The results of these studies indicate that neural circuits aimed at language processing are already functionally active in early developmental stages, and that compensation mechanisms and circuits are activated as a response to the cerebral lesion, to the detriment however, of a prolonged reorganization period, with a slow down of developmental pace which can vary depending on both individual characteristics and on the examined language aspects.

To conclude, the main result of the most recent studies on the development of language in congenital forms of hemiplegia, acquired through methodology progress (better lesion documentation with neuroimaging techniques, use of language tests that are adequate to the first stages of linguistic development, follow-up studies), can be summarized as follows:

- In children with left side congenital lesions, the development of language, even though within the range, is at the lower end and happens slowly.
- The comparison between children with right and left side lesions does not detect relevant differences, but maybe different evolution pathways, characterized by a slow down in evolution pace at least until the age of 5; after that age, there are no more differences between children with early lesions and control children (Reilly et al. 1998).

School Learning

The presence of specific disorders in the learning of written language and of mathematics in hemiplegic children with normal intellective development has been described in a very few studies (Frampton et al. 1998; Frith and Vargha-Khadem, 2001). The first study was conducted on 59 hemiplegic children of a large case study, of which 35.6% presented with learning difficulties higher than those expected on the basis of IQ, evenly distributed between right and left side hemiplegic patients in at least one of the assessed abilities (reading, writing, arithmetic). Difficulties were correlated with neurological severity (Goodman and Yude, 1996), which induced the authors to infer an existing link between learning disorder and the neurobiological abnormalities underlying hemiplegia. In the analyzed group, a high incidence of emotional and behavioral disorders was also reported (62%). The authors interpreted the high risk of learning disorders among hemiplegic individuals as evidence of the limitations of neural plasticity, which would not be compensated in more complex cognitive functions.

Such assumptions are extremely interesting, also in the perspective setting of follow-up agendas at critical ages, to monitor the process of cognitive development. However, they need to be further investigated through longitudinal research on large sample populations of hemiplegic patients.

A small patient population investigated by our group (13 children attending primary school) gave some preliminary results which evidenced, in more than half the children of the sample, the presence of specific difficulties in reading and in calculation, without any difference related to lesion side. It is interesting to observe that such difficulties were found in children at the beginning of school education but not in children attending the last two years of primary school. Data are transversal and on a small sample, therefore requiring caution in their interpretation. However, it is not possible to underestimate the striking similarity with data on linguistic acquisition, both for the presence of right and left side hemiplegic children with learning difficulties and for the initial slowdown in development pace related with the acquisition of new abilities, which are subsequently restored.

Conclusions

The examination of the many studies devoted to the neuropsychological development of children with congenital hemiplegia provides evidence for a wide variability in the results achieved, and some well consolidated data sets. The forms of congenital hemiplegia usually present a favorable outcome in terms of overall cognitive development, with the main negative prognostic factor residing in epilepsy. We believe that this is an aspect raising unanimous consensus, therefore representing a relevant data set. As for our future agenda, we consider that the study of the clinical characteristics of epilepsy and its associated neuropsychological patterns deserves further investigation.

A second aspect to highlight is related to the cost of reorganization processes: the outcome is usually satisfactory, but the time required for the acquisition of the main cognitive functions (language, visuopraxic, and spatial abilities) is much longer than in normal development. Early evaluation and follow-up on the cognitive development of hemiplegic children is therefore essential to set early and targeted rehabilitation interventions.

Neuropsychological Assessment of Hemiplegia

Neuropsychological evaluation of a hemiplegic child must include a protocol of standardized tests, different in relation to the patient's age and level of cognitive development, apart from being able to measure the main cognitive functions (language, memory, visuospatial cognition, visuopraxic abilities) (Table 8.3). Critical stages in which evaluations should be performed are pre-school age and school age. School age should also include monitoring of the different learning levels.

A basic evaluation should include at least a measurement of the overall intellectual development, through psychometric instruments previously validated on large and representative samples of the culture and the language of the examined child.

For the first four years, different intellective scales are available, producing development quotients on verbal and non-verbal ability (e.g. Griffiths or Bayley scales). After that age, other scales can be applied, such as the WPPSI and the WISC scales. The performance, starting from school age, of a problem solving test not-requiring motor output, such as Raven Progressive Matrices (1984), is also recommended. This test provides an index of fluid intelligence which can be compared with the performance achieved in psychometric scales, which instead mainly require the access to information stored in memory, reflecting a crystallized type of intelligence.

The approach of the child to the test, his adaptability to the requests of the examiner, the long level of attention required by many tests, and the capacity to face the examination without the parent's support (for children of pre-school age) are all useful markers of the child's degree of affective/cognitive maturity and autonomy.

8

Table 8.3 Functions to be
evaluated in the
neuropsychological
assessment of hemiplegia

Functions
Oral and Written Language
Receptive lexicon
Expressive lexicon
Receptive morphology and syntax
Expressive morphology and syntax
Recalling sentences
Reading
Fluency and accuracy: single words and non-words
Text comprehension
Writing under dictation of single words and non-words
Cerebral Language Lateralization
Dichotic listening test
Arithmetical abilities
Counting
Arithmetical facts
Procedures
Problem solving
Memory
Verbal working memory
Visual and spatial working memory
Verbal long term memory
Visual and spatial long term memory
Visuopraxic and Visuomotor Abilities
Drawing from model and from memory
Block design
Figure assembly
Executive Functions
Planning sequences of goal directed actions
Cognitive flexibility
Updating of information (see working memory)
Verbal fluency
Inhibition of irrelevant informations
Inhibition of response

Cognitive Evaluation of Pre-school Age and School Age Children with Tetraplegic and Dyskinetic Forms

Motor difficulties of children presenting with dyskinetic and tetraplegic forms complicate both the evaluation of the overall aspects of intelligence and the more specific neuropsychological aspects, also due to the fact that performance deficiencies are often combined with severe dysarthria or anarthria.

This has largely hindered the possibility to perform systematic research on the development of these functions at pre-school and school age, and literature on this field is extremely scarce.

Since the child's forms of interactions both with the school environment and within the family are mainly linguistic, studies performed have largely focused on this area. Dahlgren, Sandberg, and Hjelmquist (1997) investigated the metalinguistic, mnesic, and learning abilities of written language on a sample of 27 children presenting with different forms of CP, who could not use language and who employed the Bliss technique to communicate with graphic symbols (Hehner, 1982), this technique being assumed to develop symbolic functions. With individuals of same mental age (which, in the group of children with CP, was about half the chronological age), no difference was found in metaphonological abilities, both versus normal controls with equivalent mental age and versus controls with psychic delay but with the same chronological age. The performance of children with CP was instead significantly lower than that of the other two groups in sequential visual memory, in visuospatial memory, and in verbal understanding. In reading tasks, the group of children with CP was not different from normal controls, while mentally retarded children had significantly lower performance levels.

More recently, Sabbadini and co-workers (2001) proposed a large neuropsychological battery of linguistic and metalinguistic abilities, as well as mnesic, perceptive, and visuospatial abilities to a sample of eight patients with average chronological age of 16.5 years and of mental age at Leiter International Performance Scale (Levin, 1989) corresponding to 4.5 years. The experimental sample was selected on the basis of the ability to use a sensor, to maintain adequate attention and ocular fixation ability, to respect the rules of a structured task, and to understand and perform simple tasks. Performance levels of patients with CP were compared with those of the same number of controls of corresponding mental age. It is noteworthy that, while the experimental group had significantly lower performance levels than controls in visuoperceptive tests, this was not the same in all the performed tests, except the TCGB grammar comprehension test (Chilosi and Cipriani, 1995). The linguistic abilities outcome proved to be in agreement with the previous experimental studies, and was interpreted as a consequence of a mainly language-mediated environmental exposure, which supported the development of semantic and lexical components (for syntax difficulties instead, a working memory disorder is assumed).

The peculiar aspect of patients with severe motor and verbal production disorder is represented by the need to adopt modifications in the way each single test is proposed (the most frequent of which is represented by indicating a sequence of alternative answers to the patient and reporting his affirmative response), making the results less reliable due to their different collection as compared with reference values. More complex modifications of the experimental set, such as those adopted by Sabbadini and co-workers (1998) in the study on a patient with spastic tetraparesis, if on the one hand, have allowed the achievement of autonomous selection of responses to LIPS from the individual through a system of lamps controlled by a sensor, on the other hand, they worsened the issue of the validity of the collected data, as reported by the authors themselves.

This short list of references is only aimed at presenting the difficulty implied in the application of standardized tests, and the partial validity of reported performance. Based on clinical experience, we believe that collected information in the different functional domains (language, memory, perceptions), even though partially imprecise, represents the foundation and the essential precondition for a correct rehabilitation approach. An evaluation without the use of psychodiagnostic instruments would inevitably lead to overestimates or underestimates of the child's actual development level, with consequent risk of offering stimulation which is not adequate. Cognitive and specific function evaluation, even when data are to be assessed with certain caution with respect to reference values of single tests, however, enable an individual patient follow-up, through which the control of the development pace in the single functional districts is monitored and which allows adaption of the rehabilitation programme to the specific evolutionary difficulties arising.

Among the most popular and available psychodiagnostic tests, we believe the following are the most adequate to their application, if adapted depending on every child's needs: in the cognitive areas, the Leiter International Performance Scale and Progressive Matrices (PM47), in the lexical aspects of language, the PPVT, in syntax aspects of language, the TCGB, and, finally, in the visuoperceptive field, the TVPS-R.

Conclusions

The different clinical forms of CP present, as reported, a wide variability in psychological profiles and in neuropsychological functions, implying the need to offer differentiated evaluation protocols based on age and on clinical form. Studies conducted in the last decades, related with methodological evolution (e.g., a better neuroradiological documentation of lesions, availability of more refined psychodiagnostic instruments), have identified specific areas of cognitive difficulty which went unnoticed in the past. This development in the diagnostic field has not corresponded with a dissemination of a neuropsychological rehabilitation culture, different and tailored for every single individual depending on his specific characteristics. We believe that this is the main objective for the future, to be pursued through the integrated efforts of those clinicians working in the diagnostic field and the caregiving staff involved in applying rehabilitation indications. Visuoperceptive disorders, which are frequent in diplegic patients, as well as linguistic disorders characterizing the first years of hemiplegic children, and also communication deficiencies related to patients with severe motor impairment, are all fields in which a targeted action aimed at providing early compensation for the disadvantaged areas may have a significant impact on long-term development perspective.

References

Abercrombie MLJ, Gardiner PA, Hansen E et al (1964) Visual perceptual and visuomotor impairment in physically handicapped children. Percept Mot Skills 18:561-625
Aicardi J, Bax M (1998) Cerebral palsy. In: Aicardi J (ed) Diseases of the nervous system in childhood-second edition. MacKeith Press, London pp 210-239

Akshoomoff NA, Stiles J (1996) The influence of pattern type on children's block design performance. J Int Neuropsychol Soc 2:392-402

Akshoomoff NA, Feroleto CC, Doyle RE, Stiles J (2002) The impact of early unilateral brain injury on perceptual organization and visual memory. Neuropsychologia 40:539-561

American Psychiatric Association (2000) Diagnostic and statistical manual of mental disorders, 4th edition revised. American Psychiatric Association, Washington DC

Andersen GL, Irgens LM, Haagaas I et al (2008) Cerebral palsy in Norway: prevalence, subtypes and severity. Eur J Paed Neurology 12:4-13

Atkinson J, Braddick O (2007) Visual and visuocognitive development in children born very prematurey. In: von Hofsten C, Rosander K (eds) From action to cognition. Progress in Brain Research, vol. 1 64:123-149

Ballantyne AO, Scarvie Km, Trauner D (1994) Verbal and performance IQ patterns in children after perinatal stroke. Dev Psychol 10:39-50

Banich MT, Levine CS, Hongkeun K, Huttenlocher P (1990) The effects of developmental factors on IQ in hemiplegic children. Neuropsychologia 28:35-47

Barnett A L, Guzzetta A, Mercuri E et al (2004) Can the Griffits scales predict neuromotor and perceptual-motor impairment in term infants with neonatal encephalopathy. Arch Dis Child 89:637-643

Bates E, Camaioni L, Volterra V (1975) The acquisition of performatives prior to speech. Merrill-Palmer Quarterly 21:205-226

Bates E, Roe K (2001) Language development in children with unilateral brain injury. In: Nelson CA, Monica L (eds) Handbook of developmental cognitive neuroscience. MIT Press, Cambridge (Ma) pp 281-308

Bates E, Thal D, Aram D et al (1997) From first words to grammar in children with focal brain injury. Dev Neuropsychol 13:275-343

Bates E, Vicari S, Trauner D (1999) Neural mediation of language development: perspectives from lesion studies of infants and children. In: Tager-Flushberg H (ed) Neurodevelopmental disorders. MIT Press, Cambridge (Ma) pp 533-581

Bax M, Tydeman C, Flodmark O (2006) Clinical and MRI correlates of cerebral palsy: the european cerebral palsy study. JAMA 296:1602-1608

Beckung E, Hagberg G (2002) Neuroimpairments, activity limitations, and participation restrictions in children with cerebral palsy. Dev Med Child Neurol 44:309-316

Beery KE (2000) VMI Developmental Test of Visual-Motor Integration.

Booth JR, Macwhinney B, Thulborn KR (1999) Functional organization of activation patterns in children: whole brain fMRI imaging during three different cognitive tasks. Prog Neuropsychopharmacol Biol Psychiatry 23:669-682

Bova SM, Fazzi E, Giovenzana A et al (2007) The development of visual object recognition in school-age children. Dev Neuropsychol 31:79-102

Braddick O, Atkinson J (2007) Development of brain mechanisms for visual global processing and object segmentation. In: von Hofsten C, Rosander K (eds.) From action to cognition. Progress in Brain Research, vol. 164: 151-168, Elsevier, Amsterdam

Brizzolara D, Chilosi A, De Nobili GL, Ferretti G (1984) Neuropsychological assessment of a case of early right hemiplegia: qualitative and quantitative analysis. Percept Mot Skills 59:1007-1010

Brizzolara D, Pecini C, Brovedani P et al (2002) Timing and type of congenital brain lesion determine different patterns of language lateralization in hemiplegic children. Neuropsychologia 40:620-632

Carlesimo GA, Fadda L, Caltagirone C (1993) Basic mechanisms of constructional apraxia in unilateral brain-damaged patients: role of visuo-perceptual and executive disorders. Clin Exp Neuropsychol 15:342-58

Carlsson G (1997) Memory for words and drawings in children with hemiplegic cerebral palsy. Scand J Psychol 38:265-73

Carlsson M, Hagberg G, Olsson I (2003) Clinical and aetiological aspects of epilepsy in children with cerebral palsy. Dev Med Child Neurol 45:371-376

Carlsson M, Olsson I, Beckung E (2008) Behavior in children with cerebral palsy with and without epilepsy. Dev Med Child Neurol 50:784-789

Chilosi AM, Cipriani P, Bertuccelli B et al (2001) Early cognitive and communication development in children with focal brain lesions. J Child Neurol 16:309-16

Chilosi AM, Cipriani P, Pecini C et al (2008) Acquired focal brain lesions in childhood:Effects on development and reorganization of language. Brain Lang 106:211-225

Chilosi AM, Pecini C, Cipriani P et al (2005) Atypical language lateralization and early development in children with focal brain lesions. Dev Med Child Neurol 47:725-730

Chiron C, Jambaqué I, Nabbout R et al (1997) The right hemisphere is dominant in human infants. Brain 120:1057-65

Cioni G, Bertuccelli B, Boldrini A et al (2000) Correlation between visual function, neurodevelopmental outcome, magnetic resonance imaging findings in infants with periventricular leucomalacia. Arc Dis Child Fetal Neonatal Ed 82:F134-140

Cioni G, Brizzolara D, Ferretti G et al (1998) Visual information processing in infants with focal brain lesions. Exp Brain Res 123:95-101

Cioni G, Di Paco M, Bertuccelli B et al (1997) MRI findings and sensori motor development in infants with bilateral spastic cerebral palsy. Brain Dev 19:245-253

Cioni G, Paolicelli PB, Sordi C, Vinter A (1993) Sensorimotor development in cerebral-palsied infants assessed with Uzgiris-Hunt scales. Dev Med Child Neurol 35:1055-1066

Cioni G, Sales B, Paolicelli PB et al (1999) MRI and clinical characteristics of children with hemiplegic cerebral palsy. Neuropediatrics 30:249-255

Dahlgren Sandberg A, Hjelmquist E (1997) Language and literacy in nonvocal children with cerebral palsy. Reading and Writing: an interdisciplinary Journal 9:107-133

Dall'Oglio AM, Bates E, Volterra V et al (1994) Early cognition, communication and language in children with focal brain injury. Dev Med Child Neurol 36 1076-1098

Damasio H, Damasio AR (1989) Lesion analysis in neuropsychology. Oxford University Press, New York

Dax M (1865) Lesions de la moitié gauche de l'encéphale coincidant avec l'oubli des signes de la pensée. Gaz Hebd Med Chirurg 2:259-262

Decarie TG (1969) A study of the mental and emotional development of the Thalidomide child. In: Foss BM (ed) Determinants of infant behaviour, vol. 4. Methuen, London

Drotar D, Mortimer J, Patricia A, Fagan JF (1989) Recognition memory as a method of assessing intelligence of an infant with quadriplegia. Dev Med Child Neurol 31:391-397

Enkelaar L, Ketelaar M, Gorter JW (2008) Association between motor and mental functioning in toddlers with cerebral palsy. Dev Neuroriabil 11:276-82

Evans P, Elliott M, Alberman E, Evans S (1985) Prevalence and disabilities in 4 to 8 year olds with cerebral palsy. Arch Dis Child 60:940-945

Fagan JF, Shepherd PA (1991) The Fagan test of infant intelligence - Manual. Infantest Corporation, Cleveland

Fawer CL, Besnier S, Forcada M et al (1995) Influence of perinatal developmental and environmental factors on cognitive abilities of preterm children without major impairments at 5 years. Early Hum Dev 43:151-164

Fazzi E, Bova SM, Uggetti C et al (2004) Visual-perceptual impariment in children with periventricular leukomalacia. Brain Dev 26:506-12

Fedrizzi E, Anderloni A, Bono R et al (1998) Eye movement disorders and visual-perceptual impairment in diplegic children born preterm: a clinical evaluation. Dev Med Child Neurol 40:682-688

Fedrizzi E, Inverno M, Botteon G et al (1993) The cognitive development of children born preterm and affected by spastic diplegia. Brain Dev 15:428-432

Foreman N, Fielder A, Minshell C et al (1997) Visual search perception and visual-motor skill in "healthy" children born at 27-32 weeks gestation. J Exp Child Psychol 64:27-41

Frampton I, Yude C, Goodman R (1998) The prevalence and correlates of specific learning difficulties in a representative sample of children with hemiplegia. Br J Educ Psychol 68:39-51

Frith U, Vargha-Khadem F (2001) Are there sex differences in the brain basis of literacy related skills? Evidence from reading and spelling impairments after early unilateral brain damage. Neuropsychologia 39:1485-1488

Goodman R, Yude C (1996) IQ and its predictors in childhood hemiplegia. Dev Med Child Neurol 38:881-890

Goodman R, Yude C (2000) Emotional, behavioral and social consequences. In: Neville B, Goodman R (eds) Congenital hemiplegia: clinics in developmental medicine. Mac Keith Press, London

Goyen TA, Lui K, Woods M (1998) Visual-motor visual perceptual and fine motor outcomes in very-low birthweight children at 5 years. Dev Med Child Neurol 40:76-81

Griffiths R (1984) The abilities of young children. The Test Agency Lmt, Bucks

Grill-Spector K, Golarai G, Gabrieli J (2008) Developmental neuroimaging of the human ventral visual cortex. Trends Cogn Sci 12:152-62

Gunn A, Cory E, Atkinson J et al (2002) Dorsal and ventral stream sensitivity in normal development and hemiplegia. Neuroreport 7:843-847

Guzzetta A, Cioni G, Cowan F, Mercuri E (2001a) Visual disorders in children with brain lesions: 1. Maturation of visual function in infants with neonatal brain lesions: correlation with neuroimaging. Eur J Paediatr Neurol 5:107-114

Guzzetta A, Mazzotti S, Tinelli F et al (2006) Early assessment of visual information processing and neurological outcome in preterm infants. Neuropediatrics 37:278-85

Guzzetta A, Mercuri E, Cioni G (2001b) Visual disorders in children with brain lesions: 2. Visual impairment associated with cerebral palsy. Eur J Paediatr Neurol 5:115-119

Guzzetta A, Pecini C, Biagi L et al (2008) Language organization in left perinatal stroke. Neuropediatrics 39:157-163

Hadjipanayis A, Hadjichristodoulou C, Youroukos S (1997) Epilepsy in patients with cerebral palsy. Dev Med Child Neurol 39:659-663

Hagberg B, Hagberg G, Olow I, van Wendt L (1975) The changing panorama of cerebral palsy in Sweden 1954-1970 II: Analysis of the various syndromes. Acta Paediatr Scand 64:193-200

Harding CG, Golinkoff RM (1979) The origins of intentional vocalizations in prelinguistic infants. Child Dev 50:33-40

Hehner B (1982) Blissymbols for use. Blissymbolic Communication Institute, Toronto

Heller SL, Heier LA, Watts R (2005) Evidence of cerebral organization following perinatal stroke demonstrated with fMRI and DTI tractography. Clin Imaging 29:283-287

Hertz-Pannier L, Gaillard WD, Mott SH et al (1997) Noninvasive assessmento of language domincance in children and adolescnets with functional MRI: a preliminar stud. Neurology 48:1003-1012

Hood B, Atkinson J (1990) Sensory visual loss and cognitive deficits in the selective attentional system of normal infants and neurologically impaired children. Dev Med Child Neurol 32:1067-1077

Hughdal K, Carlsson G (1994) Dichotic listening and focused attention in children with hemiplegic cerebral palsy. J Clin Exp Neuropsychol 16:84-92

Humphreys P, Deonandan R, Whiting S et al (2007) Factors associated with epilepsy in children with periventricular leukomalacia. J Child Neurol 22:598-605

Inverno M, Anderloni A, Bruzzone MG et al (1994) Visuo-perceptual disorders in spastic diplegic children born preterm: correlation with MRI findings In: Fedrizzi E, Avanzini G, Crenna P (eds) Motor development in children. John-Libbey and Co Ltd, London pp 173-179

Ipata AE, Cioni G, Bottai P et al (1994) Acuity card testing with cerebral palsy related to magnetic resonance images, mental levels and motor abilities. Brain Dev 16:195-203

Isaacs E, Christie D, Vargha-Khadem F, Mishkin M (1996) Effects of hemispheric side of injury, age at injury and presence of seizure disorder on functional ear and hand asymmetries in hemiplegic children. Neuropsychologia 34:127-137

Isaacs EB, Edmonds CJ, Chong WK et al (2003) Cortical anomalies associated with visuospatial processing deficits. Ann Neurol 53:768-773

Ito J, Saijo H, Araki A et al (1996) Assessment of visuoperceptual disturbance in children with spastic diplegia using measurements of the lateral ventricles on cerebral MRI. Dev Med Child Neurol 38:496-502

Jongmans M, Mercuri E, Henderson S et al (1996) Visual function of prematurely born children with and without perceptual-motor difficulties. Early Hum Dev 45:73-82

Kirk A, Kertesz A (1989) Hemispheric contributions to drawing. Neuropsychologia 27 :881-886

Koeda T, Takeshita K (1992) Visuo-perceptual impairment and cerebral lesions in spastic diplegia with preterm birth. Brain Dev 14:239-244

Korkman M, Mikkola K, Ritari N et al (2008) Neurocognitive test profiles of extremely low birth weight fiveyear-old children differ according to neuromotor status. Dev Neuropsychol 33:637-55

Korkman M, von Wendt L (1995) Evidence of altered dominance in children with congenital spastic hemiplegia J Int Neuropsychol Soc 1:261-270

Kwong KL, Wong SN, So KT (1998) Epilepsy in children with cerebral palsy. Pediatr Neurol 19:31-36

Lansdell H (1969) Verbal and nonverbal factors in right-hemisphere speech: relation to early neurological history. J Comp Physiol Psychol 69 :734-738

Larroque B, Ancel PY, Marret S et al (2008) Neurodevelopmental disabilities and special care of 5-year-old children born before 33 weeks of gestation (the EPIPAGE study): a longitudinal cohort study. Lancet 371:813-820

Laurent-Vannier A, Chevignard M, Pradat-Diehl P et al (2006) Assessment of unilateral spatial neglect in children using the Teddy Bear Cancellation Test. Dev Med Child Neurol 48:120-5

Lenneberg E (1967) Biological foundations of language. Wiley, New York

Levine MN (1989) Leiter International Performance Scale: a handbook. Stoelting Co, Wood Dale, Ill

Levine SC, Huttenlocher P, Banich MT, Duda E (1987) Factors affecting cognitive functioning of hemiplegic children. Dev Med Child Neurol 29:27-35

Lidzba K, Staudt M, Wilke M, Krageloh-Mann I (2006a) Visuospatial deficits in patients with early left-hemispheric lesions and functional reorganization of language: consequence of lesion or reorganization? Neuropsychologia 44:1088-1094

Lidzba K, Staudt M, Wilke M et al (2006b) Lesion induced right-hemispheric language and organization of non verbal functions. Neuroreport 17:929-933

Liegeois F, Connelly A, Cross JH et al (2004) Language reorganization in children with early-onset lesions of the left hemisphere: an fMRI study. Brain 127:1229-1236

Manly T, Robertson IH, Anderson V, Nimmo-Smith V (1999) TEA-Ch Test of everyday attention for children manual. Thames Valley Test Company Limited, Bury St Edmunds England

McCall RB, Carriger MS (1993) A meta-analysis of infant habituation and recognition memory performance as predictors of later IQ. Child Dev 64:57-79

McDermott S, Coker AL, Mani S et al (1996) A population-based study of behavior problems in children with cerebral palsy. Pediatr Psychol 21:447-463

Mercuri E, Haataja L, Guzzetta A et al (1999) Visual function in full term infants with brain lesions: correlation with neurologic and developmental status at 2 years of age. Arch Dis Child Fetal Neonatal Ed 80:F99-104

Meyer M (1969) Frog where are you? Dial Press, New York

Milner AD, Goodale MA (2008) Two visual systems re-viewed. Neuropsychologia 46:774-85

Morrone MC, Guzzetta A, Tinelli F et al (2008) Inversion of perceived direction of motion caused by spatial undersampling in two children with periventricular leukomalacia. J Cogn Neurosci 20:1094-106

Muter V, Taylor S, Vargha-Khadem FA (1997) Longitudinal study of early intellectual development in hemiplegic children. Neuropsychologia 35:289-298

Nass R, de Coudres Peterson H, Koch D (1989) Differential effects of congenital left and right brain injury on intelligence Brain Cogn 9:258-266

Nass R, Sadler AE, Sidtis JJ (1992) Differential effects of congenital versus acquired unilateral brain injury on dichotic listening performance. Neurology 42:1960-1965

Orsini A, Grossi D, Capitani E et al (1987) Verbal and spatial immediate memory span: Normative data from 1355 adults and 1112 children. Ital J Neurol Sci 8:539-548

Pagliano E, Fedrizzi E, Erbetta A et al (2007) Cognitive profiles and visuoperceptual abilities in preterm and term spastic diplegic children with periventricular leukomalacia. J Child Neurol 22:282-8

Parkes J, White-Koning M, Dickinson HO et al (2008) Psychological problems in children with cerebral palsy: a cross-sectional European study. J Child Psychol Psychiatry 49:405-13

Pharoah POD, Cooke T, Johnson MA et al (1998) Epidemiology of cerebral palsy in England and Scotland 1984-1989. Archives Dis Child Fetal Neonatal Ed 79:21-25

Pirila S, van der Meere J, Korhonen P et al (2004) A retrospective neurocognitive study in children with spastic diplegia. Dev Neuropsychol 26:679-90

Reilly JS, Bates EA, Marchman VA (1998) Narrative discourse in children with early focal brain injury. Brain Lang 61:335-375

Ressel V, Wilke M, Lidzba K et al (2008) Increases in language lateralization in normal children as observed using magnetoencephalography. Brain Lang 106:167-176

Riddoch JM, Humphreys GW (1993) BORB Birmingham Object Recognition Battery Lawerence. Erlbaum Associates Ldt, Hove UK

Riva D, Cazzaniga L (1986) Late effects of unilateral brain lesions sustained before and after age one. Neuropsychologia 4:423-428

Robinson CC, Rosenberg S (1987) A strategy for assessing infants with motor impairments. In: Uzgiris IC, Hunt J, Mc V (eds) Infant performance and experience: new findings with the Ordinal Scales. University of Illinois Press, Urbana, Ill

Rose SA (1983) Differential rates of visual information processing in full-term and preterm infants. Child Dev 54:1189-1198

Rose SA, Feldman JF, McCarton CM, Wolfson J (1988) Information processing in seven-monthold infants as a function of risk status. Child Dev 59:589-603

Roth SC, Baudin J, Pezzani-Goldsmith M et al (1994) Relation between neurodevelopmental status of very preterm infants at one and eight years. Dev Med Child Neurol 36:1049-1062

Roth SC, Wyatt J, Baudin J et al (2001) Neurodevelopental status at 1 year predicts neuropsychiatric oucome at 14-15 years of age in very preterm infants. Early Hum Dev 65:81-89

Sabbadini M, Bonanni R, Carlesimo GA, Caltagirone C (2001) Neuropsychological assessment of patients with severe neuromotor and verbal disabilities. J Intellect Disabil Res 45:169-179

Sabbadini M, Carlesimo Ga, Aucoin C et al (1998) La valutazione delle competenze cognitive del paziente con grave disabilità neuromotoria e verbale: l'esperienza di una paziente con paralisi cerebrale infantile. Giorn Neuropsich Età Evol 18:111-122

Schatz J, Craft S, White D et al (2001) Inhibition of return in children with perinatal brain injury. J Int Neuropsychol Soc 7:275-284

Schenk-Rootlieb AJF, van Nieuwenhuizen O, van der Graaf Y et al (1992) The prevalence of cerebral visual disturbance in children with cerebral palsy. Dev Med Child Neurol 34:473-480

Sigurdardottir S, Eiriksdottir A, Gunnarsdottir E et al (2008) Cognitive profile in young Icelandic children with cerebral palsy. Dev Med Child Neurol 50:357-362

Slater A (1995) Individuai differences in infancy and later IQ. J Child Psychol Psychiatry 36:69-112

Springer JA, Binder JR, Hammeke TA et al (1999) Language dominance in neurologically normal and epilepsy subjects: a functional MRI study. Brain 122:2033-2046

Staudt M, Grodd W, Niemann G et al (2001) Early left periventricular brain lesions induce right hemispheric organization of speech. Neurology 57:122-125

Staudt M, Lidzba K, Grodd W et al (2002) Right-hemispheric organization of language following early left sided brain lesions: functional MRI topography. Neuroimage 16:954-967

Stella G, Biolcati C (2003) La valutazione neuropsicologica dei bambini con danno neuromotorio. In: Bottos N (ed) Paralisi cerebrale infantile. Piccin, Padova, pp 55-61

Stern RA, Singer EA, Duke LM et al (1994) The Boston Qualitative Scoring System for the Rey-Osterrieth Complex Figure: description and interrater reliability. Clin Neuropsychol 8:309–322

Stiers P, De Cock P, Vandenbussche E (1999) Separating visual perception and non-verbal intelligence in children with early brain injury. Brain Dev 21:397-406

Stiers P, van den Hout B, Haers M et al (2001) The variety of visual perceptual impairments in pre-school children with perinatal brain injury. Brain Dev 23:333-348

Stiers P, Vanderkelen R, Vanneste G et al (2002) Visual-perceptual impairment in a random sample of children with cerebral palsy. Dev Med Child Neurol 44:370-82

Stiles J (2001) Neural plasticity and cognitive development. Dev Neuropsychol 18:237–272

Stiles J, Moses P, Roe K et al (2003) Alternative brain organization after prenatal cerebral injury: convergent fMRI and cognitive data. Journal of the International Neuropsychological Society 9:604-622

Stiles J, Nass R (1991) Spatial grouping activity in young children with congenital right or left hemisphere brain injury. Brain Cogn 15:201–222

Stiles J, Stern C, Trauner D, Nass R (1996) Developmental change in spatial grouping activity among children with early focal brain injury: evidence from a modeling task. Brain Cogn 34:56-62

Surman G, Newdick H, Johnson A (2003) Cerebral palsy rates among low-birthweight infants fell in the 1990s. Dev Med Child Neurol 45:456-462

Sussova J, Seidl Z, Faber J (1990) Hemiparetic forms of cerebral palsy in relation to epilepsy and mental retardation. Dev Med Child Neurol 32:792-795

Szaflarski JP, Holland SK, Schmithorst WJ, Byars AW (2006) fMRI study of language lateralization in children and adults. Human Brain Mapping 27:2020-212

Temple C, Coleman N (2000) Children's performance on the visual objects and space perception battery (VOSP). Clin Neuropsychological Assessment 3:193-208

Teuber HL (1975) Effects of focal brain injury on human behaviour. In: Tower DB (ed) The nervous system. Raven Press, New York, pp 311-353

Thal DJ, Marchman VA, Stiles J et al (1991) Early lexical development in children with focal brain injury. Brain Lang 40:491-527

Tillema JM, Byars AW, Jacola LM (2008) Cortical reorganization of language functioning following perinatal left MCA stroke. Brain Lang 105:99-111

Uvebrant P (1988) Hemiplegic cerebral palsy: aetiology and outcome. Acta Paediatr Scand Suppl 345:1-100

Uzgiris IC (1983) Organization of sensorimotor intelligence. In: Lewis M (ed) Origins of intelligence. Plenum Press, New York

Uzgiris IC, Hunt J, Mc V (1975) Assessment in infancy: ordinal scales of psychological development. University of Illinois Press, Urbana

Van Braeckel K, Butcher PR, Geuze RH et al (2008) Less efficient elementary visuomotor processes in 7- to 10-year-old preterm-born children without cerebral palsy: an indication of impaired dorsal stream processes. Neuropsychology 22:755-764

Vargha-Khadem F, Isaacs E, Van Der Werf S et al (1992) Development of intelligence and memory in children with hemiplegic cerebral palsy. Brain 115:315-329

Vicari S, Albertoni A, Chilosi AM et al (2000) Plasticity and reorganization during language development in children with early brain injury. Cortex 36:31-46

Vicari S, Stiles J, Stern C, Resca A (1998) Spatial grouping activity in children with early cortical and subcortical lesions. Dev Med Child Neurol 40:90-94

Warrington EK , James M (1993) The visual object and space perception battery. Bury, St Edmunds: Thames Valley Test Company

Wiklund LM, Uvebrant P (1991) Hemiplegic cerebral palsy: correlation between CT morphology and clinical findings. Dev Med Child Neurol 33:512-23

Woods BT (1983) Is the left hemisphere specialized for language at birth? Trends Neurosci 6:115-117

Yokochi K (2000) Reading of Kana (phonetic symbols for syllables) in Japanese children with spastic diplegia and periventricular leucomalacia. Brain Dev 22:13-15

Emotional, Behavioral and Social Disorders in Children and Adolescents with Cerebral Palsy

9

G. Masi, P. Brovedani

Introduction

About 10% of children older than 5 years in the community can present with a mental disorder (Meltzer et al. 2000). It is well established over the past thirty years that childhood chronic disorders, such as diabetes, asthma, rheumatic disease, cystic fibrosis, and sickle cell anemia, can significantly increase the risk of mental disorders (Breslau et al. 1985; Gortmarker et al. 1990), with the emotional adjustment affected by the severity of the condition and the degree of functional limitation. Children with diseases involving Central Nervous System present the highest psychopathological risk (Weiland et al. 1992; Howe et al. 1993). When matched with disabled children with other disorders (i.e., musculo-skeletal), children with cerebral pathologies presented a two-fold higher rate of psychiatric disorders, even when IQ, social context, and physical disability were controlled for (Seidel et al. 1975).

The notion that chronic cerebral disorders strongly increase the risk of psychiatric disorders in pediatric populations is supported by a classical, rigorous epidemiologic study, the Isle of Wight study (Rutter et al. 1970). Psychiatric disorders were found in 44% of children with structural brain lesions, compared with 12% in children with non-cerebral physical disorders and 7% in children without physical disorders. Hyperkinetic disorder was 90 times higher in children with cerebral palsy or epilepsy. Even though childhood psychiatric disorders are more common in males, the gender effect was lost in this study when a brain lesion was co-existent. However, two-thirds of the children with cerebral palsy or epilepsy were free from any psychiatric disorder.

Emotional well-being, psychological and behavioral disorders, and quality of life have been explored also in children and adolescents with cerebral palsy, and these data will be discussed in this review. Most of the studies included patients with hemiplegia, usually the mildest type of cerebral palsy, while less information is available on the rate of psychiatric disorders across all forms and severities of cerebral palsies. A major limitation in most of these studies is that the assessment is not based on specific psychiatric instruments which can allow for a specific psychiatric diagnosis. For this reason, the psychopathological risk is usually reported in terms of psychological dimensions rather than psychiatric diagnoses.

A screening questionnaire should not be considered as an equivalent of a psychiatric assessment, and emotional and behavioral symptoms are not always associated with a psychiatric disorder (Goodman and Yude, 2000), even though the existing cut-offs increase the likelihood to identify a clinical problem.

Brain Disorders and Psychopathology

The analysis of the association between brain lesions and behaviour disorders during infancy and childhood presents important theoretical implications, as it can elucidate the biological underpinnings of psychological development, as well as the role of early brain plasticity. Psychiatric consequences of childhood brain disorders can be affected by different mechanisms, biological as well as non-biological. Biological mechanisms include the characteristics of brain lesions (timing, size, site, side), associated cognitive impairment (mental retardation, neuropsychological deficits), comorbid disorders (epilepsy, visual or hearing deficits). Non-biological mechanisms include the effects of impaired sensori-motor and speech skills on personality development (sense of personal identity, relationship with external and social environment), psychological effects of functional impairment, stigmatizing effect of the disorder, impact on familial relations (strength of psychological familial resources), and the environmental resources affecting quality of life. Furthermore, neurological and psychosocial variables interact, although the nature of their mutual interaction in the development of psychiatric disorders is still not clear (Goodman, 2002). A brain lesion may only amplify the effect of psychosocial adversities on psychopathological risk, or, on the contrary, biological and non-biological mechanisms may operate on independent pathways in determining psychiatric disorders (Breslau, 1990). The complexity of the relation between brain lesion and psychiatric disorders is illustrated by Lewis et al's study (1990), which reported on two identical twins with a genetic vulnerability for schizophrenia. One of them had cerebral palsy, while the other developed a shizophreniform psychosis, suggesting that brain damage does not necessarily make a genetic vulnerability more likely to be expressed.

Regarding lesion timing, early damage is less associated with clinically significant emotional and behavioral disturbances, as the brain's potential for reorganization, based on the plasticity of the newborn CNS, can partly compensate the effects of the damage, while this capacity is less effective in later occurring lesions (Trauner et al. 2001). Regarding lesion size, findings from patients with hemiplegia and/or focal lesions report less psychiatric impairment compared to unselected samples of children with cerebral palsy (Goodman and Graham, 1996; Goodman and Yule, 1997), suggesting that bilateral and/or extensive damage may be more frequently associated with a co-occurring psychopathology. Regarding lesion site, Trauner et al. (1996) compared school-aged children with anterior and posterior perinatal focal damage (stroke) and found that posterior damage was associated with social problems (assessed with the Personality Inventory for Children), while anterior damage was associated with academic difficulties. However, differences in Externalizing, Internalizing, and Total score of the Child Behavior Checklist

(CBCL) were not found between patients with or without frontal lobe involvement (irrespective of the side of lesion), whether or not IQ was used as covariate (Trauner et al. 2001).

The role of lesion side in pediatric samples is more highly debated. In the London hemiplegia study, Goodman and colleagues (Goodman and Graham, 1996; Goodman and Yude, 1997) studied about 400 children with left-or right-sided hemiplegia assessed with behaviour rating scales, and 149 of them with parent questionnaires. A high rate of psychopathology was found according to both dimensional and categorical measures assessing affective or interpersonal aspects, but it was not affected by lesion side. A similar lack of lesion side effect on psychopathological measures (Internalizing, Externalizing, and Total score of Child Behavior Checklist (CBCL) is reported in other studies including children and adolescents with unilateral brain lesions (Trauner et al. 1996, 2001; Duval et al. 2002).

An intellectual disability per se can significantly increases the psychiatric risk, including both anxiety and depressive disorders (Masi et al. 1999, 2000). According to the DSM IV (American Psychiatric Association, 1994), all types of mental disorders can be observed in these patients, with prevalence estimated to be at least 3 or 4 times higher than in the general population. In the Isle of Wight study (Rutter et al. 1970), a prevalence of psychiatric problems was found in 30%-42% of children with intellectual disability, compared with 6-7% in normal IQ children.

The role of non-biological mechanisms is also supported by the Isle of Wight study (Rutter et al. 1970), showing that children with brain lesions who developed a psychiatric disorder more frequently had a familial distress or a mentally ill mother. According to Rutter et al. (1984), the risk of psychiatric disorders in children with head injuries was related to the severity of the injury, but in the children with severe head injuries psychiatric disorders were found in 60% of children with psychosocial adversities pre-existing the trauma, but in only 14% of children without psychosocial adversities.

The causal mechanisms may be even more complex, as psychosocial pathways to psychiatric disorders may be multiple (Yude et al. 1998; Yude and Goodman, 1999; Goodman, 2002). Intensive treatments, recurrent hospitalizations, lower social opportunities, academic failure are frequently co-occurring, resulting in low-self-esteem and difficult peer relationships. Parents, peers, and teachers may have atypical attitudes toward a brain damaged child, with overprotection, rejection-or non-realistic expectations. Family disruptions may be dramatically engendered by the birth of a brain damaged child, even though family factors, including depressive suffering, parental warmth, or discord, are more likely to be consequences than causes of psychiatric problems (Goodman, 1998). Managing the psychosocial adversities, both pre-existing the lesion, or consequent to the stress, can reduce the psychopathological risk. However, it is probable that some children may develop a psychiatric disorder even in the absence of any environmental adversity. Knowing this condition may prevent the risk of self-blame or a guilty feeling in caregivers, including parents, relatives, and teachers (Goodman, 2002).

Psychopathology of Cerebral Palsy: Epidemiologic Studies

In the Isle of Wight study, about half of the children with cerebral palsy presented with psychiatric disorders (Rutter et al. 1970). Two elements which significantly increased the psychiatric risk were low IQ and specific reading deficit. The presence of comorbid seizures increased the risk of psychiatric disorders (from 38% to 58%). The typology of psychiatric disorder was not specific, except for a high rate of hyperkinetic disorders.

An epidemiologic, population-based study in the USA explored the association between behaviour problems and cerebral palsy in children, using a large nationally representative survey (n=23.586), the 1981 and 1988 National Health Interview Survey (NHIS) Child Health Supplement. (McDermott et al. 1996). The parents were asked a range of questions, including health status and behavior problems. Within this measure, children were dichotomized according to behaviour variables into those in the bottom 90th percentile and those in the top 10th percentile. The prevalence of cerebral palsy was 1.5/1.000 children (n=16) in the 1981 sample, and 2.67/1.000 children (n=31) in the 1988 sample (the increase of prevalence is probably determined by an increased survival of very low birth weight infants). In both the 1981 and 1988 samples, the differences on the behavioral scale (Behavior Problem Index) between children with cerebral palsy and those with other chronic illnesses were not significant. However, when children with a score greater than the 90th percentile were considered, problems were reported by parents in 25.5% of the 47 children with cerebral palsy, 11.9% in those with other chronic health conditions (n=6.038), and 5.4% in children with no conditions (n=5.930). Dependency was the most frequent problem in the group with cerebral palsy, and it was reported in 39.3% of children, compared to 10.9% in the group of other chronic conditions and 4.6% in the controls. Hyperactivity was reported in 25.5% of children with cerebral palsy compared, respectively, to 10.7% and 5.2% in the other two groups. The adjusted odd ratios (aOR) for specific behaviour dimensions, that is, the increased risk of specific behaviour problem among groups, revealed that children with cerebral palsy, compared with controls, had an aOR of 5.3 for any behavior problem, 17.2 for dependency, 5.2 for hyperactivity, 5.1 for headstrong, 3.5 for anxiety, and 3.0 for peer conflict (all statistically significant). Only antisocial had a non-significant aOR (2.3). Significantly lower aORs were found in the groups with other chronic conditions: 2.5 for any behaviour problem, 2.8 for dependency, 2.3 for hyperactivity, 2.5 for headstrong, 2.6 for anxiety, 1.9 for peer conflict, and 1.6 for antisocial. These findings were confirmed also when children with mental retardation were excluded from the sample with cerebral palsy, but this analysis showed that mental retardation *per se* was a significant risk factor for behaviour problems (aOR 7.9 for any problem, 11.4 for hyperactivity, 10.9 for peer conflict).

This population based study, although relying on a small sample size, describes a non-referred sample, with greater generalizability compared to more biased clinic-based samples. In summary, it confirms the increased psychopathological risk in children with cerebral palsy, even though the rate of 25.5% is smaller than that reported in other studies (including the Isle of Wight study), probably because of the differences in inclusion criteria. The high rates of dependency and headstrongness (including non-compliance at home and mood instability) may be relevant in terms of both the possible contribution of parental management practices (i.e., failure to teach skills leading to independency, inconsistencies in disciplinary practices) and possible therapeutic interventions focused on these topics.

Psychopathology of Cerebral Palsy: Clinical Studies

The London Hemiplegia Study

Hemiplegic cerebral palsy has been the most explored clinical condition. An important contribution to ascertain prevalence and predictors of psychiatric comorbidities in hemiplegic children stems from the London hemiplegia study (Goodman and Graham, 1996; Goodman and Yude, 1997; Goodman, 1998). A cross-sectional questionnaire survey was administered to 428 hemiplegic children ages 2 1/2-16 years, and 149 of them (ages 6-10 years) were individually assessed. The questionnaire survey was repeated on school age patients four years later. Psychiatric disorders were found in 61% of subjects as judged by individual assessments, and 54% and 42% as judged from parent and teacher questionnaires, respectively (Goodman and Graham, 1996). It is noteworthy that few of these young patients were being followed by child mental health services. The strongest consistent predictor of psychiatric problems was IQ, which was highly correlated with an index of neurological severity. Of note, laterality of lesion had little or no predictive power (Goodman and Yude, 1997). The conclusion of the authors was that although hemiplegic children often have clinically relevant psychiatric symptoms, these comorbidities are usually unrecognized or untreated. Regarding the type of psychiatric symptoms, about one quarter of affective disorders and conduct disorders were present in these patients, while hyperkinetic disorder was present in about 10% of the patients, and pervasive developmental disorders in about 3% (Goodman and Yude, 2000). Learning difficulties were frequently associated with a higher psychiatric risk, and hemiplegic children presented with these difficulties three times more frequently than controls (36%) (Frampton et al. 1998).

Four years later, 90% of the sample was followed up with a questionnaire (Goodman, 1998). Around 70% of children with clinically relevant psychiatric symptoms at the first evaluation were unchanged 4 years later. In addition, around 30% of children who were not psychiatric cases initially had become such 4 years later. In summary, this study supports a substantial continuity across time for most measures of psychopathology. The most relevant predictive element of later conduct and hyperactivity problems was the presence of externalizing symptoms in the pre-school years, while early emotional symptoms were not predictive of later disorders. In the school years, hyperactivity was particularly predictive of continuing psychiatric problems (Goodman, 1998).

Findings from the London hemiplegia study are not totally consistent with those of Trauner et al. (1996, 2001), considering children with focal unilateral brain injury, because the frequency and severity of psychological complications was much higher in the London patients. The inconsistencies may be partly accounted for by differences in the methodology of psychiatric assessment, as in the London study not only questionnaires were used, such as in the Trauner et al. study, but also psychiatric interviews, which may have been more sensitive in detecting psychiatric symptoms. Furthermore, Trauner et al.s' patients were classified according to neuroimaging, which clearly documented focal, unilateral lesions. In the London study, the sample was stratified according to the side of the motor deficit, without verification of the side or sites of the cerebral lesions. It is possible that some of the hemiplegic children in the London study may have had more extensive or bilateral lesions. Another possible confusing effect is that in different samples some potential determinants of later outcome and psychopathological vulnerability, such as genetic predisposition or environmental features, were not fully controlled.

The SPARCLE Study

More recently, new data on psychiatric comorbidity in cerebral palsy have been obtained from a specific analysis of behavioral and emotional symptoms in a large sample of children with all types of cerebral palsy, in different Western European countries, as part of a project investigating the role of environmental factors on quality of life in children with cerebral palsy (Colver for the SPARCLE group, 2006). Cross-sectional data on the psychiatric symptoms in about 800 8- to 12-year-old children, their predictors, and their impact on the child and family have been recently reported (Parkes J et al. 2008). Using the Strengths and Difficulties Questionnaire (SDQ) as a screening measure of emotional and behavioral symptoms (conduct, hyperactivity, emotion, peer problems), with a total difficulties score (TDS) and a cut-off score of 16 to detect "symptom caseness", 26% presented a TDS in the abnormal range compared to 10% in a British community sample. Peer problems were the most frequent (32%), followed by hyperactivity (31%), emotional problems (29%) and, less frequently, conduct disorders (17%). Mean TDS score in children with cerebral palsy (12.4) was significantly higher than in the community studies in Great Britain (8.4) and Germany (8.1). A high impact score (everyday distress in patient and parents, related to the child's mental health problems) was found in over 40% of children with cerebral palsy (compared to 13.5% in a community sample in Great Britain), and is thus considered a stronger predictor of clinical status than symptoms alone.

Predictors of pathological TDS were explored with a multivariate logistic regression. Children with severe motor limitation less frequently presented a pathological TDS (OR=0.2 to 0.4). A moderate to severe intellectual impairment was associated with a significant increase of TDS > 16 (OR=3.2) compared to children with IQ > than 70. Having no siblings (OR=1.8) or having disabled siblings (OR=2.7) was also associated with a higher psychopathological score. Severe physical pain was associated with TDS > 16 (OR=2.7). Finally, children living in a town/small city had a significant increased risk of TDS > 16 (OR=1.8). However, the final adjusted model accounted for only 10% of the variation between children with TDS > 16; impairment (motor and intellectual) accounted for only 5% of the variation. As a measure of impact of difficulties, parents were asked if they perceived emotional, behavioral, attentional, and relational difficulties in their child. Twenty-seven percent reported no difficulties, 34% reported minor difficulties, 32% definite difficulties, and 7% severe difficulties. However, 97% of parents of children with TDS > 16 reported at least minor problems. The prevalence of significant social impairment was 41%. Ninety-five percent of parents reporting at least minor problems in their child reported that difficulties were present for over a year. The child's classroom learning was the most disrupted aspect, and home life the least disrupted. In 42% of parents the child's difficulties burdened the family "quite a lot".

An interesting issue is that greater intellectual impairment and greater physical pain increased the psychopathological risk. The apparently paradoxical finding of lower psychopathological risk in children with greater functional impairment may be accounted for by the low sensitivity of the SDQ in children with severe motor impairment, as well as by the lower capacity of severely disabled children to show conduct problems. On the contrary, less severe motor disabilities may be more stressful in children who compare themselves to normal peers (always being last, never picked for sports, needing help for self-care) (Goodman and Yude, 2000).

Thus, also this study suggests that a strong proportion of children with cerebral palsy may have psychological symptoms so severe as to require referral to mental health services. Even though this study is not based on specific psychiatric instruments for specific psychiatric diagnoses, depressed mood has been found to be specifically correlated to the emotional scale of SDQ (Fombonne, 1993, 2002), which was in the abnormal range in 27.1% of children with cerebral palsy.

Peer Relationships in Hemiplegic Children

A sociometric study compared 55 children (9 to10 years old) with hemiplegia with their classmates or other matched controls according to popularity and friendship from one side, and victimization from the other (Yude et al. 1998). Even though in this study psychopathology was not specifically explored, peer relationships in school are often predictive of later psychopathology. Hemiplegic children were less popular and more frequently rejected, had less friends, and were more often victimized. Contrar to Goodman and Graham (1996), who found frequent emotional and behavioral symptoms in hemiplegic children, multivariate analyses indicated that peer problems were not totally accounted for by group differences in teacher estimated IQ or behaviour problems. It may be hypothesized that teachers may have underestimated the behavioral problems of hemiplegic children (or overestimated the problems of the normal classmates). Peer problems at school may be explained by negative attitudes of classmates, as well as by the frequent association with learning difficulties (Frampton et al. 1997). However, an associated factor may be a neurologically driven deficit in social skills. Balleny (1996) found that hemiplegic children may exhibit social and emotional immaturity, associated with a delayed maturation of a "theory of mind". This kind of social immaturity may negatively affect peer relationships in everyday life. Another psychological feature in physically ill children which may affect peer relationships and proneness to victimization is the oversensitivity to comments about the disability, as well as the tendency to attribute social difficulties to physical factors or the more visible expression of their emotions (crying, being upset) (Yude et al. 1998).

The same group (Yude et al. 1999) prospectively explored in the same sample of hemiplegic children possible predictors of peer problems. Two-thirds of the children had peer problems, and two variables were mostly related with this unfavorable development: lower IQ and teacher-reported externalizing problems (disruptiveness and hyperactivity) soon after school entry. These data suggest that this high risk subgroup of hemiplegic children with these two features may benefit from an intensive preventive program focused on school, social, and familial environment. Interestingly, peer problems were predicted neither by the degree of neurological involvement nor by the visibility of physical disability. Furthermore, teacher ratings, but not parent ratings best predicted later psychological problems, as relationships outside the family are probably more closely related to social functioning. Finally, children with emotional problems (according to teacher rating) were not more prone to later poor peer relationships, suggesting that internalizing problems are less impairing of peer relationships than externalizing problems.

Cerebral Palsy, Balance Disorders and Anxiety Disorders

Balance can be viewed as a latent factor in all daily activities, a core element of a sense of identity and of the relationship with the external world. An historical review of the co-occurrence between imbalance, anxiety, and depression is reviewed in Balaban and Jacob (2001). Anxiety disorders are reported in many patients with vestibular dysfunction (Furman and Jacob, 2001), and patients who suffer from panic attacks can also undergo vestibular sensitivity, impaired balance, or difficulties in spatial orientation (Yardley et al. 1995; Jacob et al. 1996). In both populations, space and motion sensitivity and discomfort are frequently reported (Furman and Jacob, 2001). Balance disorders and some anxiety disorders may have a common pathophysiology in the CNS, and direct connections among the vestibular nuclei, the locus coeruleus, and brainstem pathways processing visceral sensory information may provide a putative neural substrate for autonomic and affective symptoms associated with vestibular dysfunction and anxiety disorders (Sklare et al. 2001; Balaban and Thayer, 2001).

Some symptoms of anxiety and avoidance in children and adolescents with cerebral palsy can be interpreted within this framework. Patients with cerebral palsy not rarely present with balance disorders that seem out of proportion with the extent of the motor deficit, in terms of either intensity or chronicity. Additionally, these patients often show affective symptoms, either of anxiety or depression, associated with a spatial phobia, or a space and motor dyscomfort, or complaints of postural imbalance, and excessive preoccupation and disability by the balance symptoms. Perceived or real balance disorders associated with vestibular and/or visual and/or somesthethic disorders in persons with cerebral palsy can induce an excessive and impairing control of non relevant features of the external world. These features are more closely related to anxiety disorders, including separation anxiety disorder, panic attacks, agoraphobia, generalized anxiety disorder, and obsessive compulsive disorder. This psychological condition can further worsen motor attitudes and performances as well as social relatedness, in daily life as well as during rehabilitation. This is clinically relevant, as avoiding exposure to movements and environments can deprive the balance system of anxious individuals of the sensory and motor experiences necessary for extinction of phobic perception, and it reduces the opportunity to desensitize to provocative conditions.

Treatments

Since the psychiatric symptoms of childhood cerebral palsy are common, often persistent, and strongly increase the burden of the illness, they warrant specific clinical and research attention, and their prevention should be a primary target of intervention. More research is needed to define protective factors and psychosocial environments which may reduce the psychopathological risk, including social support networks for children and families, selected school placements, and behavioral interventions to increase independence.

Psychotherapy should be targeted to specific aims, including an understanding, awareness of, and feeling about the disability and its consequences in daily life. Self-control and self regulation, recognizing emotional states, problem solving techniques to understand differences in another person's point of view, and the effect of one's behaviour on others, may be possible focuses of the therapeutic process.

Parents should be always involved in the therapy. A careful interview should include questions about parents' adjustment to the child, denial of disability, self-blame, guilt, concerns, depression and dependency. Every delay in communication of the diagnosis, prognosis and treatment, and management of parental concerns can be extremely stressful, and it may increase misunderstandings and maladaptive parental attitudes, with negative impact for the child's mental development. Therapy should focus on preventive interventions, namely, in crucial moments, such as school entry, adolescence, or when facing traumatic experiences; anticipatory guidance (what to expect in the future); and crisis interventions. More specific psychotherapeutic interventions for parents, including psychological counseling and behaviour therapy, may be needed to manage depression, guilt, and dependency. There is no evidence that pharmacotherapy of psychiatric disorders in children with brain damage should be different, compared to children without brain damage, although an increased risk of specific side effects may be related to cerebral damage (Vitiello et al. 2006). Namely, increased seizures during treatment with antidepressants or antipsychotics may need an adjustment of the antiepileptic treatment. Furthermore, epileptogenic medications, such as clozapine and chlorpromazine, should be used much more carefully, with EEG monitoring. The increased risk of tardive dyskinesia in patients with brain lesions is still debated. The association with mental retardation has been ascribed to a lower efficacy of some psychotropic medications (namely psychostimulants).

9

Conclusions

Whether children with different forms of CP are at risk for specific psychiatric disorders is still an open issue. There are methodological limitations which have prevented clear conclusions on the nature of the association between brain damage and psychopathology. They include inclusion criteria (rare documentation of lesion characteristics and associated factors, such as severity of motor deficit, presence/absence of epilepsy) and measures of psychopathology which often do not allow specific psychiatric diagnosis, such as the K-SADS. Furthermore, the studies that do report specific psychiatric disorders do not take into consideration the efficacy of pharmacological and non pharmacological treatments.

All children with cerebral palsy deserve careful monitoring for psychiatric problems, with a view to preventative approaches and early intervention. Professionals and parents should be aware of the higher risk of psychological problems in children with cerebral palsy compared to their non-disabled peers. Clinical experience suggests that these comorbidities are usually unrecognized or untreated. Comprehensive health assessment and management for children with chronic neurodevelopmental disorders should be psychologically as well as physically oriented. The most severe difficulties are in peer relationships, which may have an impact on later social adjustment. Other co-occurring symptoms which reduce self-control, such as drooling, and urinary incontinence, may increase social isolation. Particular attention should be paid to a correct management of physical pain. Anxiety disorders, such as separation anxiety, may be increased by both motor limitations and parental overprotection. Inadequate and excessive limitation in daily life may increase the risk of oppositional-defiant behaviors. Higher functioning individuals are at risk for depression, as their inability to carry out tasks and their movement disorder increase frustration, in addition to the sense of being different from peers, which may become more severe with age. Acute traumatic experiences may induce brief psychotic episodes.

A still unmet need is to plan neuropsychiatric services with integrated diagnostic, preventative, and treatment programs for both neurological and psychiatric disorders, in order to define the specific psychiatric risk according to specific risk factors. Many of these issues need specialist support, which may be included in the assessment and in the rehabilitative program, to ensure that psychopathological aspects are not overlooked.

References

American Psychiatric Association (1994) Diagnostic and statistical manual of mental disorders, 4th ed. American Psychiatric Association, Washington, DC

Balaban CD, Jacob RG (2001) Background and history of the interface between anxiety and vertigo. J Anxiety Disord 15:27-51

Balaban CD, Thayer JF (2001) Neurological bases for balance-anxiety links. J Anxiety Disord 15:53-79

Balleny H (1996) Are the concepts of "Theory of mind" and "executive function" useful in understanding social impairment in children with hemiplegic cerebral palsy. ClinPsyD thesis, University of East Anglia

Breslau N (1990) Does brain dysfunction increase children's vulnerability to environmental stress? Arch Gen Psychiatry 47:15-20

Brown G, Chadwick O, Shaffer D et al (1981) A prospective study of children with head injuries. III. Psychiatric sequelae. Psychol Med 11:63-78

Colver A for the SPARCLE group (2006) Study protocol: SPARCLE – a multicentre European study of the relationship of environment to participation and quality of life in children with cerebral palsy. BMC Public Health 6:105

Duval J, Braun CM, Daigneault S, Montour-Proulx I (2002) Does the child behaviour checklist reveal psychopathological profiles of children with focal unilateral cortical lesions? Appl Neuropsychol 9:74-83

Fombonne E (1992) Parents' report on behaviour and competencies among 6-21 year-old French children. Eur Child Adolesc Psychiatry 1:233-243

Fombonne E (2003) Case identification in an epidemiological context. In: Rutter M, Taylor E (Eds) Child and adolescent psychiatry. 4th Edition. Blackwell, London, pp 52-64

Frampton I, Yude C, Goodman R (1998) The prevalence and correlates of specific learning difficulties in representative samples of children with hemiplegia. Br J Educat Psychol 68:39-51

Furman JM, Jacob RG (2001) A clinical taxonomy of dizziness and anxiety in the otoneurological setting. J Anxiety Disord 15:9-26

Goodman R (1998) The longitudinal stability of psychiatric problems in children with hemiplegia. J Child Psychol Psychiat 39:347-354

Goodman R (2002) Brain disorders. In: Rutter M, Taylor E (Eds) Child and adolescent psychiatry. 4th Edition. Blackwell, London, pp 52-64

Goodman R, Graham P (1996) Psychiatric problems in children with hemiplegia: cross-sectional, epidemiological survey. Br Med J 312:1065-1069

Goodman R, Yude C (1996) IQ and its predictors in childhood hemiplegia. Dev Med Child Neurol 38:881-890

Goodman R, Yude C (1997) Do unilateral lesions of the developing brain have side-specific psychiatric consequences in childhood? Laterality 2:103-115

Goodman R, Yude C (2000) Emotional, behavioral and social consequences. In: Neville B, Goodman R (eds) Congenital hemiplegia. Clinics in developmental medicine No. 150. McKeith Press, London, pp 166-178

Gortmaker SL, Walker DK, Weitzman M, Sobol AM (1990) Chronic conditions, socioeconomic risk and behavioural problems in children and adolescents. Pediatrics 85:267-276

Howe GW, Feinstein C, Reiss D et al (1993) Adolescent adjustment in chronic physical disorders I. Comparing neurological and non-neurologiocal conditions. J Child Psychol Psychiat 34:1153-1171

Jacob RG, Furman JM, Durrant JD, Turner SM (1996) Panic, agoraphobia and vestibular dysfunction. Am J Psychiatry 153:259-269

Lewis SW, Harvey I, Ron M et al (1990) Can brain damage protect against schizophrenia? A case report of twins. Br J Psychiatry 157:600-603

Masi G, Favilla L, Mucci M (2000) Generalized anxiety disorder in adolescents and young adults with mild mentaly retardation. Psychiatry 63:54-64

Masi G, Mucci M, Favilla L, Poli P (1999) Dysthymic disorder in mild mentally retarded adolescents. J Intell Disab Res 43:80-87

McDermott S, Cocker AL, Mani S et al (1996) A population-based analysis of behaviour problems in children with cerebral palsy. J Pediatr Psychol 21:447-463

Meltzer H, Garward R, Goodman R, Ford F (2000) Mental health of children and adolescents in Great Britain. The Stationery Office, London

Ounsted C, Lindsay J, Richards P (1987) Temporal lobe epilepsy 1948-1986: a biographical study. Clinics in developmental medicine No. 103. McKeith Press, Blackwell Scientific Publications, Oxford, London

Parkes J, White-Konig M, Dickinson HO et al (2008) Psychological problems in children with cerebral palsy: a cross-sectional european study. J Child Psychol Psychiatry 49:405-413

Rutter M, Chadwick O, Shaffer D (1984) Head injury. In: Rutter M (ed) Developmental neuropsychiatry. Churchill Livingstone, Edinburgh, pp 83-111

Rutter M, Graham P, Yule W (1970) A neuropsychiatric study in childhood. Clinics in developmental medicine No. 35/36. S.I.M.P./Heinemann, London

Seidel UP, Chadwick O, Rutter M (1975) Psychological disorders in crippled children: a comparative study of children with and without brain damage. Dev Med Child Neurol 17:563-573

Sklare DA, Konrad HR, Maser JD, Jacob RG (2001) Special issue on the interface of balance disorders and anxiety. An introduction and review. J Anxiety Disord 15:1-7

Trauner DA, Nass R, Ballantyne A (2001) Behavioural profiles of children and adolescents after pre- or perinatal unilateral brain damage. Brain 124:995-1002

Trauner DA, Panyard-Davis JL, Ballantyne AO (1996) Behavioral differences in school age children after perinatal stroke. Assessment 3:265-276

Vitiello B, Masi G, Marazziti D (2006) Handbook of pharmacotherapy of mental disorders in children and adolescents. Informa Healthcare, Oxon, Francis and Taylor, Boca Raton, FL

Weiland SK, Pless IB, Roghmann K (1992) Chronic illness and mental health problems in pediatric practice: results from a survey of primary care providers. Pediatrics 89:445-449

Yardley L, Britton J, Lear S et al (1995) Relationship between balance system function and agoraphobic avoidance. Behav Res Ther 33:435-439

Yude C, Goodman R (1999) Peer problems of 9-11 year old children with hemiplegia in mainstream schools: can these be predicted? Dev Med Child Neurol 41:4-8

Yude C, Goodman R, McConachie H (1998) Peer problems of children with hemiplegia in mainstream primary school. J Child Psychol Psychiat 39:533-541

Observing Interactions

10

S. Maestro

It is widely known that a traumatic birth, togheter with the complete set of events related to the initial intensive care provided to the newborn, will deeply impact and cause an important modification of the child's relational system. Anguish deriving from trauma, and from anxiety about the uncertainties on the infant's future development are deeply rooted in the parents' representation system, replacing the "fantasmatic" plasticity which accompanies the first stages of life of every human being. The traumatic event is like a foreign body, a sort of "intruder" in the parent-child relationship system. Later, with the child's growth and the development of processing and adaptive processes, this "intruder" is gradually substituted by what could be defined as the third pole of the system, that is the health care team. The creation of such a system establishes a complex network of relationships among all components, which are mutually dependent. An observation of the interactions therefore implies the creation of a peculiar mindset within the observer, focused on this interdependence; that means selecting within the events happening in a specific context, for example, a rehabilitation session or a control visit, such aspects of the behaviour of the different protagonists of the meeting (child, parents, therapist, clinician) that constitute a signal of the relationship which is being built. This approach to clinical practice implies a mental psychodynamic framework, according to which the relationship (i.e., the complex and articulated group of actions, emotions and fantasies that form the basis of the different relationships among human beings) represents the most suitable perspective to accept and understand the other in his complexity and fullness. Which are the instruments we need to integrate in this observation? What are, from this perspective, the risks but also the protective factors, for the psychological and emotional development of the infant with neurological lesions?

These topics will be dealt with from the point of view of the child, the family, and the health care team.

10

The Child

During the first stages of life, motricity represents an essential function in the organization of subjective experience and in the creation of different senses of the self. Through motion, the child experiments with his capacity to impact on the external environment, to generate changes, to start his first object explorations. The inner self, existential ground for the subsequent development of personality, is organized and constructed also through the child's acquisition of a full mastery of his body, his gestures, and his actions (acting self, Stern, 1985).

The image of the self, that is, the mental representation of the most significant aspect of one's own identity, is built through the processing and following integration of life experiences and fantasies related to the body. Finally, through motricity, the child experiences the first forms of separation, as a conqueror of physical distance from the other, and especially from the mother, one of the essential prerequisites to start the separation-individuation processes.

Conversely, the child with early neuromotor disorders is often obliged to give up this type of experience. Sometimes, from birth, the physical consequences of perinatal distress, tone alteration, ocular motricity impairment (so penalizing in all the relations steered by the function of gaze; see chapter 7), wake perturbations, and conditions of numbness or hyperexcitement (see chapter 9), make the child a poorly active or soliciting partner in the interaction.

It is very difficult to imagine the subjective experience of a child who cannot freely use muscular tone and posture as natural discharge vehicles of emotional tensions, but who, instead, is dominated by them. However these impaiments, which can provoke an initial mismatch between mental and body states, lead the child to look for alternative strategies for the expression of his/her relational capacity, and allows caregivers to create new paradigms to decode his interactive intentions. For too long, prejudice was the rule, and developmental models were poorly adaptable, from the emotional and social points of view, to the condition of the neurologically impaired child, and they were especially useless for the investigation of the child's strategies, strengths, and resources. For example, it is debatable how a neurologically impaired child can progress in the development of his social or interpersonal abilities.

How much can palsy of an upper limb, for example, block the onset of gestures such as requesting and declarative pointing? How can ocular motricity coordination difficulties interfere in the emergence of comprehension pointing, a precursor of shared attention (Stern, 1995)? But, most of all, through which compensatory strategies will the child organize himself? Which behavioral patterns indicate this reorganization? And how much is this organization functional to the development of social interaction with the environment? (De Gangi, 2000; Gordon Williamson and Anzalone, 2000). Research into these precursors of social development seems to be essential and preliminary to the study of affective and emotional development. Indeed, the emergence of symbolic thought, which allows us to formulate hypotheses on the organization of inner objective relations, is certainly subsequent, and therefore in the older child, allows formulation hypotheses about fantasmatic life, defensive systems, and finally about the structure of personality. Aguillar (1983) described in a very intriguing way how the impaired part of the body converts into a false container of the child's bad internal objects: "legs that do not work, a dystonic arm or a hemiplegic hand represent the bad object that needs to be exclusively repaired. This makes it difficult to achieve a mental processing of certain feelings experienced as bad, and therefore conceived as to be rejected".

This catalyst function, container of persecutory experiences of the damaged body, evolves, in the mourning coping process, from a defect in the child to an image of the self which is whole and healthy (Corominas, 1983a, b). Indeed, in children undergoing long-term treatment, we can often observe that the defense apparatus enacted against the disease deeply interferes with personality organization. Even if it is not possible to describe a unique structural analytical profile, due to the extreme variability among children, it is possible to highlight some recurrent characteristics of psychic function related to the inter-ference caused by the disease. These children, in their relationships with other individuals, may alternate seductive and provocative registers, strongly committed in their denial of the emotional and physical dependence on the adult caregiver. For example, they seldom ask for help when in need.

Expressive language is often invested in a hypertrophic way, and the ordering function of thought as well as the self-regulation of actions are often impossible to be observed. The association course may be so accelerated and chaotic as to offset motor limitations.

The contact with reality is usually preserved, although the relation with the object is superficial and approximate, as is in those individuals who aren't able to contact their own instrumental limitations.

Regression and maniacal behaviors dominate among the defenses, even though such a profile does not apply to all patients. A study focused on the emotional and psychological characteristics of dyskinetic children, reported evidence of more marked depressive traits. Therefore an explanation of personality structure and of emotional development might increase our knowledge of the child with cerebral damage, integrating the new progress achieved through the development of neurosciences

To conclude, the relational approach starts from the application of observation grids which have to be adequate to different domains of the child's development including his/her social emotions and intersubjective competences. For older children, this also means giving them the possibility to establish a relation with their inner world, and there-fore also with the suffering and the depressive feelings related to the pathological condi-tion. Indeed, sletting the sick parts free from their function of symbolic equivalent of damaged objects can restore dynamicity to mental processes and allow access to increas-ingly evolved symbolization processes. Moreover, the relational observation must focus on those behaviors that express the child's initiative to interact and communicate, evidencing his/her strengths and weaknesses.

10

The Family

Studies in the literature and clinical practice indicate that the evolutive risks of a child with perinatal disease depend, apart from biological and innate factors, also on the characteristics of his familiar environment. The incidence of different factors on the evolution of a child who presents problems at birth, such as the social and economic level of the family, the parents' age and personality, the presence of siblings, the social isolation of the family, etc., was demonstrated. Our clinical experience confirms that the treatment of the family is essential and must represent one of the pillars of the rehabilitation intervention. The main target of the therapy alliance consists of shifting parents' attention from the mere recovery of motor function to the child's global needs.

Many studies in the literature report the difficulties that parents must face, since birth, including separation, and management of care-giving that is even more difficult due to the child's physical impairment , to the uncertainties and anguish related to his /her development. In the relationship with the child with neurological lesions important risk factors also regard continuous monitoring of the child's growth, meant to discover early signs of the disease, the anxiety during follow-up visits, the complete delegation to clinicians in the evaluation of the child's condition, and the concurrent difficulty to develop the set of attitudes, behaviors and feelings which makes the parents the most naturally expert persons concerning the child. Soulé (Kreisler and Soulé, 1995) mentioned the "fragile child syndrome" to describe a particular image of the self that some of these children structure as a consequence of the feelings of precariousness and vulnerability that are massively projected on them. Stern points out the problem concerning a sort of "vacuum of representation" that parents experience when they face disability or an evolutive risk for their child. The child would then be deprived of the nourishing function of his/her parents' projections necessary for his/her mental development. As mentioned in the introduction, the traumatic event becomes the intruder in the parents-child relationship and for a long time it remains the main relational organizer. We could then hypothize that this vacuum of representation becomes saturated with anguished emotional experiences, which, in some way, hinder the creation of representations in parents, intended as mental images, dreams, and fantasies about the child's development. This first level in the parents-child relationship, which could be defined as unconscious or fantasmatic, must then be integrated in our assessments with a more concrete level, related to the actual interaction, as observed in the *hic et nunc* of the meeting. This second level is as important as the first, since it represents the bridge through which fantasies, representations, but also the anguish of the parent's experience become tangible in the relationship with the child. Therefore representation and interactions need to be explored applying different parameters. In the first case, the parents' personal histories, identifications, and internal operative work models, are analyzed, while in the second one, other aspects, such as the concrete modalities of taking care of the child, posture syntony, face to face exchanges, etc., are observed. During the first stages of the infant's life, parents are completely absorbed in the parenting process: giving physical care, adaptating to the baby's rhythms, decoding his/her self-regulation processes, understanding his/her needs, demands etc. When observing these situations it is also necessary to notice, by using the most appropriate tools, the modalities through which parents carry out these tasks. The channels employed in the mutual intentional communication, the actions facilitating the child's exploring activity, the sensitivity to his emotional signals, the enhancement of his capacities of emotion processing, represent essential parameters in the assessment of interaction.

However, in our experience, helping parents in the early processing of the traumatic event is fundamental, because such experiences engender around the child a network of projective identifications which is difficult to "disentangle". For example, it is difficult to treat an infant who continuously cries during the treatment session before dealing with the mother's anguish related to the first intrusive care-actions performed on the infant's body by the therapist's manipulations.

The child with CP certainly has less possibilities compared to healthy children of the same age, to balance the mother's projective universe: he hasn't got the help of his motricity.

In our experience, mechanisms of fusion and symbiosis are predominant for a long time in the mother-child relationship and attachment processes.

On this basis, it is possible to speculate that the feelings of guilt on one side, and on the other the lack of tolerance towards aggressive feelings which are perceived as being too dangerous towards a child who has largely frustrated the parent's narcissistic expectations, deprive the relationship of its structuring role of conflict. The mother passively suffers the child's despotic behaviour, still strenuously keeping him in a regressive and dependent condition. Helping parents in thinking about these aspects of the relationship with their child, a task we perform through different types of settings, may limit the risk of distortions in the relationship, such as, for example, forms of "maniac reparation " associated with hyperstimulation, or the identification and competition of the parent with professionals, and especially with the therapist.

The final objective is helping parents in the complex task of coping with mourning, that is the definitive separation from the ideal child, dreamt of during pregnancy, allowing them to establish a more parent-oriented and less care-oriented function. The child can then be reinvested of new fantasmatic contents. Such situations are often referred to psychological counseling because the child has developed behavioral or neurotic symptoms that represent a special point of interest to us because they indicate a restart of the mutual identification game and renewed dynamics in emotional exchange processes.

In short, the relational perspective implies inserting the child's relationship with the family within the rehabilitation project.

The Caregiving Team

The debate in the last years has led to the definition of rehabilitation as a multi-directional intervention, taking into account different aspects of the individual's life and considering the recovery of adaptative functions as a central objective. This model of intervention implies the involvement of different professional caregivers and the subsequent establishment of a therapy caregiving team. However, transforming an organizational formula into a top performing operating unit is not an easy task.

The child and the complexity of his needs may become grounds for clashes among the different professionals taking part in the rehabilitation project. For example, the needs and rules of the school environment may be extremely different from those of the therapy room and imply the application of certain strategies by the child, which are different or even opposite to those learnt during therapy. Intervention with multi-directional features implies the capacity of every single member of the team to reconsider with flexibility his /her own image of the child, and to review the therapeutic project and the possibility to make it in line with the needs of every single child, in constant communication with the other members of the team. However, to communicate this attitude, and the capacity to negotiate with one's own professional roles and cultural models is not innate and cannot be learnt through traditional training curricula. It is in fact a function that can be developed if caregivers are surrounded by the appropriate conditions to think about clinical experience. Yet, the constant relationship with the child and his family always leads the caregiver to face such issues.

A previous work about the relationship between child and therapist dealt with the observation that in the beginning of a treatment, the therapist builds in the image of an "ideal" child, a child already enabled of his possible future performance through his recovery capacities, whose collaboration and adaptability to the treatment is more or less taken for granted. Instead, the impact of the actual condition of the young patient can often be a source of stress due to the recurring conflict among subjectivity, emotionality, and the child's motivations and intervention objectives. Confronted with the characteristics of chronic disease and irreversible outcomes, the therapist may feel disarmed and may encounter difficulties in maintaining the judgment deferral which is the key to the full understanding of the child. Seeking refuge in technique, privileging action rather than thought during sessions, subdividing the young patient in a number of segments to be treated, may all represent defenses against the most frustrating aspect of the disease, such as passivity, inertia, inhibition, and negativism.

Other problems are related to the strong interference in treatment coming from the family: from the initial idealization of the therapist, to the subsequent competition in the mastering of the rehabilitation program, to the anxiety load about the child's development. Sometimes, the therapist has to "keep secret" the child's real recovery possibilities for a while, and to operate as a filter in the communication with the parents, to avoid fueling useless expectations, yet without provoking the loss of trust and effective investment in the child.

Being able to master all these aspects in the relationship with the child and with the family implies a large emotional effort that the professional may be able to offer only if adequately included and involved in the emotional responsibility towards the child. Our supervision activity is aimed at this, and during the last years we have worked on the elaboration of a language and a level of interpretation of the relationship, that integrates all these complex dynamics.

Conclusions

The introduction presented the relational approach as the most suitable to understand the individual in his complexity. Considering the issues presented (and not solved) in this chapter, it might be possible to conclude that the relational approach represents a factor complicating an already complex clinical picture, due to the chronic aspect of the disease and to the physical and mental suffering related to it. However, in our experience, embracing this complexity, of course through the use of the most suitable tools, is essential, if not directly linked to the rehabilitation prognosis, at least for successful treatment management.

In one of our works about therapist burn-out (Maestro et al. 1993), we underlined how easily the relationship with the child can turn into a highly frustrating and alienating experience (for both the partners) if the underlying dynamics are not accounted for and understood. Moreover, only through the activity of supervision and follow-up on the clinical experience is it possible to detect certain therapeutic choices that clash or collide with the patient's most impaired elements. Therefore, the possibility to reconstruct, through a teamwork discussion, the child's image as it is built up in the mind of the professionals working with him, represents one of the essential tools to provide parents with an integrated image of their child. Finally, I believe that embracing complexity allows all who are involved to take up the challenge within the approach to the chronic disease, with the target of restoring uniqueness, originality, and unpredictability to development pathways characterized by pathological events.

References

Aguillar J (1983) Psicoterapie brevi nel bambino paralitico cerebrale. In: Quaderni di psicoterapia infantile 8. Borla Editore, Roma, pp 105-127

Corominas J (1983a) Utilizzazione di conoscenze psicoanalitiche in un centro per bambini affetti da paralisi cerebrale. In: Quaderni di psicoterapia ínfantile 8. Borla Editore, Roma, pp 22-43

Corominas J (1983b) Psicopatologia e sviluppi arcaici. Borla Editore, Roma

Corominas J (1991) Psicopatologia i desenvulupament arcasi. Assaig psicoanalitic, Barcelona, Expaxs, D. L.

De Gangi G (2000) Pediatric disorders of regulation in affect and behavior. Academic Press, Los Angeles

Gordon Williamson G, Anzalone ME (2000) Sensory integration and self regulation in infants and toddlers. Zero to Three National Center for Infants, Toddlers and Families, Washington, D.C.

Kreisler L, Soulè M (1995) L'enfant prématuré. In: Lebovici S, Diatkine R, Soulé M (eds) Nouveau traité de psychiatrie de l'enfant et de l'adolescent. Presses Universitaires de France, Paris, pp 1893-1915

Maestro S, Bertuccelli B (1996) Lo sviluppo emotivo nei bambini discinetici. In: Cioni G, Ferrari A (eds) Le forme discinetiche delle paralisi cerebrali infantili. Edizioni del Cerro, Pisa, pp 98-106

Stern D (1985) The interpersonal world of infant: a view from psychoanalysis and developmental
    psychology. Basic Books INC, U.S.
Stern D (1995) The motherhood constellation a unified view parent-infant psychotherapy. Basic
    Books INC, U.S.

PART III
Classification of Spastic Syndromes and Clinical Forms

Critical Aspects of Classifications

11

A. Ferrari

Currently, cerebral palsy (CP) is still defined as a "*disorder of development of posture and movement*" (Bax, Goldstein, Rosenbaum et al. 2005). To be consistent with this definition, the only possibility to classify CP should be done by carrying out an analysis of posture and movement disorders, with movement interpreted as gesture, both assessed from a quality (nature) and quantity (measure) point of view. Consequently, the only way to measure the success of re-educational treatment is to observe if the patient has acquired a long lasting improved posture and gesture ability, differently from what would have been expected if the normal natural history of that clinical form had run its course.

Cerebral palsy: definitions

> *A persistent but non unchangeable disorder of movement and posture* (Ingram 1955)
> *A persistent but not unchangeable disorder of posture and motion, due to an organic and not progressive alteration of cerebral function, determined by pre-, peri- and post-natal causes, before its growth and development are completed* (Bax 1964; Spastic Society Berlin 1966 - Edinburgh 1969)
> *"A group of non-progressive, but often changing, motor impairment syndromes secondary to lesions or abnormalities of the brain"* (Mutch et al. 1992)
> *"A group of chronic neurological disorders manifested by abnormal control of movement, beginning early in life, and not due to underlying progressive diseases"* (Behrman et al. 1998)
> *"A persistent disorder of movement and posture caused by non-progressive defects or lesions of the immature brain"* (Aicardi and Bax, 1998)
> *"A group of disorders of the development of movement and posture, causing activity limitation, that are attributed to non-progressive disturbances that occurred in the developing foetal or infant brain. The motor disorders of cerebral palsy are often accompanied by disturbances of sensation, cognition, communication, perception, and/or behavior, and/or by a seizure disorder"* (Bax, Goldstein, Rosenbaum et al. 2005)

The Spastic Forms of Cerebral Palsy. Adriano Ferrari, Giovanni Cioni
© Springer-Verlag Italia 2010

The main principle of any classification is to place every clinical situation on the same level, separating each condition from every different one by means of common guidelines allowing us to identify and characterize it with greater or lesser detail. *"Any syndrome must be clearly defined, meaningful, reliable, and used consistently by different people"* (Colver and Sethumadhavan, 2003).

In CP, classification guidelines have always been drawn up according to the various movement disorders, namely, the different postural behaviors related to tone and the gesture performance characteristics (hypotonic, hypertonic, spastic, ataxic, choreic, atheoid, etc.), associated with their topographic distribution (tetraplegia, diplegia, hemiplegia, etc.) (see chapter 12). *"A few CP syndromes, such as choreathetosis with deafness caused by bilirubin encephalophathy, and ataxia caused by hydrocephalus have stood the test of time"* (Colver and Sethumadhavan, 2003).

Therefore, the problem of CP classification is still pending.

Probably, the difficulty in attaining an acceptable and meaningful classification for all forms of CP comes from the postulate of the classification coplanarity itself and from the arbitrary choice of guidelines. It is very difficult to think that such a complex phenomenon as CP can be exhaustively analyzed from just a single point of view, that is, through only one explorative dimension, although this might seem appealing and meaningful. The more numerous and separate points of view we manage to adopt, the more effective the observation of a complex event will be. Indeed, only if we change our point of view will we manage to distinguish the foreground from the background and to compensate the perspective deformity.

To classify CP, it is thus necessary to be able to renounce the coplanarity postulated among different forms, the homogeneity of guidelines, and the possibility to use only one point of view. This is the reason why a classification "limited" to the analysis of motor disorder (posture and gesture) and its topographic localization (tetraplegia, diplegia, hemiplegia), as in classifications currently employed (Hagberg, Bobath, Milani Comparetti, SCPE), certainly will have precise limitations.

Movement analysis allows us to access the problem of palsy (early diagnosis) in a way that is usually simple enough, convenient, precocious, suggestive and explicit, and that even later will remain the surest and most reliable starting point to measure patient progress. However, it cannot be stated that this is always the most relevant examination mode, nor the most important, nor the most precise for any situation and at any age, nor can it be stated that it is the best method for every clinical form of CP.

To solve the problem of classification and build the natural history of different clinical forms of CP, we have to learn to observe other perspectives together with that of motion. Among the most important ones are perception (see chapter 5) and intentionality (see chapter 9), which allow us to access further information that could not be collected by observing only movement.

I stand on my desk to remind myself that we must constantly force ourselves to look at things differently. The world looks different from up here. If you don't believe it, stand up here and try it. All of you. Take turns.Try never to think about anything the same way twice.

From the film "Dead Poets Society" by Peter Weir

Actually motor, perceptual, and intentional information cannot be placed on the same level, nor can they be collected from the same point of view.

An observer who merely analyzes CP from the motor perspective can only imagine or guess the presence of perceptual and intentional problems, since they are outside the applied investigative method. By changing from time to time his point of examination (3D exploration of palsy), the observer will be able to collect new and significant information, but not without having every time to re-draw the observed reality and to shift from the previously-built interpretative profile. In effect, according to the adopted point of view and classification criteria, the same clinical event could show different profiles.

Although through mental synthesis processes we manage to recognize the differences among the various perspectives, when reconstructing the overall picture of the patient, trying to explain to other people the reasons for a certain problem or a particular evolution, our considerations will be conditioned by the adopted perspective. For example, some patients will be better characterized by their postural behavior (see chapter 13: tetraplegic forms), some others by gesture ability related to walk (see chapter 15: diplegic forms) or to manipulation performance (see chapter 16: hemiplegic forms) some others will be characterized by the sensory aspects related to perceptive tolerance of surrounding space or to proprioceptive attention (see chapter 14: dysperceptive forms) some others by the intentional aspects related to participation, delegation, or renouncement (see chapter 9); some others by the neuropsychological organization (see chapter 6) or affective and relational behaviors (see chapter 10), etc.

Therefore, the "apostural" patient (the worst situation among the different forms of tetraplegia, see chapter 13) suffers from a CP form that is better recognized from the postural point of view; the "tight skirt" and the "tightrope walker" (two of the four main types of diplegia, see chapter 15) from the walk perspective; the "falling" child (the most severe among dysperceptive forms, see chapter 14) from the nature of the space perceptive problem ; the "stand-up" child (the second dysperceptive form in terms of relevance) from the baresthetic and kinesthetic awareness perspective; the "lazy" individual (the CP personality defect that is most frequently reported by the parents) from his intentional behavior (see chapter 9) and so on.

If we used only the movement perspective to classify these clinical forms, we would end up placing all of them into tetraplegic or diplegic forms, according to the importance we attribute to disorder severity rather than its somatic distribution between the upper and lower limbs, or even to the more generic bilateral form, if we followed the recommendation of Surveillance Cerebral Palsy Europe.

Of course, from the perspective of re-educational treatment, it would become extremely difficult to understand which priority problem deserves the most therapeutic attention.

The choice of criteria and aspects we consider important to classify the patient's condition into a clinical form, therefore, depend on the examiner's arbitrary decision. It would be better to judge the importance of a sign or symptom based on the computational mistake made by the individual when organizing his posture and gesture or other functions (consistency of palsy); that is to say, considering the problem from the patient's point of view rather than ours. For the child's CNS, the palsy is not simply the sum of defects of organs, structures, and systems, but rather the different functioning configuration (computational mistake), the different organization and action mode (coherence) of a system that keeps on looking for new solutions to meet the internal need to become more suitable and the external one to adapt themselves to the surrounding environment.

By adopting this CP classification method, from a certain point of view, some forms might appear impossible to distinguish, at least during some periods of development. It is difficult to distinguish the "falling" child from the "stand-up" one from the postural point of view, or the apostural tetraplegic from the akinetic one (the second most severe form of tetraplegia, see chapter 13) from the perceptive viewpoint, or the dystonic from the athetoid (one of the four main forms that compose dyskinetic syndromes). As a consequence, the same clinical form could be classified differently according to the observation method used: for example the "falling" child, defined in this way according to perceptive criteria, is also a "vertical" according to posture organization, a tetraplegic or diplegic (depending if the motor disorder is judged according to its severity or its distribution among the four limbs) according to the topographic principle, and defined as a "lazy" individual according to the criteria of intentionality and participation.

Since CP is developmental, also its diagnosis has to be developmental, and has to take this into account, considering that the natural palsy's history expresses CNS organizational competence, also elements external to the primitive lesion, such as re-education treatment, orthosis, drugs, and above all functional surgery.

Motor Perspective

The idea of a modular interactive and systematic organization of movement (Milani Comparetti et al. 1976) has currently raised both our awareness and interest in idea of the presence of single elements that can be separated and interchanged for the acquisition of procedural sequences (formulas and strategies), which allow us to control system variables (ability to act as an expression of cognitive organization of the available motor repertoire).

The first way to evaluate palsy from the motion point of view (posture and gesture) is to analyse the patient's movement repertoire (modules, combinations and sequences) and his ability to use it (formulas and strategies). The analysis of the motor repertoire represents the simplest, earliest, most convenient, and safest way to make a CP diagnosis (see chapter 4).

The repertoire concept can be correlated to what Milani Comparetti (1965) and the Bobaths (1976) in the past described as pattern analysis. These authors considered the quantitative aspect, represented by the number of movements presented by the patient as available modules with which actions can be built on (redundancy or poverty), and a qualitative aspect, related to the predominance of one pattern over others (competitive interaction), which is the condition responsible for formula stereotypy and for the impossibility to create new or complex combinations and sequences. Beside the description of the conflicting patterns characterizing clinical forms, Milani Comparetti (1978) highlighted the importance to explore, within the repertoire, the patient's preserved freedom of choice, represented by the presence of "bellini" (gracious, nice, refined) movements, which are segmental gestures, especially distal and isolated (unique) ones, allowing the child to select direction, modulate intensity, and regulate range. "Bellini" movements were considered to be relevant to prognosis, being able to elude the conflicting system of "tyrant" patterns (to measure the CNS control capacity, it is more significant to be able to move one finger rather than an entire limb). In other words, "bellini" movements could be interpreted as quality indicators.

Conversely, the concept of utilization indicates which and how much of the repertoire is easily accessible to the patient and can be easily used. Indeed, children with CP often end up using just one part of the motor repertoire they own. This aspect could be explained by the problem of dyspraxia (see chapter 6) and of perceptive tolerance (see chapter 5). The possession of some specific movements, even if considered "bellini", is not a sufficient condition and a guarantee that they will be used. In CP, repertoire and utilization can be extremely different, and this gap must influence the idea of palsy and therefore the strategy of re-educational treatment.

If physiotherapy has something to do with repertoire upgrading, in theory it should not be indicated for those people who have application problems, since increasing the number of modules and motor combinations would require on the part of the patient a greater selection and choice capacity which he will not be able to manage. Conversely, physiotherapy should increase utilization, ideally shifting it favorably from one part of the repertoire to the other.

Dyspraxia

The word "dyspraxia", as used by French authors (for example De Ajuriaguerra, 1974), refers to the concept of praxia expressed by Piaget (1936): "*Praxias or actions are not simply movements, but are groups of coordinated movements guided by an intention or directed at a specific result*". In neurology, apraxia or dyspraxia describes the inability or the difficulty to perform voluntary movements, coordinated as a sequence aimed at achieving a specific goal and not provoked by palsy, tone alterations, sensory disorders, servomotor involuntary or parasite movements, psychic disorders, mental retardation, or motor learning defects. Thus, dyspraxia does not define a movement problem, but a complex organizational disorder, characterized by the inability to reproduce intentional movements coordinated into combinations or sequences, learnt and aimed at a specific result. "*... dyspraxic children show a certain automatic-voluntary disassociation ..., while a certain motor action can be automatically or "involuntary" performed, this is not possible at intentional level, not even following instructions or imitations*" (Rigardetto and Siravegna, 1999). It is as if there was an available program, but this could not be accessed by the individual except through an automatic routine (Camerini and De Panfilis, 2003). Ideative apraxia is when the deficiency provokes the inability to formulate or recall the project from memory, while ideomotor apraxia relates to the capacity to control its implementation. "*The ideative apraxic individual does not manage to recall the gestures to be made, or invert the action order, or make with an object movements that should be made with another one, that is to say he does not know what to do*" (De Renzi and Faglioni, 1990).

This action organization disorder can be subsequent to faults that occur during the mental stage (ideation and programming), that is, during the anticipatory stage, rather than the movement execution stage, with most complex motor operations depending more on regulation systems of gesture during working progress (feedback) (see chapter 6). Otherwise, it could be provoked by the inability to stabilize into routines, and automate, the most frequent movement experiences, with a subsequent difficulty in learning new motor patterns (see chapter 8). In other situations instead, it could be produced by a mistaken sensory analysis and perceptive integration, with a subsequent alteration of the visual-kinesthetic and baro-kinesthetic engrams on which the action plan is based. It could also derive from the presence of "spatial" disorders, which can be described as the inability to correctly analyse the depth-distance ratio and transcribe it into motor coordinates (see chapter 5). Smyth (1991) stated that dyspraxic children present difficulties in movement planning, and therefore they depend more on regulation systems, i.e. on perceptive-motor feedback. This thesis relates dyspraxia to an information-processing defect during response selection operations, making the performance of a newly-acquired complex action particularly difficult. From the neurobiological point of view, the areas involved are those using the feed-forward mechanism more, i.e., the fast mechanism for the mental forecasting of the action to be accomplished (see chapter 8).

Dyspraxia is a motor learning disorder; therefore, it does not affect the development of genetically-programmed primary motor functions, but rather their use within newly acquired abilities. With regard to development age, the words *awkwardness* and *clumsiness* are proposed in the literature as synonyms of dyspraxia, to describe the difficulties met by some individuals who are normal from other points of view but not when carrying out some manual tasks, even the most normal daily activities like dressing, undressing, lacing up shoes, using cutlery, handling objects or toys, riding a bicycle, writing or drawing, or making expressive movements and highly symbolic gestures. ICD 10 includes dyspraxia among the Developmental Disabilities, classifying it within Motor Skills Disorders.

Differently from what is conceptually declared by official neurology, in the 1970s Sabbadini had already showed the existence and importance of dyspraxia as a hidden phenomenon of CP that can considerably reduce its modifiability and affect the possibility to perform re-educational treatment: "*The motor disorder of cerebral pals is the result of the interference (or sum) of several factors, probably all highly integrated executive and cognitive disorders, which not only add to "spastic palsy" (spasticity, rigidity, dystonia, ataxia), but above all influence the motor disorder or even affect it, in very relevant way compared to the central palsy*" (Sabbadini et al. 1978). By dyspraxia within palsy we therefore refer to the difficulty to decide how to accomplish a certain action (anticipatory planning), whose aim and expected result are known to the patient. "*Actually, the "executive" disorder is nothing more then the result of the sum or interference by several disorders that we could generally define as "apraxia" and "agnosia", referring to a series of "executive" and "cognitive" disorders at a high integration level*" (Sabbadini et al. 1978). Thus dyspraxia refers to cognitive elements of movement. Sabbadini (1995) talks about practognosia in order to underline knowledge-action coupling. Development dyspraxia is considered by many authors as a disorder of symbolic function (while Sabbadini prefers to consider it as a meta-cognitive disorder), with a dysmaturation base and multi-factorial origin, although its etiology is still unknown.

If palsy expresses the loss of motor modules, sequences, and combinations, dyspraxia represents the impairment of the instructions on how to build motor operations through the remaining modules, by choosing and aggregating the most suitable ones for a specific problem (anticipatory planning of the motor action). In this sense, the loss of instructions makes the problem even more severe when the patient's residual repertoire is wider, just like with a box of building blocks, where the greater the number of pieces, the more detailed the instructions and the more capable the player. If we define palsy as the loss of a certain number of pieces which does not allow the patient to achieve some performances, dyspraxia is the loss of a certain number of instructions (planning) which does not allow him to combine the available movements, neither in space nor in time, in order to achieve the expected result. The higher the number of missing pieces, the more severe the palsy, but paradoxically, the opposite occurs with dyspraxia, since planning is much more complex if the available repertoire is still broad. There are no compensatory solutions to dyspraxia, other than voluntarily reducing the remaining repertoire, renouncing the use of a part of the available modules and combinations (freezing of postures and gesture simplification), and stabilizing the adopted sequences until they become "stereotyped". Conceptually, we are now proposing the exact opposite of the primary objective in physiotherapy treatment: increasing the number of modules, combinations and sequences that are available. During development, many individuals adopt this strategy (tetraparesis, for example), by reducing along the way the repertoire and thus contradicting an initially more favorable prognosis based on the residual movement analysis. Simplification is a strategy of repertoire use, compatible with planning and action control difficulties, which has to be respected when setting up the re-educational treatment. Fixation mechanisms (or co-activation) that are used as simplification strategies could not be accepted as cost-effective in a normal condition, but they may be considered as useful in disadvantaged conditions (Giannoni and Zerbino, 2000).

For some individuals with CP, dyskinetic children for example, simplification of the repertoire is not possible, and the success of the actions is determined by trial and error, strong determination at the cognitive level and sufficient control at the emotional one, and therefore particularly difficult during early childhood. With growth and through experience, individual planning abilities will improve, although strategies will continue to by influenced by casual factors.

Motor Learning

The exact opposite to the concept of palsy is ideally represented by motor learning, that is to say, by the individual's ability to learn and preserve new and alternative motor behaviors to be used for functional tasks. Regardless of the palsy extent, the impairment, reduction, or loss of motor learning capacity represents an absolutely fundamental prognostic element. If there were no limit to motor learning, CP would not be defined as a persistent

11

and unchangeable disorder. It is not a coincidence that the equation "rehabilitation = learning" has been so successful (Perfetti, 1979). Can the learning ability of a CP child be considered as normal? Can he learn normality? Or could palsy be considered as a limited and abnormal learning condition, exercised only under particular situations by an individual who may not be particularly interested in changing? For CP prognosis the neurological examination is not sufficient, rather, as Milani Comparetti stated (1978), also the therapist's contribution is necessary, since therapy is the only way to assess the motor learning capacity preserved by the individual (prognostic treatment). Indeed, motor learning capacity influences the extent of palsy changeability and impacts on the usefulness of re-education, its length, and its intensity. In CP, the equation "diagnosis therefore therapy" is not acceptable, but it is necessary to evaluate the patient's motor learning capacity, which defines functional prognosis (see chapter 12) together with other conditions (motivation, modifiability of function architecture, perceptive tolerance, affective development, etc.). While diagnosis establishes the right to qualified care, which has to include rehabilitation physicians and therapists, prognosis allows us to make a decision on the need for re-education, its meaning, and its limitations (Manifesto per la riabilitazione del bambino – Manifesto for child rehabilitation, AA.VV, 2000).

The possibility to modify the natural history of the palsy actually depends on the learning ability of the individual. By learning we mean the genetically programmed mechanism aimed at allowing the subject to acquire what has not already been genetically provided. It is possible to learn gestures and postures, motor strategies and perceptive tactics, performances and pathways, but the individual also ends up learning non-use and bad-use, lack of attention or negligence, compensation or substitution, delegation or renouncement (adaptive recovery). The individual learns to become, but also not to be, not to do, not to give, if he is not able to overcome his fears or laziness.

Acquisition defines the individual's ability to select and preserve, rather than suppress and remove (hypothalamic areas of gratification and punishment) what he has learnt. The CP child can learn and make some things possible, but many fewer are those things he can acquire and spontaneously make probable. Only acquired learning, i.e., integrated and durable learning, can make the choice possible. In this sense, the perceptive dimension (attention and tolerance) and the intentional one (satisfaction and pleasure) are relevant. If the child's experience has been satisfactory, the operations made will be fixed in his stable memory; if the experience requires too much effort, discomfort, malaise, fear or deep disappointment, it will be removed. Rehabilitation will have to allow the child to live not just useful experiences but above all gratifying ones, since only fulfilling and satisfactory experiences will be preserved (therapy exercise as guided meaningful experience). It is not sufficient only to teach how to do something (rehabilitation as a repertoire of available spare parts), but it is also necessary to transmit the pleasure of doing it, and this is the most difficult part of physiotherapy. The acquisition is demonstrated by the individual's spontaneous use of what has been learnt. The passage from learning to acquisition allows the child to reduce the conscious control of movement and transfer to it the meaning of the action, therefore from the instrument to the aim. Saturation of acquisition, more than absolute inability to learn, leads to gradual interruption of treatment.

The peculiar aspect of acquisition is the capacity to spontaneously and voluntarily utilize what has been learnt, while progress is the capacity to disassemble in order to reassemble, to select in order to transfer, to take apart in order to rebuild according to the same rules but into new shapes, in different contexts, and for different aims. In short, progress is the capacity to transform accomplished acquisitions, modifying and generalizing them, shifting from the adopted formulas to rules which underlie mechanisms and dominate processes. This generalization capacity distinguishes learning from training, and the child through this processes is shown to be an active protagonist of his own rehabilitation and not a passive container of actions which are considered therapeutic by others. Everybody can measure the effectiveness of the therapeutic intervention by observing the child's progress. Progress, conceived as the capacity to transfer what the individual has learned in the therapy setting to the real life context, is the ultimate therapy goal and makes the difference between creating and repeating, inventing and copying.

Instead, if acquisitions remain only related to the therapeutic context, i.e., they are performed only with a therapist and only in a specific setting, treatment ends up being a closed loop, as often demonstrated by the continuous request for maintenance therapies, which shows the incapacity on the part of the patient to make progress and therefore the liability of his acquisitions.

When the patient becomes unable to make progress, therapy loses its true meaning and inevitably becomes only care to limit progressive physical degradation.

Even under the best conditions, the changes produced by therapy will not subvert the nature of the motor defect, i.e., the diagnosis, but it will change the patient's capacities in terms of ability, competence, self-determination, autonomy, independence, participation, and well-being. CP treatment thus does not imply the possibility to introduce normality patterns, but the capacity to modify in an adaptative way the patients capabilities, according to the objectives he wants to achieve. A treatment that tries to replace the patients pathological behavior with a normal motor one is impossible in its assumption.

Just think about a hemiplegic child: treatment should focus on the impaired side and the best result would be to make this side as able as the unaffected one. Instead, let us try to see the hemiplegic child as being formed by two different sides, which have to achieve different abilities to carry out tasks that can be performed by using only one upper limb or that need both limbs. We should be extremely worried if we discovered that for tasks of a certain level, the unaffected limb is actually used in the same way as the plegic one. In that case, the patient would have serious problems in the post-lesion re-organization of the CNS. Hyper-specialization of the unaffected hand, as well as its "invasion" into the operating area of the plegic one, are expressions of CSN post-lesion re-organization, of the need to look for and find new adaptative solutions despite hemiplegia: this is the expression of functional recovery.

Conversely, observing a hemiplegic child who is not able to specialize his unaffected hand but tends to use it like the plegic one, indicates a poor capacity to re-organize the CNS; therefore this has to be considered a negative prognostic marker. Hemiplegic individuals are composed of two halves and we have to deal with both of them: the unaffected half, to allow him to develop compensatory adaptative solutions, and the impaired one to allow him to assist the unaffected hand in all those activities that cannot be carried out by only one hand. In this vision, the child has to be trained not to give up any mono-lateral elementary tasks which the impaired hand is still able to perform alone.

Perceptive Perspective

As broadly acknowledged, perceptive information can be quantitatively distinguished according to its intensity (from hyper-acuity to deficiency). It is easy to understand that if an individual loses sensitivity, CNS will not effectively control what the executive systems are doing (tactile, kinesthetic, baresthetic, vestibular and visual elements are fundamental for motor control) (see chapter 5). To perform a correct movement, it is necessary to receive correct perceptive information; and to collect correct perceptive information, it is necessary to be able to make a correct movement. In CP, these conditions are impossible and on a prognostic level they affect the patient's recovery possibilities.

Segment representation is certainly correlated to motor operations, but also to the perceptive information that can be collected through them. Beyond the preserved repertoire, from the utilization perspective, the condition of a patient with severe motor impairment but with good sensitivity is better than the contrary, due to the relevance of information flow necessary to control motor performance (see chapter 5). It is extremely surprising that CP definitions do not consider this important aspect (Bax et al. 2005).

Besides a quantitative axis, or perceptive intensity, from the qualitative point of view it is possible to distinguish an attention/negligence (or indifference) perceptive axis and a pleasure/intolerance perceptive axis.

The different meaning of verbs such as hearing or listening, seeing or looking, tasting or savoring, smelling or sniffing can only be understood by making reference to an ideal attention/negligence axis. If, for example, we consider the kinesthetic and baresthetic information needed for posture control, we can observe patients who are able to perceive signals but are unable to give them the necessary perceptive attention, as in the case of a "stand up" diplegic child (see chapter 14). The "stand-up" child is able to adjust his posture if he is informed from the outside about the inadequacy of his position: therefore, he does not have insuperable motor problems nor difficulties in collecting and analyzing information, since he is able to accomplish the necessary postural correction (use of repertoire). Instead, he is unable to give continuous attention to information (deficiency of baresthetic and kinesthetic proprioceptive attention); therefore he is not able to "automate" position and maintain and adjust it if it risks being compromised or lost. "Stand-up" diplegic patients always need additional information from outside, for example "don't slouch, stand-up or keep upright", because information from inside is not taken into sufficient account, unless another perceptive channel, for example gaze, informs the child of what is happening. Only in that case can patients pay attention to what is happening at postural level and correct themselves.

Analyzing the position of baresthetic and kinesthetic information on the pleasure/intolerance perceptive axis, it is possible to understand the problem of the "falling" child (see chapter 14), who is able to perceive (intensity) and give attention to the signal but who does not have sufficient perceptive tolerance. He feels he is falling even when lying supine on the floor (illusion). The "falling" child is able to collect information, but since he cannot tolerate it, he consciously prefers not to move (intentional palsy as "defensive" modality), adopting a reactive spasticity. Also in normal individuals, perceptive conditions exceeding a certain intensity may become so unpleasant that they affect the individual's capacity to move. Marzani and co-workers (1997) confirm that if for some CP children the presence of disorders like fear of space, fear of falling, etc., seems to be connected to emotional events, other children are more affected by perceptive disorders, with different intensity levels, which are worsened by, or which worsen the difficulties of self-integration. "The issue and complexity of perceptive interpretation are clear if we consider that each perception is the result of a close relation between sensory-perceptive integrations and emotions, and it is also the result of memory and of experience processing. Perceptions accumulated continuously by a synchronic Self transform it into a diachronic Self, until subjective perceptive consciousness is built, which is unique for everybody" (Marzani, 2005).

If we ask a patient who suffers from vertigo to climb a ladder at a certain height he will refuse to go on, not due to a motor inability, but because vertigo does not allow him to achieve the preliminary perceptive consensus for this motor action. The design and planning of a movement require calibrating the perceptive information that is going to be collected, and which is necessary for the control of what is being done. If calibration indicates intolerance to the result, the consensus to the action will be missing, regardless of the fact that the motor program is feasible (see chapter 5). The statement "be careful, you are on your own", instead of improving patient's concentration on his motor performance, and therefore the result quality, ends up revoking the consensus on the action, since it makes the individual deepen his perceptive analysis. The patient who manages to stand still 10 cm from the wall but cannot do so at 50 cm certainly does not have a motor problem, but he is unable to tolerate distance, depth, and emptiness in the surrounding space (see chapter 5). The inability to tolerate this space-related information does not allow him to access what he would be able to perform from a motor perspective, due to the lack of preliminary perceptive consensus (anticipatory). Focusing on the extreme consequences of this concept, from the rehabilitation point of view, before wondering if a CP patient can carry out a certain motor action, we should ask ourselves if he can tolerate the subsequent information from the perceptive point of view. This observation should be enough to question the concept of early treatment: can the availability of motor repertoire and preliminary perceptive consensus be considered simultaneous? Can motor repertoire availability come before perceptive consensus? Is it correct to perform motor re-education before perceptive re-education? What happens if intolerable perceptions are induced in the child? It is easy to demonstrate that refusal or renouncement to move often are induced behaviors (intentional palsy). Do we have to consider the value of containment only from the psychological point of view? Or are there also precise perceptive values? In physiotherapy, besides what, how and how much (space dimension), there are also other aspects such as starting from when, how long, and until when (time dimension). To what extent is this dimension important for the stability of the recovery process? Does what the child learns generate interest (attention) and pleasure? Consequently, will it merit to be preserved (therapy as learning and acquisition of favourable stable modifications) and sought for (passion)? In our opinion, the number of things that should be transferred to the child often does not coincide with the number of things that the child is able to collect. It is not true that although physiotherapy sometimes does not work well, it is never harmful. The child who gives up is a child who has been asked to do too much or to do it too early. In some cases, starting later is a way to achieve more, and "being able to do" and "being able not to do" become strategies consistent with the natural history of the related clinical form, with the available resources, and the choices made by the individual.

Just like the "stand-up" child, the "falling" child presents with a reversed palsy, because the real paralytic is the child who is not able to stay erect, and not the child who can stand up and then loses his position or decides not to stand up in order not to suffer from the discomfort provoked by this motor performance. It is not a problem of muscle force, since it is easily demonstrable that, from the kinesthetic point of view, postures assumed by these individuals are extremely disadvantageous (the comparison with motor strategies adopted by neuromuscular patients would be sufficient to understand this). There are some diplegic patients who can walk but cannot stop, who always lean forward following the projection of their center of gravity, and who find it easier to walk fast rather than slowly, and others who arrive too fast and crash against something or someone, trying to hold on to the first thing they bump into. These children sometimes have problems of intolerance towards the space behind them, and this is why they project themselves forward: because it would be impossible to protect themselves if they were about to fall backwards. Other diplegic patients, due to the same problem, only walk if the therapist's finger touches their shoulder (one finger is sufficient to make them walk): is that finger a motor facilitation? If it were only a motor facilitation, sooner or later it would be possible to take it away. The therapist's finger is something more than a motor facilitation: it is an orientation compass, it is a counterweight for balance, it is a defense shield, it is a railing capable of reducing the backward space, it is the key that allows the patient to reach the perceptive consensus to use his motor repertoire. This is why it is so difficult to remove the finger.

To understand these clinical forms of CP, it is more important to adopt the point of view of perception rather than that of movement. Indeed, analyzing only the repertoire of motor modules, sequences and combinations, a more favorable evaluation can be made of the child's capacities, which may strongly contrast with his actual spontaneous development.

Along the pleasure/intolerance perceptive axis, we can find the individual who carries out movement as a repeated intransitive action due to a deviation of his relation behavior (generally only an added component to CP) (see chapter 10). The subjective and intransitive intrinsic pleasure generated by movement becomes such a desired aim for the individual that it overcomes any other transitive and goal directed action.

Movement, necessarily harmonious, is repeatedly generated to collect and appreciate the perceptive information that it produces. The individual does not use movement to adapt himself to environmental requests and/or to adapt the environment to his needs, but simply to draw pleasure from it. This is also an intentional palsy: movement is directed from the individual to himself and not to the environment, and the only aim is to feel pleasure. Needless to say, that in this case the motor repertoire is rich both in quantity and quality, and a good motor learning capacity is preserved.

Intentionality Perspective

Curiosity, as the need to know, as proactive behavior, and as a source of perturbations of the world, through which it is possible to collect and select information necessary to build experience, is fundamentally important for the CP prognosis. Being proactive means inducing and participating in changes, launching messages, and creating new conditions, provoking the surrounding world to better understand and judge it, improving in this way the instruments we can use to interact with it (motor development). Such knowledge tools become new categories in the relation between man and environment, testifying to the individual's awareness of his needs and to his determination to use his repertoire to achieve his aims and desires. Therefore intention constitutes a measure of the pleasure in acting, and of acting with pleasure.

A curious and proactive child obtains because he knows how to ask for things, he receives because he knows how to give, he can do because he is able to try, he learns because he can produce perturbations, and, therefore, he changes and develops. Instead, a lazy child cannot change, nor can a child who is too passive, or not lively enough, or one who is too easily satisfied, or who gets over things too rapidly, or who does not find any other interest outside himself. For an individual who cannot be curious, motivated, participating, and proactive, physiotherapy is highly questionable. Educational interventions aiming at developing interests would be preferable in such a case, instead of physiotherapy addressed at improving tools. However, the patient's curiosity is positive only if he accepts to use it within a specific domain that has been previously indicated and prepared by the therapist according to therapy objectives (setting). In CP, palsy is first of all an action problem (conceptual disorder), and only secondarily a motor disorder. If palsy has anything to do with movement, first of all it is due to a losts of pleasure, or a discomfort, or a lack of satisfaction.

The concept of intentionality also includes the pleasure and the emotion felt by the patient when performing a certain action, or the discomfort that derives from it, i.e., what he feels as well as what he is doing (success and satisfaction, failure and frustration, joy or sadness, desire or disappointment, gratification or punishment). Only those who feel pleasure in acting continue to modify their functions to achieve a result that is more and more suitable for the required tasks.

Learning does not only mean selecting and preserving, but also suppressing and removing. Success and pleasant things are preserved, while the lack of success and unpleasant experiences are removed. Perceptive and cognitive aspects play an important role in this, and they are the pre-requisite for the development of any other function.

To rehabilitate, we have to ask questions about the patient's motivations and about his learning capacity, and each time we have to wonder if what the child has done has also generated pleasure for him and sufficient satisfaction to be preserved (relation between perceptive and intentional). The child's refusal and opposition to therapy cannot be considered as an expression of relation or progress, or as a tool to build his personality or increase his self-esteem. The "if he wants it - he will achieve it" equation, which is so often supported by parents, will not allow us to achieve any development or solution if the palsy continues to be considered solely as a motor problem, as a uniquely objective aspect. The "if he wants it - he will achieve it" child, regardless of his repertoire and preserved capacity of use, reveals that he is not ready to modify himself to become more suitable to environmental requirements, and shows an insufficient willingness to modify the surrounding world to make it more suitable to meet his aims and desires. The fact that a child with CP manages to accomplish a certain task does not mean that he desires to do it. On the contrary, most of the time, the "if he wants to do it - he will achieve it" child does not want it at all (hidden palsy), and before accepting the task he negotiates an external award, which pays him back for a pleasure that he cannot feel internally, due to perceptive discomfort, fatigue, loss of pleasure, depression, fear, and fantasies, which become ghosts. But sooner or later, no award will be able to pay him back for the discomfort that he feels and eventually he will stop. It is easier to estimate that a patient will learn to walk at 8 years of age, rather than being sure that he will still be walking at 18. If he stops, will it be only due to a lack of physiotherapy and deformity relapses, or rather to a lack of interest and determination, or even a question of self identity (feeling adequate when sitting and uneasy when standing upright)? Through physiotherapy, aids, models, an adequate environment and an educated community, we can improve the "he is able" side, but what can we do to help the child desire it? We have to start thinking about satisfaction and success, creating self-confidence and self-investment, searching for pleasure within the "being able to be", "being able to do", "being able to become". The real nature of CP is linked to "he wants to": this is not just movement and not only perception, but it is related to the child's intentionality in his relation with the world and in his willingness to change.

References

AA.VV. Gruppo Italiano Paralisi Cerebrali Infantili (2000) Manifesto per la riabilitazione del bambino. Roma

Aicardi J, Bax M (1998) Cerebral palsy. In: Aicardi J (ed) Diseases of the nervous System in Childhood, 2nd Ed. Mac Keith Press, London, pp 210-239

Bax M (1964) Terminology and classification of cerebral palsy. Dev Med Child Neurol 6:295-297

Bax M, Goldstein M, Rosenbaum P et al (2005) Proposed definition and classification of cerebral palsy. Dev Med Child Neurol 47:571-6

Behrman RE, Kliegman RM, Arvin AM (1998) Nelson essentials of pediatrics, 3rd ed. WB Saunders, Philadelphia, pp 50-52

Bobath B, Bobath K (1975) Motor development in the different types of cerebral palsy. Heinemann Physiotherapy, London

Camerini GB, De Panfilis C (2003) Psicomotricità dello sviluppo. Carocci Faber Editore, Roma

Colver AF, Sethumadhavan T (2003) The term diplegia should be abandoned. Arch Dis Child 88:286-290

De Ajuriaguerra J (1974) Manuel de Psychiatrie de l'Enfant. Masson, Paris

De Renzi E, Faglioni P (1990) Aprassia. In: Denes G, Pizzamiglio L (eds) Manuale di neuropsicologia. Zanichelli editore, Bologna

Giannoni P, Zerbino L (2000) Fuori schema. Manuale per il trattamento delle paralisi cerebrali infantili. Springer – Verlag Italia, Milano

Hagberg B (1989) Nosology and classification of cerebral palsy. Giorn Neuropsich Età Evol 4:12-17

Ingram TTS (1955) A study of cerebral palsy in the childhood population of Edinburgh. Arc Dis Child 30:85-98

Marzani C, Amadei P, Clini MC et al (1997) La PCI nel bambino prematuro: l'intervento riabilitativo nel servizio territoriale. Difficoltà e prospettive. Relazione al convegno: "Diagnosi e trattamento precoce della paralisi cerebrale infantile del prematuro". Ancona 20-21 giugno 1997

Milani Comparetti A (1965) La natura del difetto motorio nella paralisi cerebrale infantile. Infanzia anormale 64:587-628

Milani Comparetti A (1978) Classification des infirmités motrices cérébrales. Médicine et Hygiène 36:2024-2029

Milani Comparetti A, Gidoni EA (1976) Dalla parte del neonato, proposte per una competenza prognostica. Neuropsichiatria infantile 175:5-18

Milani Comparetti A, Gidoni EA (1978) Semeiotica neurologica per la prognosi. VII congresso SINPIA Firenze

Mutch L, Alberman E, Hagberg B et al (1992) Cerebral palsy epidemiology: where are we now and where are we going? Dev Med Child Neurol 34:547-551

Perfetti C (1979) La rieducazione motoria nell'emiplegico. Ghedini editore, Milano

Piaget J (1936) La naissance de l'intelligence chez l'enfant. Delachaux et Niestlé, Neuchâtel-Paris

Rigardetto R, Siravegna D (1999) La riabilitazione dei disturbi minori del movimento: le disprassie. Gior Neuropsich Età Evol 20:274-283

Sabbadini G (1995) Manuale di neuropsicologia dell'età evolutiva. Zanichelli, Bologna

Sabbadini G, Bonini P, Pezzarossa B, Pierro MM (1978) Paralisi cerebrale e condizioni affini. Il Pensiero Scientifico Editore, Roma

Smyth TR (1991) Abnormal clumsiness in children: a deficit in motor programming? Child Care Health Development 17:283-94

Surveillance Cerebral Palsy in Europe (SCPE): a collaboration of cerebral palsy register. Dev Med Child Neurol 2000 42:816-24

Kinematic Classification

A. Ferrari

Cerebral palsy (CP) is considered a "persistent but not unchangeable disorder of movement and posture"; therefore, the definition given 50 years ago by Ingram (1955) and Mac Keith & Polani (1959), and subsequently divulged by Bax (1964), is still accepted as valid. In fact, also ad hoc international commission has recently reaffirmed the concept: CP is a disorder of development of posture and movement (Bax et al. 2005). In order to be consistent with this definition, the only way to classify CP would be through an analysis of posture and movement (intended from the kinesiological point of view as gesture), assessed in terms of quality (type) and of quantity (measure) (Ferrari, 1995). Actually, the most popular criterion to classify CP has always been based on the topographic (geographic) distribution of the motor impairment: tetraplegia (quadriplegia), diplegia, hemiplegia, with minor variations to these macro-categories: paraplegia, double hemiplegia, triplegia, monoplegia, reversed diplegia. Taxonomically, no importance is usually given to the location of the brain lesion (internal capsule, basal nuclei, semi-oval centre, cerebellum, etc.), to the timing of the central nervous system (CNS) damage (pre-, peri-post-natal) with the exception of hemiparetic forms (see chapter 16), to the etiology (prematurity, dystocia, neonatal asphyxia, intracranial hemorrhage, meningoencephalitis, etc.), to pathogenesis (traumatic, toxic, infective), to CNS lesion extent, which can today be quantified by neuroimaging (see chapter 3), to neurological deficits associated with palsy and their syndromic combination (epilepsy, mental retardation, sensorial deficiency, perceptive disorders, dysphonia, dysarthria, learning disabilities, behavior disorders, etc.), to both primitive and secondary associated signs and symptoms, and to their origin. Only two clinical forms have been precisely classified: choreoathetosis associated with deafness, consequent to nuclear icterus due to mother-fetus Rh-factor incompatibility, and ataxia consequent to congenital hydrocephalus (Ingram, 1984).

The criterion of topographic distribution of impaired movement (tetraplegia, diplegia, hemiplegia, and variants), although generally accepted, is anyway not exempt from criticism, since the distinction between tetraplegia and diplegia has never been completely clarified. Instead the observation that half of the neuroimages of hemiplegic children show lesions also on the homolateral hemisphere (Clayes et al. 1983) raises doubt about the assumption that the unaffected hemiside can be deemed as "completely normal" (see chapter 16).

The literature defines *tetraplegias* as those cases of CP characterized by "an equal involvement of the four limbs", and *diplegias* as forms in which the lower limbs demonstrate to be "more affected than the upper ones". However it has never been established if this comparison should be based on the existing clinical signs (tone, reflexes, muscular strength, endurance, etc.) or on patient functional abilities. According to Colver and Sethumadhavan (2003), a comparison based on clinical signs could be extremely simple in the most serious cases, but very ambiguous in intermediate situations. Moreover, some signs could vary from one day to the next and could be affected by the current mood of the child. Inter- and intra-observer diagnostic variability when assessing the same clinical sign also needs to be taken into account. For example, does "*walking with difficulties and being in need of walking aid*" mean that the lower limbs are more or less affected than the upper limbs when the child is "*not able to write neatly and needs assistance to go to the toilet*"? (Colver and Sethumadhavan, 2003).

The word diplegia, which literally should mean palsy of two limbs distributed in any way, appeared in a study made by Sach and Peterson in 1890, in which this form of CP, distributed over the four limbs, was differentiated from paraplegia, which referred to a motor impairment only affecting the lower limbs. Just a few years after this publication, Freud (1893) used the same word to indicate "a cerebral palsy of the two sides", therefore also tretraplegia and double hemiplegia, utilizing this word also for non-spastic forms. In the 1950s Minear (Minear, 1956) resumed the idea of diplegia as a bilateral form of "*paralysis affecting like parts on either side of the body*". Therefore, starting from Ingram's classification (1955), the term diplegia has been clinically applied when the involvement of the patient's homologous limbs turns out to be quite symmetric and when, relative to pathognomic signs like "hypertonia", "hypereflexia", "clonus", "weakness", etc., the involvement of the patient's lower limbs is significantly higher than that of the upper ones ("*more severe in the lower limbs than in the upper*"). But also "hypotonia", "dystonia", "stiffness" (Ingram, 1955), or "atony" (Little Club memorandum, 1959), or even "ataxia with dyssynergy and intention tremor" (Hagberg et al. 1975) and activities such as "static upright position", "walking", and "manipulation" have progressively cross over into this definition. In 1959 the Little Club, which gathered the most important researchers of CP of that time, both English and not, confirmed that in diplegia the upper limbs must be less affected than the lower ones: "*In diplegia there is affection of the muscles of all four limbs. The lower limbs are the more affected*". In 1975 Bobath and Bobath declared that in diplegia spasticity is distributed in a more or less symmetric way; children usually have a good control of their head, speech is normally not affected, and a few individuals suffer from strabismus, differently from tetraplegia, which implies poor control of the head and often severely affected speech and eye coordination. In the most unclear cases, Milani Comparetti (1965) proposed a further criterion beside the official signs, more "modern" and clarifying, based on the capacity of the patient's upper limbs to show an effective support reaction, if necessary by using orthopedic devices, such as walkers, crutches, or canes (diplegia = functionally paraparetic tetraparesis).

Nevertheless, even with such clarifications, for children with a real tetraparesis it is still possible that the lower limbs are more affected than the upper ones, so that they could be incorrectly classified as diplegic, especially if they do not present a significant mental retardation. Similarly, it can occur that true diplegic children, who are able to walk even without orthopedic devices for their upper limbs, are considered as tetraplegic only because the extent of the impairment to their lower limbs is similar, in terms of quantity, to the damage of their upper ones. From the point of view of rehabilitation results, we would then have false diplegic children who are unable to walk even with the aid of walkers, and false tetraplegic subjects who, instead, manage to walk unaided. This contradicts the broadly accepted statement according to which tetraplegia is a more severe form than diplegia, and thwarts any attempt to statistically measure the effectiveness of re-education treatments.

To further explain the differences between tetraplegia and diplegia, other clinical elements have been analyzed. Tetraplegia (see chapter 13) is usually associated with severe mental retardation; oral-facial impairment secondary to pseudo-bulbar paralysis, with subsequent impairment of mastication, swallowing, and speech; peristalsis (frequent gastroesophageal reflux) and bowel movement difficulties; high respiratory morbidity with scarcely productive cough; drug-resistant epileptic seizures that are hard to manage, and slow or stunted somatic growth. Conversely, diplegia (see chapter 15) shows a wider range of modules, combinations and motor sequences, and a functional use of fewer pathologic synergies. This means that patients have a higher freedom of choice, which should not to be interpreted as a residual normality, but as a degree of independence from primitive and pathological patterns when associating different motion modules. Compared to real tetraplegic individuals, diplegic patients show somatic hypo-development, mental retardation, speech disorders, epilepsy and pseudo-bulbar paralysis less frequently. Conversely, even if it does not generally arise, they quite often have dysperceptive disorders (such as of: spatial orienteering and walk trajectory directing, especially in the absence of adequate visual targets, coordinating eye/head movements; tolerating surrounding emptiness and spatial depth, especially backward; coping with unstabilizing inputs and loss of balance; matching information coming from different receptor systems, for example visual inputs with proprioceptive information, etc.) and dyspraxic disorders (organizing in sequence all the required movements to accomplish a targeted motor activity) (see chapter 6). For these and other reasons related to mental and emotional aspects (low self-esteem, delegation, renunciation, etc.), by assessing the quality of motor control independently from patient motor repertoire, it is possible to distinguish, among diplegic patients, children who are particularly skilled and others who are notably inhibited and clumsy. This makes the border line regarding tetraplegia even more uncertain. In diplegia, differently from tetraplegia, orthopedic functional surgery of muscular contractures and joint deformities is performed after the acquisition of upright position and walking. It is however necessary to point out that diplegic children acquire these abilities earlier than real tetraplegic ones; therefore the influence of the disproportion between the growth of muscles and long bones due to the action of spasticity is lower (Lovell-Winters, 1990; Rang, 1990; Morrissy and Weinstein, 2001). It is true that all diplegic patients will manage to walk in a more or less functional way. Nevertheless, poor motivation, insufficient force generation (Ross et al. 2002) and early fatigue, due also to the severity of secondary deformities, may lead many patients to stop walking, generally at the beginning of adolescence. Diplegic children achieve quite a good manipulation ability, especially in the sitting position (where "tetraparesis" transforms into "paraparesis"), except in the presence of dyskinetic elements. Due to difficulty in wrist control (extensors deficiency), they often show some uncertainty when performing complex activities such as using cutlery or other tools, writing, or drawing (Rudolph et al. 1996). A good manipulation competence does not always imply a good autonomy level, since diplegic children, as we have seen, can have dyspraxic and dysperceptive problems, limiting the outcomes they can achieve.

Diplegic children having a better cognitive ability, generally proportional to a greater function of the upper limbs ("*the more affected the upper limbs, the lower is intelligence*" Forfar and Arneil's: Textbook of Pediatrics, 2003), can however present other psychopathological problems (exasperated conflict, depression, anxiety, phobias, maniac behaviors, etc.). In this regard, the family's greater expectations also become important (expectation for a positive result according to the logic "*if he/she wants it = he/she will do it*) (see chapter 9). All diplegic children achieve acceptable speech, in terms of quantity, at least after early childhood, but some can have phonetic problems which do not depend on breathing function, or make semantic mistakes (see chapter 8). Due to the low incidence of pseudo-bulbar paralysis, diplegic children develop hypersialosis and sialorrhea less frequently than tetrapelegic ones. Visually, diplegia frequently includes gaze paralysis, especially with esotropy, which makes pathological motor patterns more severe, especially during locomotion (scissor pattern) and manipulation (eye-hand-mouth interaction) (see chapter 7). Apart from balance, in diplegic children all other sensorial functions are usually not severely affected (see chapter 5).

Even considering all these further specifications, as already observed by Hagberg (1989), in clinical practice, during development, the taxonomic classification of many spastic patients shifts from diplegia to tetraplegia and vice versa: "*many children change categories as they grow older*". In fact, it still needs to be clarified if the presence or absence of epileptic fits, mental retardation, and dysphagia is relevant for the diagnostic definition or if it is only an associated sign. For example, if a child with CP has all four limbs severely affected, with the upper limbs slightly less impaired than the lower ones, will it be possible to refer to the presence or absence of these other signs to classify the palsy as tetraplegia or diplegia? Since it is impossible to find a satisfactory and universally accepted solution, and troubled by the problems generated by this confusion on epidemiological case records, Colver and Sethumadhavan (2003) have recently put forth an extreme solution: the abolition of both words, diplegia and tetraplegia ("*there is no justification for separating diplegia and quadriplegia*"). Instead they joined the two forms into the macro category of bilateral palsy (*bilateral spastic cerebral palsy*), which is not totally new since it was already used by Freud more than a century ago (1897). Therefore CP would be mainly subdivided into two groups: bilateral forms and monolateral forms. Undoubtedly, this solution, certainly better than the ambiguous expression "psychomotor retardation", which is still too often employed in uncertain diagnosis, can be of help for epidemiological studies, by abolishing any uncertainty between tetraplegia and diplegia (concepts like: more or less affected, prevalent, etc.).

In a recent paper published by our group (Cioni et al. 2008) data were presented to support the proposal to maintain the distinction between spastic tetraplegia and diplegia. This idea has been validated by testing a group of 467 subjects with CP, 213 with diplegia and 115 with tetraplegia, consecutively admitted between Jan. 2005 and Dec. 2006 to the

CP-specialized centers of Pisa and Reggio Emilia. Among the spastic forms, which included the largest group of children with CP (93% in our sample), it was possible to distinguish children with diplegia and tetraplegia not only according to a different level of gross and fine motor impairment, as demonstrated with the assessment scales applied in this study (GMFCS, BFMF, MACS), but also according to other disabilities associated to the paralysis (mental, visual impairment, seizures). In fact subjects with tetraplegia strongly differed from those with diplegia, both for motor functions and for other disabilities. The main results of this study are reported in Table 12.1.

Table 12.1 Main features of 213 subjects with diplegia and 113 with tetraplegia (Cioni et al. 2008)

Type of Cerebral Palsy	Subject	Diplegia n (%)	Tetraplegia n (%)	Test	p
Mental development	Normal	105 (49%)	14 (12%)	Chi square	,000
	Abnormal	89 (42%)	95 (82,5%)		
	Missing	19 (9%)	6 (5,5)		
		Total ss 213	Total ss 115		
Epilepsy	Present	22 (10,5)	54 (47%)	Chi square	,000
	Absent	191 (89,5)	61 (53%)		
		Total ss 213	Total ss 115		
Visual abilities	Normal	94 (44%)	24 (21%)	Chi square	,000
	Abnormal	105 (49%)	89 (77,5%)		
	Missing	14 (7%)	2 (1,5%)		
		Total ss 213	Total ss 115		
GMFCS	Level 1	54 (25,5%)	2 (1,5%)	ANOVA,	,000
	Level 2	51(24%)		Bonferroni	
	Level 3	57(26,5%)	3 (2,5%)	post hoc	
	Level 4	33 (15,5%)	34 (29,5%)		
	Level 5	4 (2%)	72 (62,5%)		
	Missing	14 (6,5%)	4 (3,5%)		
BFMF		Total ss 213	Total ss115		
	Level 1	41(33,5%)			,000
	Level 2	68 (56%)	7 (10%)		
	Level 3	9 (7,5%)	11(15%)		
	Level 4	2 (1,5%)	22 (30%)		
	Level 5	2 (1,5%)	32 (45%)		
		Total ss 122	Total ss 72		
MACS	Level 1	18 (31%)			,000
	Level 2	22 (38%)			
	Level 3	15 (26%)	7 (17%)		
	Level 4	3 (5%)	13 (32%)		
	Level 5		21 (51%)		
		Total ss 58	Total ss 41		

BFMF, Bimanual Fine Motor Function; GMFCS, Gross Motor Function Classification System; MACS, Manual Ability Classification System; ss, subjects.

Our findings are in agreement with the results of a recent multicenter European study of cerebral palsy (Carr et al. 2006), where clinical and neuroradiological features of children with diplegia and tetraplegia were compared. Significant differences in the clinical picture and in brain MRI were reported between the two groups of diplegic and tetraplegic CP children.

Differently from the idea of Colver and of the SCPE group (2000) to create the macro category of bilateral cerebral palsy, our group underlines the need for professionals who work in the rehabilitation field to maintain the distinction between diplegia and tetraplegia. In rehabilitation, these terms remain indispensable clinical descriptors. In fact it can be deceiving to put into the same category children whose highest reachable target in a life-time is the control of sitting position and children who walk, run and jump, from the first years of life. From an epidemiological point of view we believe that the single category of bilateral CP forms could give more homogeneous data collected in different geographic areas. However, it has less useful application for health policies aimed at programming and organizing sanitary intervention, activities in which the distinction between diplegia and tetraplegia remains important in order to measure appropriately the rehabilitation needs and the associated sanitary and social costs as a consequence of the different motor impair-ment and of overall disability.

Moreover, the Colver and Sethumadhavan proposal is not satisfactory even for hemi-plegia (see chapter 16), which is frequently bilateral, at least as far as the lesions are concerned (Clayes et al. 1983, Cioni et al. 1999). If the presence of contralateral coordina-tion synkinesis and Raimiste's phenomenon does not contradict the hemiparesis diagnosis, should we then define the palsy as "monolateral" rather than bilateral, even if strongly asymmetric, when the child displays signs of "sympathetic" behaviors in the unaffected lower limb, adopted in order to achieve functional symmetry (for example, in fast walking and running), or movements associated in the unaffected side, or above all imitation synk-inesis, or mirror movements (see subgroups of the fourth form of diplegia, chapter 15, and hemiplegic forms, chapter 16)?

At any rate, the proposal to distinguish between bilateral and monolateral forms of CP eliminates any possibility to measure the results of the re-educational treatment, since the inclusion clinical condition of patients is not homogeneous. Therefore, another solution needs to be found.

A possibility could be represented by motoscopic analysis, based on the detection of child posture-motor disorders as proposed by Milani Comparetti (1978); another one could be the assessment of the basic functional architecture like anti-gravity organization, walk, and manipulation (Ferrari, 1997). A further possibility could be to measure the severity of impairment based on a specific motor performance like walking (Winters et al. 1987; Perry, 1992). In general, the aim is to overcome the criterion based on somatic positioning of the motor disorder (tetraplegia, diplegia, hemiplegia), to interpret its nature and deter-mine its size.

The adoption of different criteria for the nosological classification is a semiological choice. The main classification idea or concept is the possibility to put on the same level all the different situations offered by clinical practice, separating each condition from the others, through one or more homogeneous criteria that allow us to define and highlight it.

Probably, the difficulty in the creation of an acceptable and meaningful classification for all CP forms lies in the impossibility to apply the principle of coplanarity and in the intrinsic ambiguity of the adopted criteria. Indeed, it is hard to imagine that such a complex phenomenon as CP could be fully analyzed only from a single point of view, even though it might look interesting and meaningful (Ferrari, 1995). The official classification proposed by Bax (1964), based on the location of motor the disorder (tetraplegia, diplegia, hemiplegia), requires the adoption of additional criteria, such as the presence of mental retardation or epilepsy, oculomotion disorders, chewing-swallowing and speech impairments, etc. therefore losing the coplanarity of its basic criteria.

Diarchy I

> Extension pattern
> *Upper limbs*: extended shoulders, flexed wrist with ulnar deviation, closed fist, adducted thumb.
> *Lower limbs*: extended, adducted, intrarotated (crossing)

> Flexion pattern
> Upper and lower limbs in global flexion

In the natural history of this form, in inveterate cases, which are not adequately treated, a functional compromise is reached (between the two dominant patterns) in global semi-flexion. The syndrome can be tetra-, para- or hemiparetic, always with a higher prevalence in lower limbs. Typical deformities gradually arise (pes equinus, adductor hip syndrome, flexor knee syndrome, etc., all of surgical interest)

Diarchy II

> Pseudo-Moro (startle reflex pattern) supine decubitus on a rigid plane: arms outstretched position, claw hands, forced inspiration, anguished expression, semi-abducted lower limbs, and supinated feet

> Propulsion
> With the trunk inclined forward, upper limbs flexed on the shoulders, downwards oriented, intrarotated, extended elbows with forearm pronation, flexed wrists, closed fists. Extended head

The picture is worse for the upper limbs and head. The syndrome also includes: - dysphagia (mastication and swallowing disorder, loss of saliva) and dysarthria with tongue movement limited to protusion-retraction (sucking pattern). The lack of lateral movement produces a typical deformity of the oral cavity. The mouth shows spasms when opening, which are associated with the propulsion pattern or appear during motor engagement situations.
- Disorders of ocular combined movements, with a frequent prevalence of upwards conjugated movements

Motoscopic semiotics is the visual observation of postural control and movement and, more precisely, the analysis of postural and motor profiles, both normal and pathological (Milani Comparetti, 1978). By applying this technique to spastic syndromes, two different clinical forms can be identified, both characterized by "*a poverty in movement in general and particularly in normal movement*" that Milani Comparetti associated with "regression syndrome" (reduced freedom due to "excessive power by predominant pathologic profiles"). Each form imposes two profiles that represent diarchies I and II (Milani Comparetti, 1978).

Along with these spastic forms, Milani Comparetti's proposed classification includes an apostural syndrome ("postural and motor activity deficiency").

Apostural picture

Retardation in motor development = retardation in the structuring of anti-gravity primary automatisms. The child is traditionally defined as "floppy" or "hypotonic".

It can be observed in normal children or mentally retarded ones, but it can also represent an early stage or a partial aspect of cerebral palsy, whose typical patterns can be recognized despite poor motor and postural involvement. The later the manifestation of the definitive picture, the more serious the mental retardation.

A dyskinetic syndrome is also described ("interference of pathological profiles"), which appears as "a disorder in the distribution and fluctuation of muscle tone, with typically grotesque postures and athetosic movements (a subgroup is the choreoathetosic CP, where muscle tone is reduced and movements are more rapid and proximal)" (Milani Comparetti, 1978).

Dystonic-athetoid syndromes (pattern integration disorder)

This clinical picture is characterized by a disorder in pattern integration. Pattern analysis allows the examiner to recognize a continuous conflict, i.e. for the hand a continuous conflict between "avoiding" and "reaching"; for facial mimics between the pattern for acid taste and bitter taste; and among many others, the conflict between the patterns of arm extension-pronation and the asymmetric "tonic" reflex of the neck. The patterns of the II diarchy may belong to the dystonic-athetoid conflict. The disorder disappears during sleep and can vary in time. It is often anticipated by an apostural stage.

Milani Comparetti's proposal is completed by an ataxic syndrome characterized by "a defect in movement coordination with dysmetria, balance disorders, tremors and hypotonia, usually accompanied by hyposthenia and difficult to diagnose before the second year of life" (Milani Comparetti, 1978).

Ataxic picture

Dys-chronometry as integration disorder of normal functional patterns over time (it cannot be recognized on images and generally cannot be diagnosed during the first year of life).

Milani Comparetti was the first one who created a CP classification that is consistent with the international definition of "posture and movement disorder". He also studied the consequences of primitive and pathological patterns on child motor organization. His goal was not only nosological, since he aimed above all at making early diagnosis, reliable prognostic evaluation, and targeted therapeutic indication possible. The desire to measure the results obtained from physiotherapy treatment emerged clearly from his proposal: "… *in II diarchy the re-educational prognosis is limited. Generally we cannot expect to achieve autonomy in walking or in daily life activities*" (Milani Comparetti, 1978).

Therefore, with respect to the official classification of spastic forms (tetraplegia, diplegia, hemiplegia), a step forward was made, but the core problem was not solved, namely, how to clearly distinguish tetraplegia from diplegia and diplegia from hemiplegia. In Milani Comparetti's classification, tetraplegic forms have become two (diarchies I and II), while diplegic and hemiplegic forms are all included in diarchy I. Even if the latter represents a more homogeneous nosological group, it can anyway include cases of different severity, which can be associated to tetraplegia, diplegia and hemiplegia.

The declared aim of achieving an early diagnosis is undoubtedly reached, apart from cases with a prolonged apostural phase during early motor development, which can evolve towards spastic forms (more frequently towards diarchy II, especially if mental retardation is present) and dyskinetic or ataxic ones. Striving to meet the need that taxonomy used to classify CP supports therapeutic indications and allows us objective measurement of the results attained with the re-educational treatment, Milani Comparetti's proposal has yet to achieve the expected result. Since diarchies can be considered "matrixes" that heavily affect postural behaviors (in fact they are recognized through the study of postures and their variations), they cannot influence adaptive functions like walk, manipulation or speech, which are the core subjects of therapy intervention. With reference to posture organization, the influence of diarchies cannot be modified through therapeutic exercise, drugs, orthesis, orthopedic surgery or functional neurology, at least not in all patients and not in a foreseeable and verifiable way.

However Milani Comparetti managed to pave the way to a CP classification based on function analysis, starting from posture control.

In the same period in London Bobath and Bobath (1975), studying gait function in spastic diplegias, made a distinction between two patient populations:

- "*The children with a strong flexion of the dorsal column and anterior inclination of the pelvis move the trunk backwards in order to lift a leg and bring it forward in order to take a step. Therefore they launch their body forwards in order to transfer the weight (pigeon gait)*".

- *"The children who have a straight and upright dorsal column with lumbar lordosis (due to flexor spasticity of the hips, especially of the iliopsoas) will alternate the lateral flexion of the trunk from the belt upwards in order to move their rigid legs forward. While a normal person has a ductile motion of legs and a relatively stable trunk, these children show an excessive trunk mobility and stiff legs (duck gait)".*

Similarly, studying the hemiplegic gait, Winters et al. (1987) proposed to distinguish, within the same pathologic association pattern, four different impairment levels, based on the study of kinematics expressed by the patient on the sagittal plane:

- *Type 1 hemiplegia*
  Hemiplegia type 1 consists of a falling foot, which is very easily observed during the suspension stage of gait (swing phase), due to the inability to selectively control the ankle dorsal-flexors, or to hyperactivity of the triceps surae. The contact with the ground occurs flatfooted or on the toes. Since there is no contracture or retraction of calf muscles, during late stance the ankle dorsal flexion is relatively normal. The compensation for this defect is an increase in knee flexion at mid and terminal swing, initial contact and load acceptance. The swinging hip increases the flexion, with an increase in pelvic lordosis. Rodda and Graham's (2001) revision states that this gait pattern is rare, unless calf muscles have already undergone surgical release.

- *Type 2 hemiplegia*
  – 2 a pes equinus plus neutral knee and extended hip
  – 2 b pes equinus plus genu recurvatum and hyper-extended hip
  Hemiplegia type 2 is by far the most frequent type in clinical practice. A real pes equinus is observed in the stance phase of gait, due to the contracture and/or retraction of the soleus and gastrocnemius muscles and tibialis posterior and flexor muscles along the toes: there is a variable degree of forefoot fall during the swing phase due to the involvement of tibialis anterior function and ankle dorsal-flexors. During most of the stance phase, a real pes equinus is observed, with the ankle in the plantar flexion range. The coupled plantar flexors / knee extensors is hyper-active and the knee has to assume an extended or recurvatum position (Boyd and Graham, 1997). Gait speed is slower than type 1.

- *Type 3 hemiplegia*
  Hemiplegia type 3 is characterized by soleus or gastrocneumius spasticity or by their retraction, by the impairment of the dorsal-flexion angle during the swing phase and by "stiff knee gait", as a result of the contemporaneous contraction of the hamstrings and rectus femoris (Rodda and Graham, 2001), with a consequent limited flexion of the knee during swing. To compensate this defect, the patient will adopt a contralateral dynamic pes equinus, increase hip homolateral flexion, or use a sickle pattern.

- *Type 4 hemiplegia*
  Hemiplegia type 4 is characterized by a greater proximal involvement (hip flexors + adductors) and the pattern is similar to the one that can be observed in spastic diplegia (tibio-tarsic plantiflexed during swing and stance, reduced sagittal movement of the knee, hip flexion, and adduction contracture). However, as the involvement is unilateral, there will be a clear asymmetry, including the horizontal translation of the pelvis. The sagittal plane shows a pes equinus, with a flexed stiff knee, flexed hip, and antev-

ersed pelvis, with subsequent lumbar lordosis at the end of the stance phase. On the frontal plane there is hip adduction, and on the horizontal plane there is internal rotation. The incidence of hip subluxation is high (Rodda and Graham, 2001).

The idea that in order to classify the different clinical forms of CP it is necessary to overcome the univocal criterion based on topographic distribution of impairment (tetraplegia, diplegia, hemiplegia) and to analyze the function structure (architecture) equally satisfies ordinative needs (taxonomy), as well as assessment (main existing problems) and therapeutic ones (possible solutions). However, it is necessary to try to understand which motor functions are more adequate for this investigation and to decipher their architecture and above all the meaning of the different clinical forms that are included in the general "cerebral palsy" category.

First of all it is essential to consider that CP clinical forms are not only a direct expression of structural impairment, therefore of etiology, pathogenesis and lesion timing, but they are mainly the manifestation of the route followed by the CNS to "re"-construct the adaptive functions "despite" the presence of the damage. In CP, in fact, "palsy" is *the form of the function that is implemented by an individual whose CNS has been damaged in order to satisfy the demands coming from the environment*" (Ferrari, 1990). It is not the sum of the defects and deficits of the organs, structures, or systems, but rather represents "*the different functioning (computation) pattern, the different "re"-organization and action (consistency) modalities of a nervous system that keeps on looking for new solutions due to the internal need to become adequate and the external one to adapt itself to the surrounding world*" (Ferrari, 1993). Therefore it is only possible to establish general relations between lesion site, nature and size, and palsy and recovery processes. It is quite common to observe that children with very similar neuroimaging can have very different clinical manifestations of CP and on the other hand children with very similar motor behaviors can have completely different lesion histories. A very clear example of this is represented by hemiplegic forms, which show bilateral hemispheric lesions in a high percentage of cases (see chapter 16). In a few words, the "biological" idea that CP is a *development palsy* (defect semiotics) is opposed to the neuro-psychic-biological concept of *palsy development* (Ferrari, 1988), to be intended as a new dynamic relation that the individual tries to build "somehow" with the surrounding environment (resource semiotics). By understanding the rules of this process, and by studying past behaviors (anamnesis) and current behaviors (diagnosis), it will be possible to foresee the future behavior (prognosis) of the CP. Our therapies will become more efficient if they manage to tune into the patient nervous system "self-organization", by exploiting its inner consistency, to favorably deviate the organization of its adaptive functions in a stable way. Therefore re-educating the child with CP means first of all being able to set up a dialogue with his brain and not only dealing with his body.

A New Proposal

In each different clinical form of CP, the development of adaptive functions follows its own coherent logic (natural history), combined with *central factors* (top down components), as proposed in Milani Comparetti's diarchies, which are common to all individuals with the same form and of the same age and that are usually unchangeable, and *peripheral factors* (bottom up components), which are typical of the locomotor system and not necessarily identical between individuals, and *individual strategies* (coping solutions), which are quite diversified performances that can often be reproduced and are invented by the patient in "order to cope in the best possible way" (Ferrari, 2003). The sum of the central, peripheral, and individual components represents the function architecture of CP clinical forms.

Top Down Components

In CP it is possible to separately recognize the constitutive characteristics of the motor performance and the operating modalities used by the structure that organizes them. The more serious the palsy, the more recognizable they are. The performance includes all patient motor behaviors: from modules to synergies (see chapter 4), starting from the lowest integration level, the monosynaptic reflex, and arriving at the highest one, that of specialized gesture, through reactions, primary motor patterns, secondary automatisms, etc. Instead, the organizing structure includes information collection and processing, comparison and integration of sensations into perceptions, recognition of perceptions and their storage as representations and final elaboration into life experiences (see chapter 5); action design and planning (see chapter 8); simultaneous and sequential control capacity; the possibility to automate the perceptive-motor patterns which are at the basis of the most repeated performances, to avoid conscious control; memory in all its forms and above all learning and acquisition ability. To simplify the understanding of the proposed model, it is possible to imagine that, when constructing a function such as locomotion and manipulation, the different types of motor performance act as ingredients, while recipes used to mix them together show how the operating systems are used by the organizing structure. We have already explicitly used this paradigm when we mentioned Milani Comparetti's "bellini" (gracious) movements (see chapter 11) as quality indicators of the child's motor repertoire, and freedom of choice or motor equivalence (see chapter 4) as indicators of the properties and efficiency of the organizing structure. Since young children have limited CNS abilities, the recipes will be elementary and mainly based on the assembly of simple components, such as pre-formed elements like reflexes, reactions, and primary motor patterns. The use of these will progressively decrease, and give way to "specialized" tailor-made movements, that is to say movements learnt and adapted through the integration with the environment and improved on through experience, shaped in intensity and duration, combined into complex formulas and produced in a time tested, pre-cabled sequence, with a guaranteed result (see chapter 6).

The development of manipulation gives us an example of how the CNS acts when accomplishing a motor function. The basic ingredients to "build" it when the child faces this endeavor are mainly genetically pre-formed elements: grasp, release, magnet, avoiding, limb support reaction (extension in quadrupedic antigravity and flexion in bipedic antigravity, see chapter 13), and flight reaction, all combined in elementary synergies. So, for example, it is easier to hold an object in the hand, moving it closer in a centripetal pattern, than to release it following centrifugal movement. Of course, "outside pattern" movements can be present from the beginning; they are more isolated and differentiated, as, for example, the singular movement of the thumb or index finger, freeing them from a closed hand. To make manipulation sufficiently effective, all the basic elements will have to be present and the organizing structure will have to be able to make them interact according to a partial and provisional predominance logic that Milani Comparetti (1965) called competitive interaction. If the grasp is totally absent, we will not be able to grasp anything, but even when this reaction is excessively present (fist closure) we will not be able to manipulate because, paradoxically, the hand is already committed to grasping itself, in particular its own thumb. If the magnet reaction is missing, we will not be able to follow, reach and hold a moving object, and if the avoiding reaction is missing we will not be able to rapidly move away from a contact that might be dangerous. The organizing structure has the task to make decisions on the most suitable combination form (recipe) on the basis of the collected information (tactile, proprioceptive, visual). As a consequence, the grasp and magnet reactions might be combined with the support reaction (under extension) when a child is crawling and holding a toy in his hand, or (under flexion) when the child is drawing and contemporarily supporting himself on the homolateral elbow. Instead, the release and avoiding reaction might need to integrate with the flight reaction in order to protect the hand or the whole upper limb from a harmful surface (something that burns, freezes, stings, hitches, stains, etc). When the limb support reaction (under extension) has to occur rapidly, the support reaction combines with the hand release like in a parachute reaction (or protective extension), while, during the sit up maneuver the support reaction under flexion must be combined with the grasp reaction. When the child launches an object in the air, the hand opening (shift from the grasp to the release reaction) has to occur immediately after the end of the extension of the entire limb, just like its closure during a flexion movement, when he catches a flying object. This is a more complicated task for the organizing structure: not only deciding about the quantity of each ingredient, but also establishing how ingredients have to arrive or leave the scene, what in cinematographic terms would be called fading. When building a tower, in order to lift and delicately place the pieces, the child has to be able to combine grasp and release, magnet and avoiding, support and flight, and so on. The appearance of these capacities shows the ability level that has been reached by the organizing structure: it will not be the object that adjusts itself and lets the fingers close around it, but rather the hand that progressively differentiates and anticipates and adapts itself to the object characteristics in order to reach the action target.

In normal individuals, the mutual influence of constitutive elements (ingredients) and the properties of the organizing structure (recipes) within the involved function can only be recognized when this function appears, while in children with CP both are visible during their whole lives. This situation, which could be defined as still primitive, can be worsened by pathological patterns of CP and the laws that regulate them, namely the pathological organization (see chapter 4). The function will be more impaired if the individual ingredients (primitive and pathological) become less numerous and more aggressive, and if the properties of the organizing structure become more limited and rigid. Milani Comparetti's diarchy II shows one of these extreme situations, where the propulsive reaction and the startle reaction are the two "tyrants", both with a low excitability threshold in relation to endogenous and exogenous stimuli and both able to extend their influence to the whole body, "globalizing" the pattern.

The presence of clearly pathological reflexes, reactions, primary motor patterns and secondary automatisms that cannot be related to any normal developmental stage, such as the adduction and intrarotation of the shoulder, elbow flexion, forearm pronation, wrist flexion, and fist closure in some hemiplegias, is accompanied in CP by the alteration of some normal behaviors which are sometimes insufficient or excessively inhibited, such as the lack of parachute reaction of the upper limbs. More often they are exaggerated in terms of size, or they are still present after the natural physiological remission when the organizational period has finished, such as in the automatic walk for some forms of tetraplegia (see chapter 13) and the support reaction during the flexion of the upper limbs for some forms of diplegia (see chapter 15).

The primitive and pathological patterns on which functions are based represent the intimate nature of the CP motor defect. As we have seen, the properties of the organizational structure have to be added to them: first of all the motor learning ability in order to acquire new adaptative behaviors and the ability to make learnt sequences automatic so that the performance can shift from voluntary to spontaneous (with or without conscious thinking).

The defects and deficits of the top down components are the least changeable part of the CP. Therapists still define as a "prognostic treatment" (see chapter 11) the measurement of the possibility given to the child, who is therapeutically guided through proper facilitations and sometimes inhibitions, to be able to re-organize the function by modifying its architecture (selection of ingredients and choice of recipes) within the freedom of choice offered by the cerebral palsy.

Is it possible for a clinical form to transform into another? If we recognize the main task of top down elements within the function architecture and accept the very low possibility to change them through the therapeutic instruments so far available, we will have to infer that clinical forms represent stable categories, with internal differences, but which cannot be modified so as to lose their nosological identity. However we are ready to admit that some of the signs used to identify clinical forms can be ambiguous, especially in young children, and that during long periods of motor development we do not have sufficient visual perceptives to recognize and foresee the most significant differences between one form and the others.

Bottom Up Components

As well as "central" components, in CP, similarly to what happens in other childhood disabling diseases, the locomotor apparatus (LA) has its own "peripheral" characteristics, which the CNS has to take into account when building adaptative functions. Some of these characteristics, like secondary deformities, are direct consequence of mistakes made by the CNS which are amplified by somatic growth; some others, like the structural characteristics of muscles, connective tissue, and to a certain extent of bones, are a direct consequence of the lesion but not of the palsy (Romanini et al. 1989; Ito et al. 1996; Marbini et al. 2002; Lieber and Friden, 2002; Lieber et al. 2004; Novacheck, 2003; Dan and Cheron, 2004).

Strength, elasticity, and endurance of striated muscle, weakening of the connective tissue especially of capsules and ligaments, bone deformity, etc., are not to be underestimated when determining function architecture. Hip luxation, for example, cannot be exclusively attributed to the predominant motor pattern (scissor pattern) or to the imbalance between dominant flexor and adductor muscles and weak extensor and abductor ones. In fact, given the same pattern, the hips of tetraplegic children often luxate, the hips of diplegic ones can do so as well, while those of hemiplegic children never luxate. It is necessary not only to consider the strength of the hip muscles, but also the intrinsic resistance of the joints the shape of the femur and the pelvis bone structure. Therefore, it is clear that also hip joints can luxate in those individuals whose lower limbs have a frog pattern (especially if spasms in extension are present, see chapter 13), although in a different direction (frontally, or laterally and/or posteriorly). The therapeutic repercussions of luxation attributed to some muscle (hypertonia), to the joint itself (instability), or to bones (acetabular hypoplasia, distortion of inclination and declination angles) cannot obviously be the same.

Recent studies on the structure of CP spastic muscle have demonstrated the presence of 2c type fetal fibers, disproportion of fiber types, myopathic degeneration phenomena, denervation/reinnervation and alteration of rheological properties of the mesenchyme (Castle et al. 1979; Lieber and Friden, 2002; Delp 2003). The micrographies obtained from muscles of spastic individuals showed an increase in the variability of fiber size, an increase in the number of round fibers, moth-eaten fibers and in some cases an increase in extracellular space (Lieber et al. 2004). The severity of spasticity is correlated to the rise in collagen content (Booth, 2001). Although composed of cells that have a shortened resting sarcomere length and a higher intrinsic passive stiffness, spastic muscle contains extra cellular matrix whose mechanical resistance is lower than normal (Lieber et al. 2004). Muscle cells of spastic individuals have a higher deformability module, which is a consequence of the remodeling of structural components like titin and collagen (Frieden and Lieber, 2003). The average size of spastic muscle cells is only a third of normal ones (Lieber and Friden, 2002); spastic muscle is not able to match its length to the lengthening of the relative bone levers (Lovel-Winters, 1990; Rang, 1990), therefore it is less able to add new series of sarcomeres as a response to somatic growth (Lieber and Friden, 2002), etc.

During the building of adaptative functions between the CNS and LA, there are continuous reciprocal influences. A clear example can be clubfoot. A child, who is otherwise normal but born with a stiff clubfoot (supinated and equinovarus), will achieve upright position and walk with no delay, but he will do it following a different pattern. Since there is no reason to think that "peripheral" foot alterations should correspond to equivalent "central" alterations of the organization of upright position and walk, we have to conclude that it is clearly the foot deformity that "guides" the brain towards the most suitable solution for its structural characteristics. What should we think of pes equinus in a CP child or, more in general, of his spasticity? For neurologists, talipes equinus is undoubtedly a central sign, a "top down" sign, which is pathognomonic of the current clinical form and developmental stage. Instead, for orthopedic surgeons it has a specific peripheral, "bottom up", meaning, since with chemical inhibition or surgical correction, significant changes in the function architecture can be achieved. And what should the rehabilitator think? He agrees with both of them, in the sense that pes equinus can effectively be an expression of the CNS organizational strategy and therefore be a top down element, since its correction would be detrimental, for example, due to the abatement of the standing reaction. On the other hand it can testify to the influence exercised by the locomotor apparatus on the CNS, and therefore be a bottom up element. In this case its correction obliges the CNS to reset the function architecture, by applying advantageous changes that are similar, but not identical, to the ones that occur in the child with congenital clubfoot after surgical correction. Obviously there is some overlap between central and peripheral components, so that it is important not just to decide what to correct, but also when to correct (organizational level maturation), and above all how much to correct (function modification limit).

Therefore, spasticity is both a "central" and a peripheral sign that is able to affect the CNS's choices, similarly to what happens in a muscular dystrophic child due to weakness. A clear demonstration of this aspect is provided by the syndrome of Segawa et al. (1976), which is a progressive palsy provoked by the exhaustion of central mediators and sensitive to substitutive treatment with levoDOPA. The presence of a worsening spasticity progressively forces the child suffering from this rare syndrome to adopt motor behaviors similar to those of diplegic individuals, up to the loss of gait. After substitutive therapy is adopted, the clinical picture dramatically reverses, with the patient progressing from the wheelchair to walking ability in a few days.

In conclusion, during the building of adaptative functions, the CNS is also widely influenced by the structural characteristics of the locomotor apparatus, which it has contributed to modify both at a primitive level, throughout tissue growth and typing, and at a secondary one by pathological motricity.

Coping Solutions

The third factor to be considered in order to understand function architecture is represented by the coping solutions adopted by the child to "cope in the best possible way". Since they are individual performances, coping solutions cannot be outlined in a general context, but some "tricks" are quite common and can be used as examples. In the tetraplegic child's walk, for example, we can observe gesture simplification and posture freezing (see chapter 13); in the diplegic child's gait (see chapter 15) we can see sequence acceleration, swinging movements of trunk and upper limbs, shifts in joint fulcrum and overall point of balance, etc. In the hemiplegic child's manipulation (see chapter 16) we can notice the visual support of the plegic hand (second information), the use of subsidiary pincers (mouth, chin, armpit, elbow, tights, etc.), the evocation of pathological synergy proximally originated in order to pick up the object, and the activation of servomotor movements in order to release it, etc.

Bottom up components and especially coping solutions are responsible for the interindividual differences that can be observed between individuals that belong to the same clinical form of CP, and for intra-individual modifications that occur during development for the same compensation strategy (internal coherence) and after the most aggressive interventions (drugs and functional surgery). They can be widely influenced by re-educational treatment carried by specialists, who, after abandoning the normality model, should be able to observe the best "tricks" discovered by the most able CP individuals and teach them to the less able ones.

Conclusions

In CP spastic syndromes the basic motor functions that are more suitable to be explored for taxonomic aims are:
- The antigravity function (posture organization) in tetraplegia forms
- The mature gait pattern in diplegia forms
- The manipulation modality in hemiplegia forms

From a prognostic point of view, since not all tetraplegic children can sit down autonomously and reach an upright position, even with devices, posture architecture can be considered as the most significant function to be explored in order to classify and measure the results that have been obtained with the re-educational treatment. Instead, all diplegic children can walk (although some of them later stop), but with extremely different modalities and conditions. Gait architecture can therefore be a significant element to differentiate the various clinical forms of diplegia and above all to choose modalities and tools for re-educational treatment.

The same criterion could also be valid for hemiplegic individuals, as already demonstrated by Winters et al. (1987), but since no hemiplegic child (apart from hemiplegia "plus") shows difficulties in spontaneously acquiring upright position and walk, in our opinion it is preferable to classify the clinical forms of childhood hemiplegia by analyzing manipulation architecture.

A classification which is organized on the analysis of the architecture of basic motor functions such as postural control, locomotion, and manipulation is surely in line with the current CP international definition of "posture and motion disorder". However in order to be relevant for the therapeutic project and the measurement of the results obtained by re-educational treatment, the assessment should not simply consider only the motor elements (modules, praxes, and actions, see chapter 4), but it should be extended to include perceptive features (sensations, perceptions, and representations, see chapter 5) and intentional aspects (see chapters 8 and 9).

In the chapter on tetraplegic forms we will analyze the different aspects of antigravity organization in CP children, which include the absence of a true reaction to the body weight, the primitive defense in flexion the horizontal antigravity reaction typical of four legged animals and finally the organization of verticality. In the chapter dedicated to diplegias we will successively analyze different walking patterns, starting from the most severe form (forward leaning propulsion) up to the mildest ones (distal diplegia and double hemiplegia). Finally, in the chapter devoted to infantile hemiplegias, the different strategies of manipulation will be analyzed, following inversely a progressive scale of severity in order to comply with the proposal of Winters et al. regarding hemiplegic gait classification.

12

The following box lists the main top down and bottom up components of the anti-gravity function, gait, and manipulation. Only a few examples of coping solutions will be given.

Antigravity function

Top down components
> Body weight support reaction
> Righting reaction
    axial cranio-caudal
    rotatory - derotative
> Fixation mechanisms
    disto-proximal
    proximo-distal
> Egocentric, allocentric or geocentric spatial reference
> Others

Bottom up components
> Muscle strength and endurance
> Soft tissue stiffness
> Joint ROM and deformities
> Bone geometry
> Segment weight
> Others

Coping solutions
> Spatial head position
> Eye movements
> Functional compromise between global synergies
> Gesture simplification
> Joint freezing
> Use of grasp to facilitate posture control
> Others

Gait function

Top down components
> Body weight support reaction
> Step central pattern generator
> Static and dynamic balance
> Orientation and direction
> Topographic memory
> Others

(*cont* ➤)

(*cont*)

Bottom up components
> Muscle strength and endurance
> Soft tissue stiffness
> Joint ROM and bone deformities
> Segment weight
> Others

Coping solutions
> Gesture simplification
> Sequence acceleration
> Trunk and arm swing movements
> Selection and succession of rotation fulcra
> Choice of points of balance
> Others

Manipulation function

Top down components
> Orientation
> Direction
> Reaching
> Anticipation and grasping
> Exploration and manipulation
> Transport
> Release
> Others

Bottom up components
> Muscle strength and endurance
> Joint ROM and bone deformities
> Others

Coping solutions
> Visual support of the plegic hand activity (supplementary information)
> Use of subsidiary pincers (mouth, chin, armpit, elbow, tights, etc.)
> Proximal-originated evocation of the pathological synergy to close the plegic hand
> Implementation of servomotor movements to release the object
> Passive loading of the plegic hand by the unaffected one
> Others

12

References

Bax M (1964) Terminology and classification of cerebral palsy. Dev Med Child Neurol 6:295-7

Bax M, Goldstein M, Rosenbaum P et al (2005) Proposed definition and classification of cerebral palsy. Dev Med Child Neurol 47:571-6

Bobath B, Bobath K (1975) Motor development in the different types of cerebral palsy. William Heinemann Medical Books, London

Booth CM, Cortina-Borja MJ, Theologis TN (2001) Collagen accumulation in muscles of children with cerebral palsy and correlation with severity of spasticity. Dev Med Child Neurol 43:314-20

Boyd R, Graham HK (1997) Botulinum toxin A in the management of children with cerebral palsy: indication and outcome. Eur J Neur 4:S15- S22

Carr LJ, Tydeman C, Bax, M (2006) Clinical findings from a multicentre European cerebral palsy study; can we distinguish quadriplegia from diplegia? Dev Med Child Neurol; suppl. 107, vol. 48, 4-5

Castle ME, Ryman TA, Schneider M (1979) Pathology of spastic muscle in cerebral palsy. Clin Orthop Rel Res 142:223-32

Cioni G, Lodesani M, Coluccini M et al (2008) The term diplegia should be enhanced (II): contribution to validation of a new classification system. Eur J Physic Rehab Med 44:203-211

Cioni G, Sales B, Paolicelli PB et al (1999) MRI and clinical characteristics of children with hemiplegic cerebral palsy. Neuropediatrics 30:249-255

Clayes V, Deonna T, Chrzanowski R (1983) Congenital hemiparesis: the spectrum of lesions. A clinical and computerized tomographic study of 37 cases. Helv Paedriatic Acta 38:439-455

Colver AF, Sethumadhavan T (2003) The term diplegia should be abandoned. Arch Dis Child 88:286-290

Dan B, Cheron G (2004) Reconstructing cerebral palsy. J Ped Neurology 2:57-64

Delp SL (2003) What causes increased muscle stiffness in cerebral palsy? Muscle Nerve 27:131-2. Review

Eliasson AC, Krumlinde-Sundholm L, Rosblad B et al (2006) The Manual Ability Classification System (MACS) for children with cerebral palsy: scale development and evidence of validity and reliability. Dev Med Child Neurol 48:549-54

Ferrari A (1988) Paralisi cerebrale infantile: problemi manifesti e problemi nascosti. Gior Ital Med Riab 2:166-170

Ferrari A (1990) Interpretive dimensions of infantile cerebral paralysis. In: Papini M, Pasquinelli A, Gidoni EA (eds) Development, handicap, rehabilitation: practice and theory. Excepta medica, International Congress Series 902, pp 193-204

Ferrari A (1993) Dal concetto di lesione a quello di paralisi. In: Cristofori Realdon V, Chinosi L (ed) Un bambino ancora da scoprire. Marsilio Editore, Venezia, pp 111-117

Ferrari A (1995) Paralisi cerebrali infantili: appunti di viaggio attorno al problema della classificazione. Giorn Neuropsich Età Evol 15:191-205

Ferrari A (1997) Proposte riabilitative nelle paralisi cerebrali infantili. Del Cerro editore, Pisa

Ferrari A (2003) In tema di postura e di controllo posturale. Giornale Italiano Medicina Riabilitativa, vol. 17 n 1:61-74

Freud S (1897) Die infantile Zerebral Laehmung. In: Notnagel ab Specielle Pathologie und Terapie. A Holder Inc, Wien 2 pp 1

Friden J, Lieber RL (2003) Spastic muscle cells are shorter and stiffer than normal cells. Muscle Nerve 27:157-164

Hagberg B (1989) Nosology and classification of cerebral palsy. Giorn Neuropsich Età Evol 4:12-17

Hagberg B, Hagberg G, Olow L (1975) The changing panorama of cerebral palsy in Sweden 1954-1970. Acta Paediatrica Scand 64:187-199

Himmelmann K, Beckung E, Hagberg G, Uvebrant P (2006) Gross and fine motor function and accompanying impairments in cerebral palsy. Dev Med Child Neurol 48:417-23

Ingram TTS (1955) A study of cerebral palsy in the childhood population of Edinburgh. Arc Dis Child 30:85-98

Ingram TTS (1984) A historical review of the definition and classification of the cerebral palsies. In: Stanley FJ, Alberman ED (eds) Spastics international. Oxford Blackwell Scientific, pp 1-11

Ito J, Araki A, Tanaka H et al (1996) Muscle histophatology in spastic cerebral palsy. Brain Dev 18:299-303

Lieber R, Friden J (2002) Spasticity causes a fundamental rearrangement of muscle joint interaction. Muscle Nerve 25:265-270

Lieber R, Steinman S, Barash I, Chambers H (2004) Structural and functional changes in spastic skeletal muscle. Muscle Nerve 29:615-627

Marbini A, Ferrari A, Cioni G et al (2002) Immunohistochemical study of muscle biopsy in children with cerebral palsy. Brain and Development 24:63-66

MacKeith RC, Mackenzie ICK, Polani PE (1959) The little club: memorandum on terminology and classification of cerebral palsy. Cerebral Palsy Bulletin 5:27-35

Mc Intosh N, Helms PJ, Smyth RL (2003) Forfar & Arneil's textbook of paediatrics, 6th edition. Churchill Livingstone, London

Milani Comparetti A (1965) La natura del difetto motorio nella paralisi cerebrale infantile. Infanzia Anormale 64:587-628

Milani Comparetti A (1978) Classification des infirmités motrices cérébrales. Médicine et Hygiène 36:2024-2029

Minear WL (1956) A classification of cerebral palsy. Pediatrics 18:841-845

Morrissey RT, Weinstein SL (2001) Lovell and Winter's pediatric orthopaedics, 5th ed. Lippincott Williams & Wilkins, Philadelphia

Novacheck TF (2003) Cerebral palsy pathomechanics. Lettura al congresso internazionale: Il cammino del bambino con paralisi cerebrale infantile: architettura della funzione e strategie di recupero. Reggio Emilia, November 12

Palisano RJ, Rosenbaum PL, Walter S et al (1997) Development and reliability of a system to classify gross motor function in children with cerebral palsy. Dev Med Child Neurol 39:214-223

Perry J (1992) Gait analysis: normal and pathological functions. Slack Inc Thorofare, New York

Rang M (1990) Cerebral palsy. In: Morrissy RT (Ed) Lovell and Winter's paediatric orthopedics, 3rd ed. JB Lippincott, Philadelphia pp 465-506

Rodda J, Graham HK (2001) Classification of gait patterns in spastic hemiplegia and spastic quadriplegia: a basis for management algorithm. Eur J Neurol 8:98-110

Romanini L, Villani C, Meloni C, Calvisi V (1989) Histological and morphological aspects of muscle in infantile cerebral palsy. Italian Journal Orthopaedic Traumat 15:87-93

Ross SA, Engsberg JR (2002) Relation between spasticity and strength in individuals with spastic diplegic cerebral palsy. Dev Med Child Neurol 44:148-57

Rudolph AM, Hoffman JIE, Rudolph CD (1996) Rudolph's pediatrics, 20th ed. Appleton & Lange

Sachs B, Petersen F (1890) A study of cerebral palsies of early life. J Nerv Ment Dis 17:295-332

Segawa M, Hosaya A, Miyagawa F (1976) Hereditary progressiva dystonia with marked diurnal fluctiations. In: Eldridge R, Fahn S (eds) Advances in neurology. New York Raven Press 14, pp 215-233

Surveillance Cerebral Palsy in Europe (SCPE): a collaboration of cerebral palsy register. Dev Med Child Neurol 2000; 42:816-24

Winters TF Jr, Gage JR, Hicks R (1987) Gait patterns in spastic hemiplegia in children and young adults. J Bone Joint Surg Am 69:437-41

Wright J, Rang M (1990) The spastic mouse and the search for an animal model of spasticity in human beings. Clin Orthop Relat Res; (253):12-9

Tetraplegic Forms

13

A. Ferrari, M. Lodesani, S. Muzzini, R. Pascale, S. Sassi

The literature defines tetraplegia (quadriplegia), or tetraparesis, as those cases of cerebral palsy (CP) characterized by:

- "Equivalent" involvement of all four limbs
- Difficult somatic growth
- Often severe mental retardation
- Frequent visual disorders (gaze paralysis, reduced visual acuity, visual agnosia, etc.)
- Possible hearing deficiency (deafness, intolerance to particular types of noise)
- Oro-facial impairment, secondary to pseudobulbar palsy, with consequent disorders of mastication, deglutition, facial expression and speech
- Epilepsy with fits difficult to control (infantile spasms, etc.)
- Severe periventricular leukomalacia with poroencephalic cysts as typical cerebral lesion.

In this complex neurological setting, the analysis of antigravity organization (CP = posture and movement disorder), as described in chapter 12, is usually sufficient to differentiate the main clinical forms of tetraplegia.

A short introduction to postural organization, its mechanisms and main disorders must be conducted before the principal tetraplegic forms are described.

Postural Analysis

Posture represents a specific mutual relation among all the constituent segments of the body, conceived as a unit that can be fractionized, relative to egocentric space coordinates, having the trunk of the individual as point of reference (Ferrari, 2003). However, in clinical practice, by posture we mean the ability of the individual to keep a certain *position* in the geocentric space, the one related to the force of gravity.

Space frames of reference

> *Egocentric frame*: the body of the individual is the point of reference, especially its longitudinal axis (idiotropic vector)
> *Allocentric or esocentric frame*: the external space is the point of reference
> *Geocentric frame*: its reference is the vertical line, i.e. the direction of gravitational force, and the horizontal line, i.e. the tangent planar to the earth's surface

In the genesis process of space knowledge, children at first use the egocentric frame of reference, constituted by their body, its positions, and its movements. By doing so, children process body coordinates that are taken as reference for the production of personal (active and passive) movements in space. This first frame of reference depends on the neurofunctional unit that is first developed, the body axis (the trunk), and on postures originating from it.

The second frame of reference, the allocentric one, comprises objects and events coming from the external world, which counterbalance errors the first frame might have produced.

Progressively, the ability to apply relevant information to recognize if the repetition of similar events happens in the same space emerges: this is the third frame of reference, corresponding to a *cognitive map* (Neisser, 1976) or an *inner model*, acquired at 18 months together with the maturation of symbolic functions and of mental representation skills, allowing the child to represent the mutual relations among the elements of the external world.

The *support reaction* expresses the capacity of the individual to oppose the action of gravity applied to body mass (weight). During motor physiologic development, a support reaction can be evoked starting from the 18th week of pregnancy (Milani Comparetti, 1976) up to approximately the second month of neonatal life.

This first "immature" expression of the support reaction, also called the André Thomas static reaction (1952), subsequently disappears (period of "astasia" or loss of the support reaction), only to reappear in a "mature" and definitive form between the seventh and tenth month of neonatal life. In fact, the André Thomas static reaction, which can be observed in pre-term infants and in the first months of life, is not really a support reaction, but rather the expression of the motor behavior implied in the ejection mechanism employed during delivery and therefore destined to disappear, once the function has followed its course. "*The so-called support reaction is likely to be an extension reaction aimed at facilitating the delivery of the foetus from the uterus, in that the foetus can actively participate in its ejection by pushing against the uterus vault .... The foetus, by setting its feet against the uterus vault, starts the ejection contractions and also extends, passing from the so-called foetal position to a globally extended position, with the upper limbs along the sides allowing its passage through the narrow delivery channel*" (Milani Comparetti, 1976).

Being independent from the coordinates of geocentric space, the André Thomas static reaction acquires different names consequent to the different examination positions:
• Creeping "reflex" according to Branco Lefevre
• Propulsive reaction according to Milani Comparetti

- Alternate creeping reaction according to Bauer.

"Forward progression is not an awkward attempt of locomotion on the horizontal plane, but a perfect mechanism to allow a subaqueous to emerge from the narrow passage of the delivery channel" (Milani Comparetti, 1976).

During the first year of life, the absence of the André Thomas static reaction, its preservation after the fifth month, its overall disorganization, or its exaggeration into a stereotypical pattern may evidence the existence of important neurological disorders, especially of CP. The André Thomas static reaction may be reduced or absent in "hypotonic" children (those with flaccid upper limbs) and in those with spinal cord lesions (presenting with tonic upper limbs), while it may be increased in "hypertonic" children, who respond to the test with an extension-adduction overreaction (scissor pattern) and standing on their toes (digitigrad pattern), or present with asymmetric posture indicating hemiparesis. In children with tetraplegia and spastic diplegia, the static reaction reverts into being positive before the sixth month or never stops being positive (abolition of the astasia period). A chronological mismatch in neuromotor development between the fourth and the sixth month in case of upright position possibility without acquisition of autonomous sitting position must always draw the clinician's attention. *"The straightening is very intense, with marked adduction, sometimes such as to trigger a scissor pattern. This increase in extensors tone may not be evident on first test, but it can be favored by subsequent flexion-extension movements of the lower limbs in plantar support, with consequent intense contraction of extensor muscles. ... In case of marked hypertonia of the muscles of the posterior plane, sometimes even from the neonatal period, every attempt to bring the child in sitting position during the examination produces an inevitable movement of generalised straightening in opisthotonus"* (Amiel-Tison and Grenier, 1985).

In case of CP, after the first year of life, to broadly analyze the possible modifications of the support reaction, at least relative to upright standing and the sitting position, mistakes of different type can be detected:
- quality mistakes: "primitive" support reaction
- quantity mistakes: – hypertonia (antigravity overreaction)
  - hypotonia (insufficient antigravity reaction, hypo-posture- capability).

The term *primitive support reaction* groups a heterogeneous cluster of postural behaviors in which the child clearly presents with a general ability to analyze and react to gravity by standing upright and holding that position, but through quite improper mechanisms such as freezing and distal fixation.

Under physiologic conditions, antigravity muscles are defined as those opposing the angular movement produced by supporting joints against the gravity applied to the weight of mobile segments. A competent antigravity behavior implies the central nervous system (CNS) ability to analyze weight force effects, for every joint station, and to counteract them through one or more isometric, synergic and simultaneous muscle contractions. The resulting strength must have the same point of application, intensity and direction of gravity, but the opposite sense. For this reason, the CNS must single out antigravity and progravity muscles involved in every posture and calibrate the required intensity of muscle contraction to generate force with respect to the body's mobile segments.

In the primitive support reaction, the CNS seems unable to single out the activity of antigravity from that of progravity muscles. Consequently, agonist and antagonist muscles operating on the same joint are simultaneously activated (pathological co-contraction), breaking the Sherrington principle of mutual inhibition, resulting in a joint "freezing" of the mobile segment, temporarily effective from the point of view of posture (and not of gesture) but detrimental from the ergonomic one. Due to a broader extension of the support, to a reduced presence of mobile segments, to a better overall stability, and to the subsequent improved static balance, the individual in sitting position may not need to implement "freezing" mechanisms and therefore appears more relaxed, or even "floppy" (unstable).

Hypertonia can be defined as a pathological support reaction or a support overreaction, developed along the so-called "extension pattern" (extended hips, tendency to intrarotation and thighs crossing, extended knees and talipes equinus), even if, at a closer look, none of the lower limb joint stations is totally extended. The hips still maintain a certain degree of flexion, usually not resolving in walking and associated with pelvis anteversion; the knees are never fully aligned, not even during vertical shift to the opposite limb (zenith cross); the feet, despite talipes equinus, show some metatarsus-phalangeal dorsiflexion components. By applying hypertonia in extension, the patient acts as if trying to disproportionately respond to his/her weight.

Also hypertonia in flexion, of both cerebral and spinal cord type, might cause the patient to crouch, assuming a fetus-like position (flexor pattern). In such cases, antigravity behavior, if persistent, is ascribable to a primitive flexion defense of akinetic tetraplegia.

The increased tone, referred to when describing hypertonia in extension or in flexion (hyper-tone), is not a "muscle" tone, that is the number of motor units still active in a muscle at rest which can be checked through the passive stretching of the muscle, but a "postural" tone, involved in maintaining the mobile segments of the body in a specifically defined mutual relation.

In sitting patients, the inhibition, at least partial, of hypertonia in extension can be achieved by introducing one or more elements of flexion, such as the forward bending of the head, forced flexion of the hip joints below 90 degrees, forced flexion of the knees below a right angle, dorsal flexion of the feet or plantar flexion of the toes. Such measures usually are insufficient if hypertonia in extension does not present in a stable fashion but as sudden spasms. Among all suggested expedients, the most effective "key" to control posture is definitely hip flexion below 90 degrees through an appropriate inclination of the seat surface and a matching 45 degree belt that secures the pelvis to the wheelchair.

Conversely, *hypotonia* represents an insufficient reaction to gravity due to "central" movement programming and/or planning mistakes, of motor or perceptual origin (top down, see chapter 12), rather than "peripheral" performance defects (bottom up, see chapter 12). This phenomenon is also rightly called *hypo-posture*, highlighting its temporal dimension (rapidly depleting support reaction), and, but not so correctly, *flaccidity* (sluggishness, weakness) to stress its quantitative dimension. The terms hypotonia, hypo-posture and flaccidity are often confused in clinical practice. Hypotonia can be better recognized with the patient in a sitting rather than a standing position. The patient adopts a generally flexed position: the head tends to bend forward, the trunk becomes progressively kyphotic, the shoulders undergo further depression and antepulsion, elbows are flexed, forearms show pronation, and the wrists are flexed with loose semi-extended fingers. At the lower limbs level, the pelvis appears as retroverted, thighs are slightly adduced, sometimes even slightly rotated outwards, knees are slightly flexed, and the feet are dropped and continuously slide off the wheelchair footboard due to the incapacity to keep knees properly flexed. The posture is not in the least stable and the individual tends to progressively intensify its overall flexion even without external destabilizing forces. A possible way to facilitate the support reaction in such patients is to incline the wheelchair's level surface forward to induce an active trunk straightening starting from the lumbar hinge (sitting position in active lordosis). This remedial action is effective but cannot be applied forever, due to the antigravity activity required by trunk erector muscles.

Straightening reactions are automated movements developing from the first year of life and guided by vestibular, visual, and tactile information. Their aim is to keep or recreate the head, trunk and limbs alignment in the egocentric frame. They are subdivided into *axial straightening* and *rotation-derotative straightening*. In spastic syndromes, axial straightening follows a cephalo-caudal direction and proximal-distal progression (Gesell, 1940) and, in a developmental pattern, anticipates the *rotation-derotative straightening*. The latter can be strongly impaired, giving an "en bloc" feature to trunk movements for the difficulty encountered in turning rightwards and leftwards from any initial position. In dyskinetic syndromes, the rotation-derotative straightening prevails on the axial one, the latter developing in a caudal-cranial rather than cranial-caudal direction. This results in the capacity to turn rightwards and leftwards, sometimes even to a more than normal extent, but also in the difficulty for the patient to completely extend the trunk and to keep the head, ideally representing the last link of the chain, straight and aligned especially in sitting and upright standing positions. The "reversed" characteristic of dyskinetic diplegia derives from this.

Fixation indicates the stability relation between body axis and limbs. *Distal fixation* (more primitive, with fixed limbs and mobile body axis) implies the stabilization of the central axis achieved in a centripetal and not centrifugal direction, i.e. from the limbs to the trunk rather than from the trunk to the limbs. Overall, to control biped standing position with hands holding stable supports, for example parallel bars, even distal fixation may be effective. However, to manipulate with two hands without pressing the trunk against a support and, most of all, to be able to walk, an essential prerequisite the patient must acquire is *proximal fixation* (more mature, with mobile limbs and fixed body axis), without which abandoning parallel bars or walking frames is impossible. To employ solely crutches or walking canes or, even more, to walk without the assistance of his upper limbs, the patient must have previously acquired the ability to fix the trunk on the supporting lower limb while the contra lateral one is moving, and at the same time to push the walking aids towards the ground instead of pulling the trunk towards them, as happens when clinging. If a proximal fixation is lacking, at every step, the pelvis shifts horizontally towards the supporting limb, while the trunk tends to bend towards the opposite side. The effects of a lack of proximal fixation can be detected even in sitting position: when performing a transitive movement with an arm, for example grasping a far object, the patient ends up shifting the trunk in the same direction as the hand and contemporaneously grasping with the other the armrest of the chair. Obviously, if the patient tried to manipulate with both arms, the trunk would lose stability, leaning towards any spatial direction.

> Distal fixation on hands and feet: walking with parallel bars or anterior or posterior weighted walking devices is possible
> Proximal fixation: characterized by thigh extension-adduction; walking is possible with four points canes, walking canes or antebrachial crutches
> One leg fixation: upper limbs canes can be abandoned; upper limbs can show defense, parachute, or balance movements
> Normal mature fixation: upper limbs can perform swinging walk movements

While in spastic syndromes a distal fixation can be clearly recognized at the start of the standing position, with support (parallel bars and walking devices) then progressively transforming into proximal fixation to allow walking with mobile support (four points canes, walking canes, antebrachial crutches), in dyskinetic syndromes fixation is fluctuating, sometimes being disto-proximal (the patient grasps the support with the hands while the body axis continues to move in an unstable way) then totally distal, then proximal again, etc., with consequent severe posture instability.

Posture Organization Disorders

According to Haeckel's (1892) theory, ontogenesis, i.e., the genesis of every single individual, recapitulates phylogenesis, i.e., the same evolutive history of the species the individual belongs to from the appearance of life on earth up to the present. From the water environment of the early period, with fish-like motor organization, the progenitor of man gradually moved onto the emerged land, becoming first amphibious and then a quadruped mammal. Relatively recently, in the evolutionary process, he acquired the ability to be supported by only the posterior limbs, becoming biped and devoting the anterior ones to more important tasks such as grasping and manipulation. This developmental path is sometimes testified to by the presence of embryonic malformations in the fetus, manifesting the primitive presence and the original function of organs that have now disappeared or that have been completely transformed (for example the fusion of both lower limbs to form a single fin, or sympodia, the presence of branchial pouches at the sides of the neck, palmate fingers or toes, excess mammary glands, double uterus, etc.). Our quadruped past history is easiest to demonstrate: the structure of the hip joints is, in fact, fully centred when the thigh is flexed at 90 degrees and slightly abducted, exactly as in four-legged mammals; the structure of the spinal column makes it more suitable to be employed as a beam rather than a pillar, therefore being more exposed to scoliosis and backache; but what confirms Haeckel's theory most is the metameric innervations, still dating back to the times of our past development. As in four-legged mammals, the part of the body that is the furthest from the head is the gluteus region (the circumanal area, since man lost his tail long ago) and not the foot plant as one might think considering an erect man.

The phylogenesis of mankind also includes the history of human posture evolution, conceived as an adaptive solution enacted to face the progressive change of the characteristics in the surrounding environment. No trace is left, in a healthy individual, of the long transformation process of posture, because all the antigravity development, from birth onwards, takes place following a strategy aimed at making man a biped animal. However, under pathological conditions, when this developmental path is already strongly disarranged in fetal life or in case of regressions to neurologically previous (or archaic) behaviors, traces of postures preceding the current vertical one can be detected. CP is the most recognized among such pathological conditions. It consists of four different models of posture organization: apostural or aquatic ability, stereotyped posture in flexion or primitive antigravity defense, quadruped or horizontal trunk antigravity, and biped or vertical trunk antigravity.

Apostural Form

This is the most severe form of posture disorganization or "regression" identifying the condition of those children who have no antigravity reaction at all. Posture organization can be compared to a sort of "floating" (in water, due to a lack of emptiness and to weight reduction by a third, a weaker antigravity reaction is needed).

Defense in Flexion

This is the typical antigravity behavior of the fetus, momentarily recognizable also in the newborn, still without an organized support reaction. It is characterized by an overall flexion behavior independent from body orientation in the surrounding space (geocentric frame). It recalls the so named fetal position.

Quadruped Antigravity

According to Haeckel's theory, this posture should be interpreted as a block of the ontogenetic development in which antigravity organization has stopped at the quadruped ability level: the body axis is horizontal and acts as a beam, while the four limbs perform as columns.

Biped Antigravity

This posture behavior implies the vertical position of the body axis, through the use of the supporting lower limbs, as in quadruped antigravity, and of the upper ones to perform grasp and manipulation. The pelvis acquires an intermediate weight bearing function, while vertebrae become the new pillar (backbone).

Evolution of the Support Reaction

The key element to recognize the four forms of antigravity organization is upper limb behavior, especially that of elbows and hands:

- In the apostural form, the upper limbs, totally incapable of a support reaction, hang at the side of the trunk, usually extended or semi-extended with open hands.
- In defense flexion crouching, similar to the fetal, position prevails (adduced shoulders, flexed elbows and wrists). Hands are slightly more closed but still passive.
- The shift to quadruped antigravity organization appears with acquisition of the extension response in prone position (adduced arms, extended elbows, flexed wrists and semi flexed fingers, with hands acting more as a support structure, i.e. hoof, than a tool to grasp and manipulate). However, initial manipulative abilities are possible, mostly far from the median line (hit, push, press, etc).
- The achievement of biped antigravity is shown by elbow flexion and fist clench, expressing grasp and the antigravity lifting ability of the trunk towards the hand, and also the ability to grasp and draw objects towards the body to manipulate them.
- A fifth possibility, typical of the normal mature antigravity organization, is the extended position of the upper limb along the side, free from posture tasks. If the upper limb needs to be used as a support, due to difficulties with one or both lower limbs, the movement will take place again in extension (support to walking cane).

The lower limb behavior is less relevant, presenting as extrarotated in extension in the apostural form, intrarotated in flexion in primitive defense and intrarotated in extension both in quadruped and in biped antigravity forms.

Antigravity Behavior and Tone Variations

Within the different antigravity behaviors, the terms hypertonic and hypotonic can define the degree (quantity parameter) of the support reaction. The features of posture organization should not be mistaken by tone variations. In this regard, it is interesting to observe how the apostural patient initially presents as a hypotonic (flaccid) individual, who may remain apostural and even becoming progressively hypertonic (stiff), as often happens during the aging process. With reference to a structure/function relation considering structure, flaccidity and stiffness should connote two opposite patient groups, while following function, flaccid and stiff individuals present some similarities as to their inability to organize an antigravity postural reaction. Stiffness might represent the evolution of a previous flaccidity in a uniform organized postural behavior, i.e., aposture.

Topographic Distribution

Furthermore, it can be stated that all apostural individuals, if classified on the basis of the somatic distribution of their impairment (topographic taxonomy), result as being tetraplegic.

The same can be stated for quadruped antigravity, while biped antigravity includes one form of tetraplegia, all forms of diplegia and, obviously, all forms of hemiplegia (since the unaffected hemiside allows the child to achieve an upright position).

The sole analysis of antigravity organization is therefore sufficient to classify tetraplegic forms, but not diplegic and hemiplegic ones. To differentiate the main clinical forms of diplegia, gait analysis should be applied. For infant hemiplegia, apart from lesion type and timing, the features of manipulation should be examined along with gait patterns, to achieve at functional diagnosis.

However, dyskinetic syndromes might emerge from transient apostural pictures, inevitably being cases of tetraplegia, or be organized in pictures of asymmetric diplegia (double hemiplegia), reversed diplegia and, ultimately, hemiplegia (hemidystonia).

Main Forms of Tetraplegia

According to the above description, four different main clinical syndromes can be identified based on the prevalence of one of the following features:
1. Apostural behavior
2. Antigravity defense in flexion
3. Quadruped or horizontal trunk antigravity
4. Biped or vertical trunk antigravity

A possible variant of horizontal trunk antigravity is tetraparesis with subcortical automatisms, while able-bodied tetraplegic represents a rare variant of vertical trunk antigravity.

The identification of the clinical forms of tetraplegia proposed by our classification, with the corresponding signs and symptoms allowing us to connote and differentiate them, is the result of the longitudinal observation of a very large number of patients referred to the national child rehabilitation centers of Reggio Emilia and Pisa.

To construct the individual's natural history, a clinical analysis is carried out for each patient in association with periodic video recording over a long period of time, following an agreed upon protocol. The video-recorded material is then submitted to board appraisal to allow taxonomic framing. Further essential information is also provided by parents and external members of our team, such as nurses, surgeons and anesthesiologists on one side and orthopedic technicians on the other. The collected material is periodically assessed by other experts and by the consensus of clinicians and physiotherapists of other Italian rehabilitation centers through national and international continuing education courses on CP, jointly organized every year by our two centers.

1. Apostural Behavior

Taxonomically, apostural behavior must be considered the first form of CP, being characterized by the absence, or by the extreme deficiency, of posture and motor patterns.

Indeed, this peculiar form of tetraplegia clinically represents the situation of a halt or greater regression of motor development associated to cerebral palsy.

The apostural child is deprived of the possibility to complete motor related fetal development and to reach the ability to be born into and to live in (gravitational) an extrauterine environment. His motricity is anchored to the "aquatic organization" of the intrauterine environment, in which segments virtually have no weight and move against constant resistance; the body is at the same time weightless, slowed, restrained and held, and movements are retained and harmonious. In such an environment, neither space orientation can be developed, except for the central-periphery direction, nor can the straightening, support, defense, parachute and balance reactions be completed.

A distinction can be made between an **apostural stage** (transient apostural behavior) and a true **apostural form**. The apostural stage may be concluded with the organization of an antigravity reaction, which represents a neurological progress even in its most primitive and pathological expressions (tetraplegia with antigravity defense in flexion, quadruped tetraplegia, dyskinetic tetraplegia or, rarely, ataxic tetraplegia). An un-resolving apostural stage characterizes the proper apostural form (see later). The longer the apostural condition lasts, the worse the prognosis will be (evolution towards proper apostural form, dyskinetic forms, or, in extremely rare cases, ataxic form).

Apostural Form (Proper)

A prognosis of apostural tetraparesis is made when the child, even at the age of three or five, presents with no antigravity organization.

The deficiency characterizing this form of CP lies in the inability of the CNS to analyze and react to gravity but not so much to muscle tone variations. Indeed, some apostural individuals become progressively stiffer without losing their apostural condition. However, apostural children usually present as flaccid, hypotonic and hypokinetic. In supine position (Fig. 13.1), they have an extended and laterally inclined head, semi-open mouth, adduced upper limbs, with slightly intrarotated or extrarotated semiflexed elbows, open hands, adduced and extrarotated thighs, semi-extended knees and talipes equinus-varus-supination. In lateral decubitus (Fig. 13.2), they adopt the so-called fetal position, but keeping the head extended or inclined and with semi-open hands. From the prone position they are better able to control their autonomic status, crouching in flexion and "knowingly" adopting immobility and indifference towards the environment. With the organization of stiffness, hands tend to clench in a fist, with an increase in flexion of the elbows and knees, while head extension, body axis hypotonia, and the need for postural retention remain unchanged.

To posture variations passively imposed from outside, the apostural child can react "like a little rag doll", if they are slow and delicate, or with a "startle-spasm-dystonia", if they are rough and sudden. Spasms start from the head and progress in extension-torsion along the body axis, with upper and lower limb adduction. Sometimes spasms are spontaneously evoked by the individual, as a defense or in general as communication, to draw attention or to express discomfort. At any rate, it is evident that the child is unable to

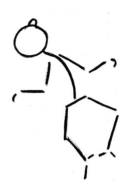

Fig. 13.1 *Proper apostural form: supine decubitus*
Extended and laterally inclined head, semi-open mouth,
adduced upper limbs, slightly intrarotared or extrarotated
semiflexed elbows with open hands, adduced and extrarotated
thighs, semi-extended knees, talipes equinus-varus-supination

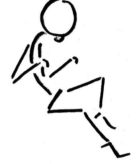

Fig. 13.2 *Proper apostural form: lateral decubitus*
Extended or inclined head, upper and lower limbs in triple
flexion, open hands, talipes equinus-varus-supination

tolerate movement of any form, both imposed from outside or produced by himself.

The child with apostural tetraplegia seems to be forced to swing between two possible choices:

No movement:

- "time out", according to Bottos (1987, 2003), hypotonia, hypokinesia, indifference to the environment;
- quest for "rest" (well-being of resting without moving);
- conscious choice of immobility ("intentional" palsy).

Maximum contraction:

- to stop movement someway: startle, spasm (in extension-torsion), dystonia (in the literal sense, as passage from an apostural hypotonia condition to a stiffness hypertonia condition);
- as defense and closure towards the surrounding environment (effective but rapidly depleting solution).

Quite a recurrent anamnestic finding is the early and extended (lissencephaly, bilateral schizencephaly, etc.) or lesional malformation damage, especially in severely pre-term children. Already from the 32nd week of pregnancy, the child develops what Milani Comparetti (1965, 1978) defined as *amphibious ability,* or motor potential of the fetus, aimed both at development in the uterine environment (water ability), and at the possibility to be born and to survive in the extrauterine environment (antigravity ability). The apostural child retains water ability, with a consequent halt in the development of neonatal adaptive functions (organizing an effective antigravity straightening and support reaction and achieving an adequate autonomic control). The apostural child can achieve better control when dressed and well retained (in somebody's arms, cradled in a hammock, lying on a soft and comfortable surface, folded in a blanket, etc.) rather than naked and exposed to air and space, conditions that lead the child to further crouch in a flexion defense pattern (similar to fetal position) or to initiate a series of startles in rapid sequence.

The protection of a simple cloth sheet can already lead to the interruption of generalized spasm reactions in extension-torsion, with adduction of the upper and lower limbs, tachycardia and polypneic phenomena, and conditions of psychomotor restlessness. In older and stiffer individuals, the retention action is performed by posture units allowing a semi-lying position, being especially soft and comfortable.

Even in the most retained postures, the head is hardly ever aligned, not even with the placement of an occipital headrest support, but flexed forward and laterally inclined, or inclined and hyperextended, with depressed and antepulsed shoulders, semiextended elbows and passive hands close to the trunk. Pelvis retroversion and major back kyphosis favor the triple flexion of the lower limbs, which in supine and semi-sitting positions must be supported at the popliteal fossa level to prevent a sideward falling, with the consequent appearance of a wind blown deformity of the lower limbs.

Other Typical Features

Autonomic control: there is a persistent difficulty in organizing the different biorhythms (i.e., sleep/wakefulness, hunger/satiety, activity/rest, open/close mindedness, body temperature, heart rate, respiratory rate, etc.), from which derives the great difficulty of the child in adapting to the changes in the external rhythm of his/her micro-environment life and to the different behavior of the caregivers (see family holidays). Patients struggle to reach and keep a state of quietness as expression of frame "stability" (in which quietness is not inactivity but tolerance, it is not inertia but inner commitment, it is not renunciation but availability, it is not inhibition but aware expectation). The apostural child always remains extremely fragile and vulnerable. Even the most basic functions for survival, such as respiratory and heart rate, struggle to remain stable. Indeed, the child continues to respond to any endogenous or exogenous stimulus with panic reactions.

Mental functions: the apostural child faces difficulties in defining his/her borders and in separating the inner self from the outer self (construction of the inner self), therefore considering the adult caregiver as an "auxiliary self", a sort of "total prosthesis" in which the child mingles and blends, often forever. Corominas (1993) defined this "parasite condition" as an extremely primitive form of mother-child symbiotic relation. Also Marzani (2005) in this regard makes reference to an undifferentiated self / external world and asserts that "*all children with pre-, peri- or post-natal cerebral damage, implying tone-posture and/or motor impairments, mostly severe, face an extension of the normal period of physiologic and mental fusion and a troubled separation-individuation process, often difficult to recognize. This is worsened by birth-related conditions and consequent events (low weight, placement in incubator, respiratory, food and sleep disorders), with the mother's inability to feed the child, and unavoidable interference on mother's skills derived by depressive feelings or by narcissistic delusions"*.

Since these individuals always present with severe reductions of intellectual perform-ance, caregivers might experience a deep feeling of helplessness that impairs their ability to achieve full emotional involvement towards the child (see chapter 9).

Communication: apostural children employ the change of state as a means to communicate with the environment. Compared with the basal condition of apathy, described by Fava Viziello (2003) as "living death", the discomfort produces whining, while situations of refusal may be expressed not only through an inconsolable and often unbearable crying, but also as sequences of startles and spasms in extension-torsion. The crying, at first scarcely organized, requires time to finally achieve the meaning of targeted message.

Epilepsy: in apostural children, epileptic fits may be difficult to control. Among the possible forms of epilepsy are infant spasms, generalized forms, forms requiring complex treatment and continuous adjustments of drug combinations, drug-resistant forms, etc.

Perceptual tolerance: the apostural child struggles in orienting remote receptors, selecting afferent signals, calibrating the intensity of incoming stimuli, and integrating different pieces of collected information into coherent perceptions (see chapter 5). Among his sensations, an absolute prevalence of proprioceptive and enteroceptive can be observed.

Sight: these children usually present with complex sight and oculomotor defects (see chapter 7). The gaze is often roving and disturbed by nystagmus, sometimes with hyperfix-ation, and by typically persistent optical defense reactions, sometimes forever. Even in the most favorable cases, ocular dyspraxia is severe and impairs the achievement even of a minimal eye-hand-mouth coordination.

Hearing: hypersensitivity to noise (startle) and discomfort to excessive silence coexist. Parents soon discover the tranquilizing effect of a soft background sound transmitted close to the child's head, such as that produced by a tape recorder playing, without pause, chil-dren's songs or melodic music.

Taste: children with apostural tetraparesis show intolerance to (hot, cold) temperature and to strong tastes, reduction or absence of taste exploration, poor adaptation to new nipples, mostly those with a small hole, and to metal cutlery (softer plastic cutlery is preferred); they usually do not like the pacifier.

Breathing: usually it is superficial and frequent, with recurrent secretions of the upper airways and scarce or unproductive cough (crackling breathing). The picture is worsened by the concurring ciliry depression induced by treatment with antiepileptic drugs.

Food: usually, these patients present with suction-swallowing problems, persistence of non-nutritive suction, sometimes pseudo-rumination, favored by esophageal reflux, inappetence, repeated vomiting, dehydration, and deficiency and malnutrition problems with consequential severe slowdown of somatic growth. Swallowing difficulties and severe inappetence contribute to induce anxiety in the mother at meal time, preventing her from establishing a positive relation with the child. PEG (percutaneous endoscopic gastrostomy) can improve the situation both from the organic and from the relational point of view.

Secondary deformity: unlike other forms of tetraparesis, a possible anterior dislocation can appear at hip level, due to excessive extension-extrarotation of the thigh. The vertebral column may be deformed in kyphoscoliosis, mostly if the lower limbs acquire a wind blown deformity.

Proper apostural tetraparesis

> *Sitting position*: not achievable
> *Upright standing*: not achievable
> *Horizontal locomotion*: not achievable
> *Walking*: not achievable
> *Manipulation*: not achievable
> *Food*: with nipple or spoon for blended and semi-liquid food
> *Psychic functions*: severe mental retardation
> *Speech*: absent
> *Connotative element*: floating reaction (semiextended elbows and knees)

---

2. Tetraplegia with Antigravity Defense in Flexion (Akinetic Tetraplegia)

These children, after a prolonged *apostural stage* lasting two to three years or more in which they show no ability to analyze and react to gravity, select **monopostural defenses in flexion** as the only organization option (antigravity defense typical of fetuses and newborns, not a proper support and straightening reaction).

In this form of tetraplegia, the dominance of the flexor pattern ideally relates to the first mode of antigravity organization in extrauterine life, when the infant feels the need to crouch (centripetal reaction) to improve autonomic control and to protect himself from external stimuli that can be too strong or too threatening compared to the child's inner world.

This feature of stability and the child's concentration on the inner environment, which is functional during the first weeks of life, become a permanent solution for these tetraplegic children. They keep their posture in flexion unchanged irrespective to any space posture changes they undergo (supine, prone, on the side, supported, etc.) (Figg. 13.3, 13.4). The stereotyped (monopostural) posture behavior exposes the severity of the clinical picture.

Fig. 13.3 *Tetraplegia with antigravity defense in flexion: supine position*
Extended or inclined head with semi-open mouth, antepulsed shoulders, flexed elbows, flexed wrists, extended fingers, kyphosis and scoliosis. Lower limbs with wind blown deformity (especially when dyskinetic elements are present), talipes valgus-pronation in dorsal flexion (also possible talipes varus-supination and consensual deviations)

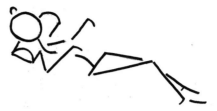

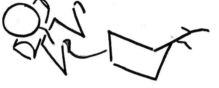

Fig. 13.4 *Tetraplegia with antigravity defense in flexion: position on the side*
Same pattern as observed in supine position

These tetraplegic patients have the lowest movement capacity (**akinetic**), they cannot fix on the medial axis, and they are never really able to reach either true antigravity straightening or real support competence, not even when they become stiffer. To contain them, once they grow older, extremely wrapped posture holding systems, wrap-around padded seats, a thoraco-lumbo-sacral corset posteriorly prolonged under the glutei with a five points harness system, tilting or reclining wheelchairs, etc., are needed. This form of CP appears more frequently in severe pre-term infants and in term infants who suffered from a severe perinatal asphyxia.

The impairment of primary biologic activities and superior psychic functions is always severe. These children experience enormous difficulty in adapting to new situations and even to the slightest changes to already known conditions. Unlike apostural children, who prefer their "environment niche" to being held, tetraplegic children with antigravity defense in flexion prefer to remain cradled by an adult, spending most of their waking time and sleep in that position. Even when they are fast asleep, they require constant physical contact with the adult caregiver's body.

Regarding postural development, neither axial straightening nor rotatory-derotatory posture is present.

The support reaction remains insufficient or rapidly depleting even when initial flaccidity disappears and a slowly progressive stiffness develops. Obviously, no form of locomotion is developed, neither horizontal nor vertical. Even though defense in flexion is a pattern organized on the grasp reflex, no manipulative competence is developed in this form of tetraplegia. Children do not like putting their hands into their mouth or sucking their finger, even if they are favored to do so by their "fetal" position.

Other Typical Features

Autonomic control: this remains unstable as shown by the frequency of vasomotor disorders, digestive difficulties, recurring respiratory diseases, and unjustified temperature changes. Environmental control and the ability to adapt to new situations are extremely limited.

Mental functions: generally there is severe mental retardation. Adhesive and symbiotic behavior with one of the caregivers, usually the mother or one grandparent, are required to satisfy the child's need of holding and the adult caregiver's desire to feel at least useful, if not essential, towards the child.

Communication: the family intensely creates a profound relation with the child, who proves to be able to establish contact (tonic dialogue). The child, even without developing any form of evolved communication (lack of speech), can anyway express his/her emotional state (pleasure, discomfort, pain) and be in tune with the familiar caregiver who usually looks after the child.

Epilepsy: the control of (generalized) fits can be difficult and constant adjustments of complex combinations of antiepileptic drugs.

Perceptual tolerance: children affected by this form of tetraplegia do not tolerate being handled (they usually react by stiffening to passive or assisted mobilization). Conversely, they calm down with rhythmic and repeated rocking movements. For this reason, they especially like being cradled. Over time they achieve a certain ability to adapt to recurrent and habitual environmental stimuli (noises, smells, hygiene procedures, feeding, etc.).

Sight: the patient presents with nystagmus, especially horizontal but also vertical or rotatory, sometimes with erratic gaze, and commonly with visual acuity reduction, oculomotion disorders, and other visual disorders of central origin (see chapter 7).

Hearing: hypersensitivity to loud and sudden noises is frequent, even when such noises are recurrent or habitual. Children show pleasure in listening to nursery rhymes, cradle songs, lullabies, melodic music, etc.

Taste: a frequent sign is intolerance to temperature and to strong tastes.

Breathing: breathing is usually frequent and superficial. Due to ciliary hypomobility (worsened by antiepileptic drugs) and the reduced coordination between compression of the chest bellows and glottic opening, cough is scarcely productive and secretion stagnation is common, especially in the upper airways (crackling breathing). Persistent non-nutritive suction and pseudo-rumination of saliva concur to increase the frequency of respiratory infections.

Food: mastication is totally lacking or severely impaired, swallowing is often difficult (gavage during the first periods of life and later a soft nipple with a larger hole). The contact of the spoon with the mouth often triggers a "reflex" bite. Dentition, influenced by the persisting suction reflex, shapes as malocclusion. Due to the poor oral hygiene, favored by hypersialosis and sialorrhea and especially by antiepileptic therapy, the teeth rapidly deteriorate. A common event is vomiting, before feeding, of dense saliva and previously swallowed bronchial secretions which frees the stomach and prepare thes child to eat the meal.

The esophageal reflux commonly appears due to cardia incontinence and dyssynergic peristalsis. Persistent constipation with frequent formation of scotomas is usual. Growth is difficult and hypo-somatic features become characteristic in this form of tetraplegia.

PEG improves food intake pattern and child growth as much as the overall care activities.

Secondary deformity: the head is kept in a forced posture (extended, reclined, rotated on the side, seldom flexed). A common feature is a dorso-lumbar kyphosis with developmental characteristics, followed by progressive scoliosis, fed "from below" in case of monolateral hip dislocation, pelvic obliquity, and wind blown deformity of the lower limbs ("passive" scoliosis), or "from above", in case of forced head rotation ("active" scoliosis), favored by an incoercible lateral gaze shifting.

Wrist hyperflexion can reach dislocation of the first bone row of the carpus. Hands are thin and they often rest on a surface on the backside. Fingers are flexed but not clenched in a fist. Due to the prevailing muscle activity in flexed-adduction of the thighs, it is possible to observe hip dislocation (postero-lateral migration) either only on one side (more severe) or, more commonly, bilaterally (less severe).

Feet usually present with either valgus-pronation or varus-supination, sometimes consensual (one feet is valgo and the other is varus). Rather than talipes equinus, feet talism with eversion can be present (pronation, abduction, dorsiflexion). Immobility, absence of load, and food intake deficiencies favor osteoporosis and osteomalacia. When growing up, such patients may display pain to the rachis and to the main articulations due to immobility, deformity, osteoporosis and cartilage atrophy.

Tetraparesis with antigravity defense in flexion

> *Sitting position*: not achievable
> *Upright standing*: not achievable
> *Horizontal locomotion*: not achievable
> *Walking*: not achievable
> *Manipulation*: ineffective
> *Food*: with a spoon and finely minced food
> *Psychic functions*: mental retardation
> *Speech*: tonic dialogue with the caregiver
> *Connotative element*: defense in flexion (stiffly flexed elbows and knees)

13

3. Tetraplegia with Horizontal Trunk Antigravity

"Horizontal" trunk antigravity is typical of those animals that were raised against gravity and became quadruped. To achieve this result they lost the peculiar body axis mobility of amphibians and developed the proximal fixation of the trunk on the legs necessary to support themselves. In this form of tetraplegia, the four limbs are dominated by an extension pattern, since also the upper limb only performs a support function, as if it were an anterior leg, rather than grasp and manipulation tasks.

Unlike tetraplegia with antigravity defense in flexion, in which elbows and knees present as steadily flexed, in horizontal trunk antigravity the organization of the support reaction drags the four limbs from flexion to extension. This clinical expression may be preceded by a more or less durable stage of apostural behavior, in which elbows and knees present as semiextended due to the persisting floating reaction.

Figures 13.5 and 13.6 show the dominant reactions of this form of tetraplegia in supine and prone position. The conflict between startle reaction and propulsive reaction constitutes the second diarchy theorized by Milani Comparetti (1978) in his classification proposal.

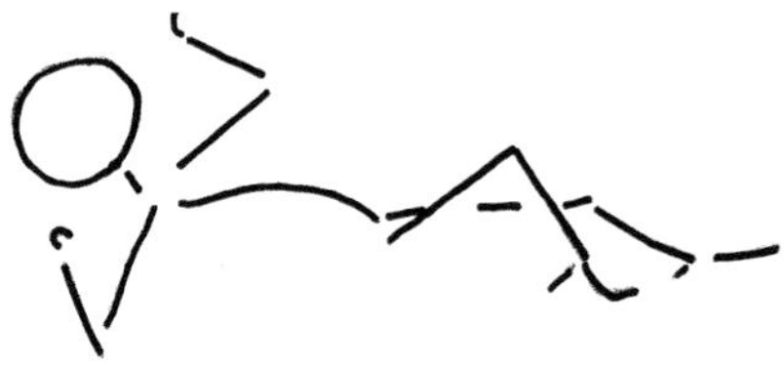

Fig. 13.5 *Tetraplegia with quadruped antigravity: supine position*
*Startle reaction or pseudo-Moro reflex
- extended head
- upset face, open mouth
- "crosswise" arms
- contracted but open hands
- lifted chest in forced inspiration
- semiabducted lower limbs
- semiextended knees
- talipes varus-supination (rarely valgus-pronation)
(Milani Comparetti, 1978)

Fig. 13.6 *Tetraplegia with quadruped antigravity: prone position*
*Propulsive reaction
- inclined head with open mouth
- trunk extended or in torsion
- antepulsed and depressed shoulders
- extended arms, pointing downwards
- semiextended elbows
- forearm pronation
- semiflexed wrists
- open or semi-open hands
- slightly adduced semiextended and
  intrarotated thighs
- semiextended knees
- talipes varus-supination or valgus-pronation
(Milani Comparetti, 1978)

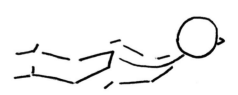

A warning sign of this form of tetraplegia is retropulsion of the head and the upper part of the column. The asymmetric tonic neck reflex (ATNR) is powerful but, due to the lack of an evident asymmetry in the evolution of limitations and of secondary joint deformities, its influence on the organization of pathological motricity does not seem to be as important as it was considered in the past (Bobath and Bobath, 1975).

Due to the strength of the rotatory-derotatory straightening, the trunk preserves an "en bloc" characteristic, adequate to protect it from scoliosis, unless a hip monolateral dislocation with secondary pelvis obliquity occurs.

The main motor patterns of this form are as follows:

Supine Position

Lower limbs often show intermittent and jerky "cycling" sequences, tracing back to the neonatal stepping reflex (central pattern generator). Some individuals also attempt retropulsive crawling. The upper limbs develop some reaching movement, of ballistic type, with a proximal start and usually targeted downward and sideward. The hands, unable to reach the medial line due to the strength of the ATNR, show some ability in adapting the grasp but they still have limited competence in manipulation. Commonly, individuals with this form of tetraparesis can lift their head from a flat surface, but they are unable to completely turn on their side.

Prone Position

Spasms in extension and trunk torsion starting from the head and followed by mouth opening are common. When the patient tries to turn in the prone-supine position, the adducted upper limbs are trapped below the chest, stopping complete rotation. Sometimes, a slight forward progression, usually described as "reflex crawling", is possible, as expression of a targeted, but not functional, application of the propulsive reaction.

Sitting Position

To lift the gaze, the child must bend the head forward and intensify dorsal kyphosis to avoid the relapse of startle. Under ATNR influence, elbows flexion takes place under the shoulder line, contrary to what usually happens in supine position. The most suitable posture systems for these patients are extra folding wheelchairs with five point harness system to prevent the pelvis from sliding forward, sometimes also with shoulder straps, padded neckrest, and foot support and reclined backrests equipped with gas dampers or with other dynamic systems to absorb such spasms in extension.

Upright Standing

Craniocaudal axial straightening is blocked in quadruped organization and does not allow the child to achieve autonomous upright standing. Assisted verticalization incites head hyperextension and trunk retropulsion, usually engendering automatic walking. At any rate, the support reaction tends to prevail over the spinal central pattern generator (CPG) for locomotion, unlike in subcortical automatisms and in vertical trunk tetraparesis (see below).

Other Typical Features

Mental functions: children affected by this form usually achieve separation-individuation (see chapter 9). However, they often maintain psychological dependence on the caregiver and they soon give up autonomously applying the scarce cognitive and motor performance they have maintained. In order to feel more secure, they often employ projective strategies, withdrawing in the illusion to be able to dominate the environment through the influence they exert on other people. As observed by Marzani (2005) *"These children are often very close to their parents, other toddlers or teachers; they build up the illusion of having no motor constraints by letting themselves be moved by others, pretending and intensely developing imitation".*

Communication: children with horizontal trunk tetraplegia often present with features of dysarthria and dysphonia, but their speech is quite understandable, especially when there is no severe reduction of intellective performance.

Epilepsy: epileptic fits, mostly generalized, are common. The response to antiepileptic drugs is sometimes unsatisfactory.

Perceptual tolerance: children accept movement and sometimes even seem to like it. They fear noise, strong or sudden light, and unexpected or sudden stimuli, which lead them to respond with the startle reaction.

Sight: visual disorders of central origin are usually present (see chapter 7) such as gaze palsy, especially horizontal nystagmus, persistence of optical defense reaction, reduction of visus, etc.

Hearing: intolerance to noise is often present, lasting long and triggering the startle reaction. This happens also for familiar noises which are well known, repeated, expected, and also self-provoked. The child struggles to develop a habituation process to the stimulus. Lower tones are better tolerated than higher ones.

Taste: children like all tastes but they may experience difficulties in adapting to very hot or very cold food.

Breathing: the tendency to mucus hyperproduction, typical of previous forms, is also common in tetraparesis with horizontal trunk antigravity, but with lower intensity. Episodes of bronchospasm are still likely to occur. Respiratory morbidity, especially in infant communities, is still higher in peers.

Food: children acquire the capacity to chew solid food, with a prevalence of vertical crushing movements organized around the bite reflex. The problem of hypersialosis and sialorrhea remain evident and is favored by the onset of malocclusion (open bite) due to prominence of the mandibular arch over the maxillary one and to palate bowing. Esophageal reflux is less frequent than in previous forms.

Secondary deformity: hip posterolateral dislocation is common, mostly monolateral, with consequent negative impact on the spinal column alignment, and sometimes bilateral, therefore overall less damaging. The pelvis, retroverted in a primitive stage, may become anteverted after surgical lengthening of the hamstrings, if not associated with a release of the hip flexors, especially of the deep muscles. Due to subrotular ligament failure, rotulae tend to rise, especially if standing on a static table or a kneeling position is performed. The prevalent feet deformity is equinus-valgus-pronation, with anterior and inferior talus dislocation and dislocation of the peroneus longus tendon to the front of the lateral malleolus.

Tetraparesis with horizontal trunk antigravity

> *Sitting position*: not autonomously conservable
> *Upright standing*: not achievable
> *Horizontal locomotion*: sometimes crawling from prone position
> *Walking*: not achievable
> *Manipulation*: ballistic grasping movements and primitive grasp patterns
> *Mastication*: open bite
> *Psychic functions*: possible mental retardation
> *Speech*: dysarthria and dysphonia, but with possibility of verbal communication
> *Connotative element*: quadruped antigravity (elbows and knees extension)

Tetraplegia with Subcortical Automatisms

These tetraplegic children have a quite rare variant of the horizontal trunk antigravity form which is interesting in order to formulate the prognosis for walking (differential diagnosis in comparison to diplegias) and to show both a relevant support reaction and a strong spinal central pattern generator of walking. However, these children are unable to match these two mechanisms properly because the step generation ends up strongly prevailing over the support reaction. In assisted walking, with the caregiver supporting them from the shoulders, the patients alternatively move both lower limbs forward without truly accepting the load and displace them too far from the vertical trunk projection, pushing the

13

trunk backward (retropulsion) and rotating it on the longitudinal axis (twisting). The upper limbs are still unable to support the load but they hint at organizing an antigravity reaction in flexion (Fig. 13.7). Parachute and balance reactions are lacking, while grasping defense reactions, even though poorly effective, can be performed.

During walking, these tetraplegic children are unable to follow a trajectory but they are able to get oriented and directed. If they are given walking devices, such as an anterior two wheel walking frame with posterior glutei support and a forearm rest board with hand grips, these patients tend to assume an excessively forward tilted trunk, with flexed hips, semiflexed knees, and feet in equinus-valgus-pronation (Fig. 13.8). They exhaust the support reaction very rapidly and are unable to guide the device and to calibrate the forward movement of all four limbs and trunk. Indeed, while the upper limbs push the walking frame too forward, the lower limbs are always too backward, conversely to what happens in case of walking supported from the shoulders by the caregiver.

These children frequently demand to be helped in walking while supported from the shoulders, an activity in which they achieve high levels of excitement and pleasure. This condition contributes to generate in the patient and his family the mutual illusion that

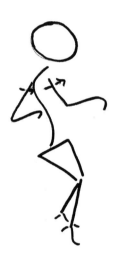

Fig. 13.7 *Tetraplegia with subcortical automatisms: assisted walking*
Head in vertical position or in slight retropulsion, trunk in hyperextension or retropulsion, semiflexed upper limbs at elbow level, with usually open hands, flexed, adduced and intrarotated thighs, sometimes crossed, semiextended knees, talipes equinus-valgus-pronation with large recruitment of plantarflexor muscles

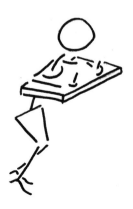

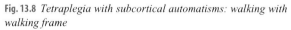

Fig. 13.8 *Tetraplegia with subcortical automatisms: walking with walking frame*
Flexed head, trunk in antepulsion, support of forearms with unstable grasp, flexed, adduced and intrarotated thighs, sometimes crossed, semiflexed knees with depletion of support reaction, talipes equinus-valgus-pronation

independent walking, even with supporting devices, could be a therapeutic goal that is at some point attainable.

When they organize a horizontal locomotion, they can perform hare-like crawling movements with adduced and even alternatively advanced extended upper limbs and lower limbs that are asymmetrically flexed to the hip and advanced almost simultaneously, with mild joint excursion. Overall movement speed on the ground remains quite reduced, but the performance is much better than expected just by observing gait.

In sitting position, patients with this form of tetraplegia can control and orientate their head, free the gaze, and manipulate (with difficulty); however, they tend to pull the trunk backwards (retropulsion) when lifting their hands at shoulder level. They retain, for a long time, elements of hypo-posture (dorsal kyphosis). Hip dislocation, especially monolateral, may occur if the flexion-adduction interference subsequent to the gait pattern is not controlled on time. Common features are patella lift and talipes equinus-valgus-pronation deformities, with medial talus dislocation, tibia extratorsion, and knee deforming stress in flexion-valgismus.

Intellectual performance is generally reduced, with dysarthric and dysphonic speech that is quite understandable. From a psychic point of view, these children can achieve separation-individuation. However, the relationship with the adult remains adhesive. Patients require to be attended in all activities and, in interactive activities, the adult caregiver still needs to perform also part of their role.

4. Tetraplegia with Vertical Trunk Antigravity

"Vertical" trunk antigravity is typical in evolved mammals, such as arboreal monkeys, that abandoned quadruped posture and acquired biped posture by modifying the support reaction on the anterior limbs and by changing their organization from extension (pull) to flexion (grasp). They preserved the support reaction in extension typical of horizontal trunk antigravity in the posterior limbs, but adding hip extension and a better capacity in the proximal fixation of the thighs to the trunk to allow the one leg stage of the gait cycle.

In this form of tetraplegia, the support reaction of the upper limbs shows a characteristic response in flexion organized in a grasp, even if decreased, at least in part, by the learning of behaviors in extension induced by physiotherapy.

A certain degree of manipulation activity can be achieved. However, when grasping, the hand tends to open insufficiently with regards to the object's dimensions, due to the impairment of the anticipatory pre-adaptation ability. The same thing happens in releasing. The grasp can be cluster type, interdigital, or lateral with thumb-forefinger-middle finger. Despite the inclination to keep hands clenched in a fist, grasp is insecure and exhaustible.

Due to the uncertainty of the proximal fixation (flexion-adduction of thighs with pelvis anteversion and shoulder antepulsion with elbow flexion) and to the difficulty in arm abduction and in complete elbow extension, patients experience less difficulty in performing movements from periphery to body axis than in the opposite. Compared with performance achievable in upright standing, in sitting position upper limb function appears to be remarkably better (as in diplegia).

13

> *"Upper limbs are often kept adduced due to the predominance of pectoral muscles, of teres major and minor muscles and of latissimus muscle of the back; elbows are semi-flexed; wrists are in partial flexion and pronation and fingers are unable to perform a satisfactory voluntary action."*
> J. Little (1862) quoted by Majoni (2003)

In the lower limbs, the prevailing pattern is of thigh flexion-adduction-intrarotation with knee semi-extension and talipes equinus-valgus-pronation, but with a marked component of adduction-intrarotation (scissor pattern) compared with the usual pattern of tetraparesis with horizontal trunk antigravity.

When starting to assume the standing position, patients perform a distal fixation (hands and feet), keeping for some time an unstable body axis. Gradually, they learn a proximal fixation, enhancing the pathological scissor pattern. Spasticity in flexion-adduction also increases in knee position (W-shape), in crawling, and in posture changes from and to the sitting position and the upright standing position. For this reason, in these tetraplegic children, functional orthopedic surgery on lower limb deformities, at least in the first stage (adductors and medial hamstrings), results in anticipating the acquisition of walking (differential diagnosis with diplegia).

The development of the "interference" pattern of thigh flexion-adduction in the patient's motor activity, "neurologically" testifies to the evolutionary process of the support reaction and the achievement of proximal fixation abilities, even though "orthopedically" it would damage the joint stability of the coxofemoral joints.

In general, being unable to organize complex movement combinations, patients with this form of tetraparesis tend to reduce their repertoire in order to improve utilization (adaptive simplification of gesture, freezing of posture). This element implies a more difficult expression of a reliable motor prognosis to the family when diagnosis is communicated.

Figures 13.9, 13.10, 13.11, 13.12 describe the dominant reactions in supine and prone position in this form of tetraplegia. The conflict between extension and flexion pattern constitutes the first diarchy theorized by Milani Comparetti (1978) in his classification proposal.

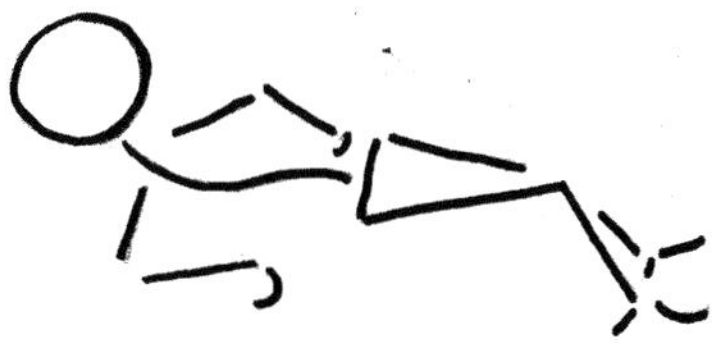

Fig. 13.9 *Tetraplegia with biped antigravity: supine position, extension pattern*
Head in slight flexion and antepulsion, shoulders antepulsion and depression, slightly abduced and intrarotated retroflexed arms, flexed elbows, forearm pronation, flexed wrists with ulnar deviation, clenched fists, adduced or enclosed thumbs, semi-extended trunk with lumbar hyperlordosis, semiflexed hips with pelvis anteversion, adduced and intrarotated thighs (sometimes even with scissor pattern), semiextended knees, talipes equinus-valgus-pronation, grasp reaction to toes (plantar grasp). Milani Comparetti (1978)

Fig. 13.10 *Tetraplegia with biped antigravity: prone position, flexor pattern*
The support takes place on all of the forearm with flexed elbow. Hands can be more or less clenched in a fist. Sometimes wrist hyperflexion causes the patient to rest the closed fist on the dorsal surface, instead of the palmar one. Lower limbs are adduced and intrarotated with flexed knees and talipes equinus-valgus-pronation. Milani Comparetti (1978)

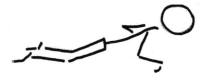

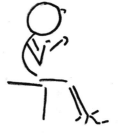

Fig. 13.11 *Tetraplegia with biped antigravity: sitting position*
Functional compromise of Milani Comparetti between the behavior of the upper limbs and trunk, controlled by flexion, and that of the lower limbs controlled by extension

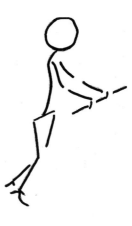

Fig. 13.12 *Tetraplegia with biped antigravity: upright posture*
Kyphotic and also flexed trunk, adduced and intrarotated thighs, talipes equinus-varus-supination

The main motor pattern of this form are as follows:

Sitting Position

The trunk is kyphotic with head antepulsion and shoulder depression. The load shifts on the sacrum, with evident pelvis retroversion and lumbar kyphosis, at least until a surgical lengthening of hamstring muscles is performed. Antigravity straightening is favored by head extension (with tilting) and by vertical gaze lifting.

Upright Standing

Overall, the trunk remains kyphotic, but lumbar lordosis can appear as a compensation to hip flexion and pelvis anteversion. In the upright standing position, patients are hardly ever symmetric: one knee is usually more flexed than the other and talipes equinus is more evident on one side than on the other (differential diagnosis with double hemiplegia).

Horizontal Locomotion

Crawling is achieved also before the age of three years in a flexion-adduction-intrarotation pattern of the lower limbs favoring coxofemoral joint distress. After the age of three, children can have hare-like movements or creep, without completely releasing the lower limbs, which tend to remain bound together during forward movement. A delay in achieving horizontal locomotion implies a negative impact on gait prognosis.

Walking

Walking is always acquired quite late and is slow, hard and discontinuous, due to the patient's, inability to "adjust" the operating motor program; they need in fact to periodically slow down and re-start, so they are unable to achieve fluency.

They experience difficulties in combining the support reaction with the spinal central pattern generator of walking and to distribute the load between the upper and lower limbs. If walking aids for the upper limbs are too high, they bend the elbows, while if they are too low, instead of extending the elbows, they rather bend the knees. In this form of tetraplegia therefore, upper limb function is indeed the true "passport to walking". Patients experience difficulties to release the two muscle girdles, even though they are able to rotate the trunk en bloc, by properly taking advantage of the head facilitation. Therefore, evolutive scoliosis remains a quite rare event, even in case of monolateral hip dislocation (an event which instead is quite frequent).

These tetraplegic individuals move forward by dragging on tiptoes (ineffective clearance) for the following reasons:

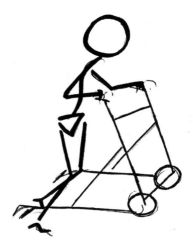

Fig. 13.13 *Tetraplegia with biped antigravity: walking with walking frame*
Trunk antepulsion, scissor pattern of lower limbs.

- If they increase flexion of the swing limb, they reduce the support reaction in the stance one.
- If they increase the extension of the stance limb, they inhibit the gait pattern of the swing one.

The conflict between support reaction and spinal central pattern generator of walking is evident also in the transition from walking with a walking frame, in which patients try to hang on, therefore with a prevailing gait pattern, to walking with crutches, in which the support reaction with dragging tiptoes usually prevails (Fig. 13.13).

If they try to walk faster, they considerably increase the overall recruitment, worsening the whole performance.

Due to the simultaneous presence of a support talipes equinus and of a swing one, the feet are dragged on the floor, more frequently in valgus-pronation. The head can rotate from one side to the other at each step to facilitate the release of the lower limb that needs to be pulled forward.

Patients need to visually control their position and the advancing direction by properly targeting with gaze the surrounding space.

Walking, usually acquired between three and six years of age, is often dropped during adolescence both because it lacks functionality compared with an orthopedic wheelchair in terms of effort employed and because secondary deformities of the pelvis and lower limbs inevitably become more severe with growth.

Other Typical Features

Superior cortical functions: intellectual performance is usually preserved and more developed than in other forms of tetraplegia (see chapter 8). During school activities some patients may present with gaps in logical-mathematical skills.

Communication: due to the extended hypertonia of mouth and speech muscles, speech may be slightly impaired, especially in conditions of emotional involvement.

Epilepsy: epileptic fits are common but the response to antiepileptic drugs is usually satisfactory.

Perceptual tolerance: dysperceptive disorders are quite common, especially those related to the upright standing position and walking with devices.

Sight: gaze palsy is common, especially in exotropia, with reduction of visual acuity and ocular dyspraxia (see chapter 7). Sometimes reductions of the visual field are reported.

Hearing: tolerance to noise and hearing acuity are usually satisfactory.

Taste: no report of particular problems.

Breathing: usually major problems are not reported. Some children during the first years of life may present with episodes of bronchospasm.

Food: mastication and swallowing are adequate. Problems related to hypersialosis and sialorrhea may persist in some patients.

Secondary deformity: as a consequence of the antigravity pattern in flexion, the shoulders usually present with depression and antepulsion, elbows are in flexion, with forearm pronation, wrists are flexed and fingers are more or less in grasp. The trunk is commonly kyphotic, with the head in antepulsion.

The pelvis, due to the prevalence of the iliopsoas, may present with anteversion and compensatory hyperlordosis, or rarely with retroversion if the hamstrings prevail. Thighs are flexed-adducted-intrarotated with a tendency to, a usually monolateral, posterolateral dislocation of the heads of the femur, and secondary pelvis obliquity, on the dislocation side. The necks of the femurs are valgus and intrarotated (anteversion), with subsequent rotula "strabismus" of proximal origin. Knees, as a result of femurs intrarotation and of tibiae extratorsion, are deformed in valgismus. Rotulae may rise (anterior cause) contributing, together with hamstring contracture (posterior cause) to knee flexion and consequent reduction of the support reaction (crouch gait). Feet are usually deformed in equinus-valgus-pronation, with talus medial dislocation and plantar arch flattening.

Tetraplegia with vertical trunk antigravity

> *Sitting position*: on sacrum with trunk kyphosis and knees semi-extension
> *Upright standing* : possible with upper limbs devices
> *Horizontal locomotion*: possible creeping, crawling and their variants
> *Walking*: possible with upper limbs aids
> *Manipulation*: possible with difficulty
> *Mastication*: effective
> *Psychic functions*: usually preserved
> *Speech*: sufficiently understandable
> *Connotative element*: antigravity reaction in flexion to upper limbs and in extension to lower ones (scissor pattern)

Able Tetraplegic

This rare clinical form, a variant of tetraplegia with vertical trunk antigravity, is characterized by the ability to express distal "slow" isolated and selective "unique" movements in manipulation (for example, some patients can even embroider) (Fig. 13.14), despite the severity of the spasticity and the use of clearly pathological motor patterns. Such individuals can even "beat" a rhythm with repetitive movements of their hands or fingers on a table.

The child soon acquires good control of the head, presenting with neither severe gaze palsy nor mastication-swallowing related disorders, showing good intellective ability, with adequate speech and satisfactory facial expression. Antigravity organization is of vertical type, but usually the patient is unable to acquire autonomous walking ability, not even with walking devices used by his upper limbs . Deformities of the upper and lower limbs soon become extremely severe, in contrast with the patient's motor control, and require repeated functional orthopedic surgery operations. Hip dislocation is frequent, while scoliosis is rare, due to the strongly "en bloc" characteristic preserved by the trunk. A severe deformity in flexion of the elbows, wrists, and fingers is usually present.

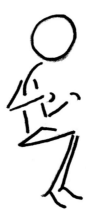

Fig. 13.14 *Able tetraplegic*
Antepulsed and depressed shoulders, slightly adduced and intrarotated arms, flexed elbows with forearm pronation, flexed wrists with ulnar deviation, usually clenched fists with free first finger, stiff lordosis with pelvis anteversion, adduced-intrarotated thighs, flexed knees, extratortion of tibias, talipes equinus-varus-pronation

This clinical form of tetraparesis is important from the rehabilitative point of view since it clearly demonstrates how spasticity and motor control are not strictly interrelated or always equivalent.

Incidence of the Different Forms of Tetraplegia in a Hospital Based Series

During a two year study period, 467 subjects with CP were recruited by our leading national centers of Pisa and Reggio Emilia (Table 13.1). Their age ranged from 2.0 to 21.7 years (mean 7.8 ± 4.1); 262 were male. A large prevalence of spastic CP forms was found (434 subjects, 93%) versus dyskinetic (24 subjects, 5%) and ataxic ones (9 subjects, 2%) (Cioni et al. 2008).

As also reported in the previous chapter (see chapter 12), among the spastic forms that include the largest group of children with CP (93% in our sample), it is possible to distinguish children with diplegia and tetraplegia, not only according to a different level of motor impairment, as demonstrated with the assessment scales applied in this study (GMFCS, BFMF, MACS), but also according to other disabilities associated to the paralysis (mental retardation, visual impairment, seizures). The use of the GMFCS, according to Morris and Rosenbaum (2003), underlines the existence of two different categories, as we found subjects with diplegia mainly of levels I – III and subjects with tetraplegia in levels IV and V (see results shown in Table 12.1 chapter 12).

In the same population of subjects we also evaluated the incidence of the proposed forms of tetraplegia as indicated in this chapter. Moreover we also explored the incidence of some of the features of each form. In particular we assessed the level of GMF-CS, mental functions and sensory activities (visual and auditory) and epilepsy. These findings are reported in Table 13.2.

Table 13.1 Distribution of the main types of cerebral palsy, classified according to Hagberg et al. (1996; 2005)

Type of Cerebral Palsy	n (%)
Spastic CP	434 (93%)
Tetraplegia	115 (25%)
Diplegia	213 (46%)
Hemiplegia	106 (22%)
Dyskinetic CP	24 (5%)
Dystonic	17 (3.5%)
Choreo-athetotic	7 (1.5%)
Ataxic CP	9 (2.0%)
Total	467

Spastic diplegia was diagnosed in 213 subjects (115 male, mean age 7.9 ± 3.9, range 2.0-21.7 years). This group was the largest in this series (46%), whereas 115 subjects had tetraplegia (25%) and 106 hemiplegia (22%).

Table 13.2 Incidence and main features of the four different forms of tetraplegia

		Apostural tetraplegia (2 ss)		Akinetic tetraplegia (15 ss)		Horizontal tetraplegia (15 ss)		Vertical tetraplegia (27 ss)		Non-classifiable tetraplegia (2 ss)	
		ss	%	ss	%	ss	%	ss	%	ss	%
GMF-CS	1st level				/		/		/		/
	2nd level				/		/		/		/
	3rd level				/		/	3	11	1	50
	4th level			2	13	3	20	20	74		/
	5th level	2	100	13	87	11	73	4	15		/
	missing				/	1	7		/	1	50
Cognitive behavior	n.n.				/	4	27	6	22		/
	borderline				/		/	6	22		/
	mild retardation			1	7	5	33	5	18		/
	moderate retardation	1	50	1	7	1	7	1	4		/
	severe retardation			10	67	2	13	7	26	2	100
	very severe retardation	1	50	1	7	1	7		/		/
	missing			2	13	2	13	2	7		/
Visual functioning	n.n.				/	2	13	8	30		/
	mild compromised	1	50	8	53	9	60	18	67	1	50
	severely compromised	1	50	4	27	1	7		/	1	50
	missing			3	20	3	20	1	4		/
Auditory functioning	n.n.	2	100	9	60	14	93	25	93	2	100
	mild compromised			6	40	1	7		/		/
	severely compromised				/		/	2	7		/
Presence of epilepsy		1	50	13	87	3	20	6	22	2	100

ss, subjects

Vertical tetraplegia was the most common form of tetraplegia in our hospital based series and the apostural one the rarest. Only a few cases were unclassifiable. GMF-CS indicated an increasing severity level from the apostural form to the vertical one. This was also true concerning the incidence and severity of mental retardation, visual impairment, and the presence of epilepsy. These preliminary data seem to confirm the applicability of the suggested classification system of tetraplegia.

13

References

Amiel-Tison C, Grenier A (1985) La surveillance neurologique au cours de la première année de vie. Masson, Paris

André-Thomas, Saint-Anne Dargassies S (1952) Etudes neurologiques sur le nouveau-né et le jeune nourrisson. Masson, Paris

Bobath B, Bobath K (1975) Motor development in the different types of cerebral palsy. William Heinemann Medical Books, London

Bottos M (1987) Paralisi cerebrale infantile. Diagnosi precoce e trattamento tempestivo. Ghedini editore, Milan

Bottos M (2003) Paralisi cerebrale infantile: dalla guarigione all'autonomia. Diagnosi e proposte riabilitative. Piccin editore, Padua

Cioni G, Lodesani M, Coluccini M et al (2008) The term diplegia should be enhanced (II): contribution to validation of a new classification system. Eur J Physic Rehab Med 44:203-211

Corominas J (1993) Psicopatologia e sviluppi arcaici. Borla editore, Rome

Fava Viziello G (2003) La presa in carico del bambino con patologia disabilitante cronica. In: Bottos M (ed) Paralisi cerebrale infantile: dalla guarigione all'autonomia. Diagnosi e proposte riabilitative. Piccin editore, Padua, pp 353-359

Ferrari A (2003) In tema di postura e di controllo posturale. Giorn Ital Med Riab 17:61-74

Gesell A, Halverson HM, Thompson H et al (1940) The first five years of life: a guide to the study of the preschool child, from the Yale clinic of child development. Harper, New York

Haeckel EH (1892) Storia della creazione naturale. UTET Editore, Turin

Hagberg B, Hagberg G, Orlow I (1996) The changing panorama of cerebral palsy in Sweden, VII. Prevalence and origin during the birth period 1987-1990. Acta Paediatrica 85:954-960

Himmelmann K, Hagberg G, Beckung E et al (2005) The changing panorama of cerebral palsy in Sweden. IX. Prevalence and origin in the birth-year period 1995-1998. Acta Paediatr 94:287-94

Majoni A (2003) Semeiotica preoperatoria e tecniche di intervento. In: Bottos M (ed) Paralisi cerebrale infantile: dalla guarigione all'autonomia. Diagnosi e proposte riabilitative. Piccin editore, Padua, pp 295-342

Marzani C (2005) Psicopatologia e clinica dei disturbi mentali nella paralisi cerebrale infantile. In: Ferrari A, Cioni G (eds) Le forme spastiche della paralisi cerebrale infantile: guida allo sviluppo delle funzioni adattive. Springer-Verlag Italia, Milan

Milani Comparetti A (1965) La natura del difetto motorio nella paralisi cerebrale infantile. Infanzia Anormale 64:587-628

Milani Comparetti A (1976) Dalla parte del neonato: proposte per una competenza prognostica. Neuropsichiatria Infantile 175:5-18

Milani Comparetti A (1978) Classification des infirmités motrices cérébrales. Médicine et Hygiène 36:2024-2029

Morris C, Rosenbaum PL (2003) Describing impairment and disability for children with cerebral palsy. Electronic Letter to editor. Arch Dis Child 2003; 30 May

Neisser U (1976) Cognition and Reality. Cambridge University Press, New York

Dysperceptive Forms

14

S. Alboresi, V. Belmonti, Al. Ferrari, A. Ferrari

Introduction

In over thirty years of clinical observation of cerebral palsied (CP) children, especially among premature babies with bilateral motor damage, we have repeatedly found a group of patients with a unique combination of clinical characteristics which, we believe, could represent a specific group within the CP categorization. For convenience, we have termed them "dysperceptive" and we have been studying their behavior in a fairly large group of patients in order to see if some phenomena, unmistakably observed in single cases, were recognizable, also in different degrees, in larger groups. We have maintained the term "perceptual disturbance or dysperception" for the first and most interesting hypothesis that the errors performed by these children could happen during the collection, interpretation, and re-elaboration of information, especially of "the sense of movement", even if other fascinating theories can be found especially in the field of psychology. These complex behaviors, for example fear, can be observed during clinical examination or physiotherapeutic treatments. In addition, parents and older children often describe some specific situations, which are recurrent and typical, that take place in everyday life in different settings (at school, on holiday, with friends, etc.), often underlining the limitations produced by these phenomena regarding motor independence and quality of life. These signs can be observed in CP children with diverse motor damage (diplegia, tetraplegia, but not hemiplegia) and at different development levels. In order to explore consistency and recurrence of the more important or frequent dysperceptive signs, describe them in detail and collect evidence by suitable instruments, we have been and are still employing video recording sessions (natural history of these signs).

In chapter 5 we analyzed the three levels of sensation, perception, and representation and formulated some different hypotheses concerning the origin of dysperception that could explain some of these phenomena. Obviously we are just at the beginning of the long process necessary to test and accept or refuse a new scientific hypothesis, but we are convinced of the absolute importance of these aspects for CP interpretation and treatment and would like to draw the greater attention of the scientific community to them.

From the motor point of view, dysperceptive children belong to the category of bilateral CP and should be classified as either diplegic or tetraplegic (we have never observed these signs in true hemiplegic forms). In diplegic forms the perceptual components are milder and with a generally more favorable evolution than the analogous situation occurring in tetraplegic ones, where the expression of these components are more severe and often insurmountable. Taking into account only motor aspects, we do not consider that, in addition to the disturbance of posture and movement, some patients also have other significant disturbances which can interfere with motor performance. While classic diplegias and tetraplegias usually present with prevalent motor aspects in every stage of their evolution, in the corresponding CP dysperceptive forms the perceptive disorders are by far more important than the motor ones. Consequently, if we base our diagnostic framework only on the analysis of motor problems (classifying the child on his posture/movement patterns as tetraplegic - mainly with vertical trunk antigravity - or diplegic), we will not be able to explain the real difficulties of the child and, thus, our long-term prognosis will be misdirected and overly optimistic. For this reason we have decided to describe these forms of cerebral palsy in a separate chapter, rather than in those devoted to tetraparesis or diplegias, because we think the key to their interpretation lies fundamentally in perception and not in movement.

For a comprehensive analysis of the influence of perceptive disorders on motor organisation see chapter 5, and for classification issues see chapters 11 and 12.

Clinical Features of Perceptual Disturbances in Diplegias (Semiotics)

The hypothesis of the existence of two groups of diplegic children, one with prevalent motor problems and the other with prevalent dysperceptive ones, is becoming more and more convincing. The diagnosis of diplegic forms with dominant perceptual disturbances, analogously to what happens in the corresponding forms with prevalent motor problems, is performed through the observations of some specific key clinical signs in the perceptual domain during the standard clinical examination or, in our case, more precisely, through a specific assessment protocol created in order to detect the key perceptual disturbance features. The systematic use of this assessment tool on many children with diplegia has allowed us to distinguish when and how children with "dysperceptive" forms are different from those with "motor" ones. In these two groups the studied sign was considered statistically significant if present in over 70% of the individuals. Beside direct observation of the signs, we also collect indirect descriptions through a semi-structured questionnaire administered to parents. This has further confirmed the important differences between the two groups in "spontaneous" behavior in various life settings (home, school, holidays, etc.).

Our study is mainly a qualitative type of research given that it uses assessment tools that emphasize verbal descriptions. In the future, in order to satisfy also quantitative aspects, we will need to enhance our research project by increasing the number of enrolled and instrumentally tested diplegic subjects. The final aim remains, obviously, to improve the comprehension of the problems of CP children and, separately, to test the results of therapeutic treatments for the two categories of motor disorders, with and without associated perceptual disturbances, using evidence based medicine practices.

It is well known that clinical research into developmental age is very complex and presents many limits in the application of the scientific method. This is due to both the variability among subjects with the same clinical phenotype and the spontaneous changes that occur in the same individual during the period of observation (natural development).

Through the use of video recording, following standard shared protocols, it is possible to greatly reduce inter-observer variability, compare subjects, and document significant changes over time. The systematic video recording of many CP children has allowed us to create a database transforming initial descriptions of meaningful signs observed in single cases into systematically designed operative definitions, that is, a neutral, pragmatic, atheoretic description with the aim of obtaining a common language among professional workers.

According to the type of selected patients attending our leading national centers, research has been performed on diplegic children between the ages of 4 and 17. All the enrolled subjects had a well established rehabilitation history and a long term relationship with the center. All the children had already acquired the upright position and were able to walk with or without devices, and did not present any severe visual or hearing impairment or important cognitive, behavioral or attention disturbances. Furthermore they had not undergone any functional surgery or botulinum toxin injection during the previous year.

A selected group of examiners performed the assessment over a period of at least one year. In general terms, we can note that the most typical behaviors were related to different stimuli, particularly the surrounding space and type of posture and gesture being performed.

A short list of operative descriptions of the main clinical signs is as follows:
- startle reaction
- upper limbs in startle position
- averted eye gaze
- frequent eye blinking and closing
- facial grimaces
- freezing of posture
- verbal expressions

The Startle Reaction

To startle means to undergo a sudden involuntary movement of the body, caused by surprise, alarm, or acute pain (Simpson, 1989).

According to Meinck (2006), we can define startle as a "stereotypical response to a sudden and unexpected stimulus (acoustic, visual, tactile, vestibular); similar in all mammals. The response is composed of motor, autonomic, and emotional components. The motor component is an involuntary, brief and jerky movement that cannot be suppressed by will" (Koch, 1998).

A lot of information can be found in the international scientific literature on the startle reaction and this phenomenon has been specifically studied in CP subjects. Studies on the physiologic startle reaction suggested that the bulbo-pontine reticular formation could be the probable matrix of the human startle generator; this area is subjected to a sophisticated and complex modulation by upper centers (other nuclei of the brainstem, limbic system, cortical areas, etc.) (Mirte J et al. 2006).

The motor startle pattern has been quantified with surface EMG and described by video recording. The main experimental setting to study the startle reaction (SR) is the auditory startle reaction (ASR). In this setting, the SR is analyzed through the activation pattern detected by a surface EMG after a sudden auditory stimulus (orbicularis oculi muscle, sternocleidomastoid, spinal extensors, finger extensors) matched with a video recording analysis. It is necessary to carefully control the stimulus parameters (intensity, presence of a pre-stimulus, repetition rate, location) and the posture (presence of voluntary contraction), because it has been demonstrated that both the physiologic and pathologic SR are influenced by many different factors, such as attention, posture and movement.

The heterogeneity of SR causes and the complexity of its modulation suggest that a variety of mechanisms contribute to amplify the SR. This exaggerated SR can be distinguished from the physiologic one since it can be evoked by ordinary, weak, and expected (not sudden) stimuli (ineffective under normal condition) because it presents a lower threshold, greater extension pattern, resistance to habituation after repeated stimulation and reduction after pre-stimulus (Brown P, 1991, 2002; Nieuwenhujizen PH, 2000).

We can observe this exaggerated SR (according to response intensity and frequency) in many neurological pathologies: hyperekplexia literarily means to startle excessively (hyperstartling) and this term has been introduced to define a specific hereditary disorder.

The primary acquired exaggerated SR (symptomatic hyperekplexia) is a clinical sign of cerebral or brainstem disorder without specificity for etiology or lesion site. The pathological SR observable in CP can be allocated in this category. Pyramidal lesions can explain the phenomenon from a neuroanatomical point of view. In fact in CP corticospinal motor pathways can exert inhibitory effects on the ASR (Mirte J et al. 2006).

An interesting review on startle syndromes has been made recently by Mirte, who states that the SR is a bilaterally synchronous shock-like set of movements. The most prominent features are forceful closure of the eyes, raising bent arms over the head, and flexion of the neck, trunk, elbows, hips and knees (Mirte J et al. 2006).

We have compared this literature data with our own video recordings in order to achieve an operative definition of the SR sign.

Startle Reaction: Operative Definition

What can we observe?

Startle reaction is a sudden and involuntary movement, executed almost immediately (milliseconds) after an efficacious stimulus, with an "opening" motor pattern which can be seen in the upper limbs (in their maximum range of motion flexed at the shoulder, usually with the elbow flexed at 90°, a flexed wrist and abducted-extended fingers); sometimes in association with head extension, anguised facial expression (grimace), wide-open or shut eyes, open mouth, and forced inspiration position of the chest. SR is an involuntary behavior that strongly limits the acquisition of motor abilities since it produces important perturbations of posture and gesture which can not always be modulated or blocked by the child.

The SR sign can be observed in different contexts and postures and following different kinds of stimuli. It is not truly a reflex but a reaction, that is, a complex behavior modifiable by the child. In some occasions, for example, SR can be inhibited by hand grasping. This aspect can be interpreted as a strategy used by the child to overcome the imbalance produced by the SR itself. Is grasping therefore a coping behavior? When this strategy is inadequate to inhibit SR, it is impossible for the child to use grasping to support himself with devices or to drive a powered wheelchair. In this sense, grasping can be considered a coping solution.

In the sitting position, lower limb movements, given their response variability, are less significant in recognizing the SR pattern than upper ones. In the most evident expression, lower limbs are semiabducted, with extended knees and equinus-varus-supination of the feet. If the child is seated and tightly holding onto the armrests with a forward leaning trunk, there is often a triple flexion (ankle, knee, foot) response of the lower limbs with increased flexor pattern and loss of foot ground contact.

In older children, SR can still be partially expressed: we can recognize the residual SR pattern at hand level. It consists of sudden movements of fingers that abduct and extend rapidly, with a subsequent hand opening, occurring immediately after the stimulus. Normally it is a bilateral and symmetric sign, but if the child is grasping something with only one hand, we can see the SR pattern on the opposite upper side. The SR can threaten balance and compromise postural control (both sitting and standing) and gesture (walking, manipulating, etc.).

When?

Many different stimuli can produce the SR; here is a short simple list:

- auditory stimuli (normal intensity – low threshold - familiar or unknown)
- vestibular stimuli (sudden shift of the center of gravity, postural perturbations produced by the subject himself or by others)
- visual stimuli (object or person moving quickly forward or away from the child)
- tactile stimuli (loss of physical contact with objects and persons)

Among the different sounds, dysperceptive children can show SR with very common noises such as the telephone, door bell, vacuum cleaner, or pets, especially barking. The essential condition in order to produce SR is the fact that the stimulus must be sudden and unexpected rather than loud.

Not only child-independent stimuli can produce SR, but also stimuli directly produced by the child himself and theoretically foreseen (i.e., the child lets an object fall voluntary, but the noise or the sight of falling provokes SR) or linked with a wrong anticipation of the consequences of an event (i.e., the child touches an object and believes it is going to fall, so he will have a SR even if the object actually does not fall).

Sometimes we observe SR even in a child simply lying supine on a mat. In this situation the child's behavior is surprising, because it is impossible to fall and consequently feel unsafe or threatened, given the great postural stability.

The SR and the upper limbs in SR position during walking can be observed almost in every diplegic child with perceptual disturbances; analyzing a group of 41 diplegic subjects walking with hands free from any kind of grasping (without devices or adult hand) these two signs distinguished the two groups of diplegic children with and without perceptual disturbances.

Our studies confirm the variability of this sign in clinical observations, but we have been able to find SR even when its characteristics are less evident. In order to recognize this sign we must pay particular attention to time. In fact it occurs an instant after the efficacious provocative stimuli. Finally, the SR description is a gestalt pattern and not a kinesthetic one; the single element can be involved in the SR in slightly different ways and with variable characteristics (i.e., the wrist is usually flexed but can be seen also in neutral or extended position).

Upper Limbs in Startle Reaction Position: Operative Definition

What can we observe?

This sign consists of a typical static position (posture) of the upper limbs in which it is possible to easily recognize the influence of the dynamic SR pattern (gesture).

In sitting position, the child maintains his upper limbs in slight abduction, with flexed and abducted shoulders, opened hands, and flexed or aligned wrists. The upper limbs are usually kept in this "opened" position also during activities like manipulation, in which greater adduction towards the trunk is normally required. The difficulty in keeping the upper limbs lowered and alongside the trunk, together with flexion or hyperflexion of the wrists with generally abducted and extended fingers, is the main distinguishing element of the presence of SR. In addition, sometimes we can observe also a slight arm adduction, with abducted and pronated forearms and partially extended elbows. In this case, arm adduction improves manipulation ability. Upper limbs in SR position can be observed also during walking, especially in the initial learning phases, and during postural changes, mainly moving towards the standing position. In the latter, the sign is observable in particular when the awareness of exposure to the surrounding space is greater. In some cases it is even possible to detect the sign in this supine position.

Averted Eye Gaze: Operative Definition

What can we observe? Gaze is intentionally oriented away from the target of the ongoing function (the object of grasping, the direction of walk, etc.) towards other unrelated or insignificant targets.

When?

This sign can be seen during both the manipulation-praxis function and walking. This could underline a common standard strategy utilized for different situations and functions.

For example, the diplegic child can use this strategy during upper limb reaching movement toward a target: the child looks at the object to localize it before starting the gesture, then, during the reaching phase, looks elsewhere, thus eliminating visual control of the current action. Another typical situation in which we can observe the use of this strategy is climbing down stairs. At each step, the eyes are deliberately turned laterally or towards a target which has nothing to do with the current movement, the general action, or control of the surrounding environment.

Frequent Eye Blinking and Closing

What can we observe?

Eye blinking observable in diplegic children with perceptual disturbances differs from that of healthy subjects, being characterized by a prolonged and intense eye closure or by an increased blinking frequency.

When?

This sign can be observed in relation to many of the stimuli that can produce the startle reaction; however it is a separate sign because it can be seen also without the SR motor pattern. The eye blinking can occur after sudden stimuli, as in healthy subjects, but in CP children the phenomenon can take place also after well known, self produced, foreseen, or weak stimuli. Furthermore, we can sometime observe this sign without any visual or acoustic stimulus, as a consequence of an expectation of what is about to happen. For example if a child is playing with a toy that has a cause-effect system, he could start blinking repeatedly before activating the device, i.e., pushing the start button.

Facial Grimaces: Operative Definition

What can we observe?

Facial grimaces of a child usually express anguish or fear. It is a reaction that involves mimic muscles, eyes (wide open or tightly closed), and mouth.

When?

Similar to what happens in the startle reaction, facial grimaces can be produced by loud or unexpected sounds or by visual stimuli of fast traveling objects moving towards or away from the child. Facial grimaces can be caused if the distance of the child from the ground increases (i.e., sitting on a high stool rather than a chair), or during motion generated either by the child or by others, or if the surrounding space becomes increasingly emptier. Facial grimaces in CP are a pathological expression of severe anguish relative to harmless stimuli.

Freezing: Operative Definition

What can we observe?

The child freezes one or more body joints to avoid or reduce movement. This produces an interruption of ongoing motor activity and anxious glances at everything that is happening in the surrounding space. In this situation, the child frequently verbally expresses uneasiness and implores the caregiver to come nearer. The child shows great difficulty or refusal to incline the trunk in sitting position (shifting the center of gravity) and lifting the upper limb such as for the task of leaning over and reaching a distant object). During tests, this behavior becomes very evident during reaching activities executed in a sitting position or during a task of visually following a ball thrown quickly toward the child, in both the sitting or standing position. The trunk and the head are petrified or blocked in rigid and fixed positions that inhibit the child from using his motor repertoire at all. In extreme cases, we can interpret the choice of immobility as an extreme need for steadiness.

When?

We observe this sign when the enclosure of surrounding space disappears. This is due to loss of contact or to the presence or closeness of reference objects and people. During activities that require leaning, freezing is usually directly proportional to depth perception of the surrounding space and/or height of the support base which the child is sitting on.

Verbal Expressions: Operative Definition

What can we observe?

Use of language to express uneasiness in particular situations or tenacious refusal to perform required tasks by the CP child. The most common verbal expressions are: I am falling, help me, hold me, catch me, I can't do it, etc.

When?

These expressions are typical in older children. The conditions and stimuli in which the phenomenon can be observed are more or less the same as those that determine the previous signs.

How to Detect Clinical Signs of Perceptual Disorders

The clinicians that work with diplegic children must carefully investigate signs (startle reaction …) and symptoms (fear, anxiety ...) due to dysperception. Observation (without prejudice) should be sufficient in order to detect their presence/absence. The following assessment tries to attribute a meaning to these signs, determining if they are defects or compensation strategies.

In cerebral palsy, none of these signs, per se, is pathognomonic for perceptual disturbances, and some of them might even be recognized in normal subjects, but with significantly qualitative differences. In fact it is unusual to observe a startle reaction in healthy subjects, perhaps occasionally after a very intense and sudden noise (i.e., when two trains on parallel tracks pass each other). But we all agree that the same reaction for a recognizable ordinary noise (i.e., a pencil that falls on the floor) is not so physiologically acceptable. So it is necessary to establish standardized and reproducible conditions for clinical observation

An evident progressive reduction of support reaction efficacy in diplegic and tetraplegic children is a very important and frequent clinical behavior. This problem is often associated with perceptual disorders. A possible hypothesis suggests that these children, due to their notable postural instability, have a consequently greater fear of falling.

According to Alain Berthoz (1997), we consider the "sense of movement", i.e., the perception of body position and motion, a determinant factor in motor control. An alteration of this sense might clarify some particular behaviors observable in dysperceptive CP children.

It is possible that errors in multiple sensory integration can be present among CP disorders. Sensations, originally segregated on the basis of their physical properties, could lead to ambiguous interpretations of reality. In the effort to achieve more coherence, the subject may learn how to suppress incoherent information. An example of this can be averted eye gaze" while walking down a set of stairs as a compensatory strategy of a probable visuo-kinesthetic conflict (Berthoz et al. 1999).

The existence of visuo-perceptive disorders in diplegic children is well documented, but neuropsychological tests do not allow us to study the more complicated integration problems regarding movement (visuo-kinesthetic collimation). For more information about collimation defects, see chapter 5.

Concerning the difficulty in multisensory integration, we can identify other perceptive processes that, when affected, seem to worsen the functional ability of these children: for example, the ability to use more appropriate frame references for a specifically requested action, or the possibility to access opportune representations of motor action organization, especially in terms of postural anticipatory adjustments.

For perception, the brain uses several reference systems relative to the task at hand and to the sensory indexes available at the moment and most suitable for the sought out result. Body scheme represents the sum of these reference systems (Berthoz, 1997).

Actions are coded in relation to different reference systems that correspond to different spaces concerning body or environment (ego-allo-geo-centric). The choice of the reference system depends on the type of action, and during the same action there may be a shift from one reference frame to another. Clinical observations of CP dysperceptive subjects suggest a possible difficulty in this process. This hypothesis could explain the difficulty these children have in starting to walk, letting go of stable supports, and the relative facilitation allowed by the close physical presence of a caregiver (behind, next to, in front of the child), or by visual references such as a wall corner or a piece of furniture on which to fix gaze. The caregiver, parent, or therapist seems to function like an external reference that the child relies on for simple tasks like standing in the middle of the room.

The activation of the subjective vertical also seems to be affected in different situations, in particular when the subject is exposed to empty space. This aspect could be interpreted as an error of multisensory integration. In fact subjective vertical is the final synthesis of different types of vertical coming from the various sensorial systems (visual, vestibular, proprioceptive, tactile, etc.). If a caregiver walks slowly away from a standing diplegic child with perceptive disorders, that child will usually start to gradually slant in the same direction.

A recent research area concerning perceptive impairment explores anticipatory postural adjustment (APA) in diplegic children in the sitting position during a reaching task. In an experimental set-up, some parameters of the stimulus are modified (stool height, object reaching distance, reaching direction). The behavior of the child is evaluated through the observation of videotapes (qualitative analysis) and by the displacement of the center of pressure (COP) as detected by a force plate placed under the stool (quantitative analysis). Preliminary results seem to confirm the clinical observation of the freezing strategy of posture and give us interesting information about APAs. These are practically absent in the majority of subjects with perceptual disorders, whereas they are constantly present in the control group of diplegic children without dysperceptive disorders.

APAs are based on preventive representations of actions we are about to do. When APAs are lacking, postural control is carried out only through feedback mechanisms during movement. We can image the subject with perceptual problems as being surprised by the loss of balance as a consequence of his own movements (Adkin et al. 2002; Ferrari et al. 2008b).

In chapter 5, the functioning of the process of perceptual transcription of motor programs was analyzed. According to that theory, we may also justify many other phenomena observable in dysperceptive children. If there is an error in perceptual transcription (corollary discharge), simple actions, feasible from a motor point of view, may be mentally inhibited because they are considered potentially dangerous: the CNS in this case rejects the consensus to act. The lack of action consensus may even be linked to an anticipatory simulation of a threatening perception that could appear during the action. Examples of this phenomena are frequent eye blinking and startle reactions before the occurrence of the triggering factor, therefore anticipating the justified reaction to the relatively disturbing stimulus. With regard to this aspect, neurophysiological research has recently demonstrated the existence of bimodal neurons with a tactile and three-dimensional visual perceptive field, whose depth corresponds approximately to the arm length (peripersonal space). This space codification is needed in order to execute actions in the peripersonal area. According to this hypothesis, if we think that in normal subjects there is a codification of space in motor terms (Fogassi, 2005), it is probable that subjects with central motor disturbances can have difficulties in analyzing and coding their own movements, the space surrounding them, and the reciprocal relations between movement and space.

Memory of previous movement perceptions (located in hippocampus, prefrontal and parietal cortex) is an essential guide for future actions (Berthoz, 1997).

Why does action inhibition continue in children with perceptive disorders even after they have directly experienced the same situation or activity many times, verifying that it is not effectively dangerous? Can these phenomena be interpreted as a result of a cognitive disorder characterized by difficulties in experience elaboration and learning process?

Fear and negative experiences in these children concerning movement, open space, and depth and height from the ground might be interpreted also psychiatrically, and we could place these phenomena among the various manifestations of anxiety. A harmful event produces anxiety and may generate a lifetime negative experience, so it is difficult to understand if anxiety and panic are the "primum movens" or the consequences created by a series of negative incidents.

This interpretation does not conflict with other hypotheses, because experiencing intolerant sensations leads to a continuous negative reinforcement regarding action and movement.

General psychopathology recognizes some perceptual disorders and could explain some types of illusion and hallucination that some children seem to experience (see chapter 5). Also for this reason, it is easy to foresee that much work has yet to be done in order to better understand the nature of perceptual disorders in CP children.

Clinical Aspects of Perceptual Disorders

Many years ago two characteristic CP dysperceptive forms were identified: the falling child and the stand-up child (Ferrari, 2000). In the following pages, we will review this original subdivision, which can still be considered helpful in clinical evaluation in severe cases of CP.

1. The Falling Child

The falling child cannot perceptually tolerate the depth of the surrounding space and does not react properly to the force of gravity. The child frequently experiences the feeling of losing posture control, being dragged down by his own body weight; he feels and believes to be endlessly falling, even if he is aware of lying flat on the floor. As if in a nightmare, he lives the sensation of his body breaking up and spreading out. The child seems to believe the whole world is slipping though his fingers; as a consequence, the child tries desperately to grab onto any real or imaginable object.

The falling sensation, felt also in supine position, is not the result of previous catastrophic experiences, but a distorted perception, between illusion and hallucination, associated with an understandable state of anxiety.

The falling child cannot tolerate externally induced postural changes and often even self-induced ones; he manifests distress and fear through repeated startle reactions and quite often expresses this sensation with the words "I'm falling! I'm falling!". Movement is better tolerated in confined spaces (i.e., in a wrap-around stroller or in an electronic wheelchair with belts) or in tight physical contact with the caregiver's body (holding).

This conflict with space usually disappears in water, where the child can better express his motor potential, maybe because water acts as an enclosed, defensive, protective, and supportive element (water is an old acquaintance, since it greatly reduces the sensation of emptiness and heaviness). The falling child has trouble in defining the borders of his own body, in keeping the intrapersonal (autonomic) world separate from the extrapersonal (contextual) one, in distinguishing the space which can be perceived from that in which motor activities can be performed. The perceivable space, in fact, is wider than the performing one. The surrounding space is experienced and internalized (memorized) in a distorted way, as if the individual were not able to keep his body well contained inside his

14

skin. The skin of the falling child is an insufficient container and he looks for substitutes, inside and outside himself, such as muscle tone, the caregiver's body, or a "pleasant ecological nest", appropriately built in the surrounding environment:

- Internally (inside) → spasticity ("muscle" skin, defensive shield): it allows better posture and emotional stability, but it turns out to be so rapidly exhaustive that the child quickly tires. This spasticity is similar to the features of hypertonia that derives from the pathological support reaction, but it over-reacts to antispastic drugs and is difficult to "calibrate" with functional orthopedic surgery. It can be diminished by application of orthosis, usually AFO and KAFO, or supporting devices such as wrap-around padded seats and thoraco-lumbo-sacral corsets.
- In body contact → clothes: these children never like to be completely undressed. In fact their naked body induces a feeling of anguish and despair. Simple motor performances, such as turning over, possible if the child is covered with only a thin sheet, become impossible if the child feels too exposed to the surrounding space and vulnerable to the perception of emptiness.
- Externally (outside) → an adult body, particularly that of the mother, becomes an instrument for physical and psychological holding (containment) for the falling child.

"The tactile, visual, acoustic sensations etc., evoked by environmental inputs, must be transformed and "mentalized", so that they can be "contained", "tolerated" and not become devastating. In the endouterine life, the environment itself functions as a "container", while in extrauterine one there are no "physical" enclosures and the child has to face environmental inputs no longer mediated by the uterus. The activity of the mind must be that of containing inputs and subsequently to "mentalize" them. This is possible in children without severe neurological deficiencies only if this containment is guided by the maternal "rêverie" (Bion, 1962) which acts as a "filter", as a mediator, between environmental inputs (therefore also physical sensations) and the mind of the child" (Ferrari Ar, 1992).

Commonly, these children have sufficient cognitive abilities but, as they grow older, they face great difficulties in being separated from the mother. With the adult, especially the mother, they have a binding relationship of fusion/confusion, in a situation that can be defined as more parasitic than symbiotic. In the arms of the caregiver, the falling child becomes more courageous and interested in acting and interacting with the surrounding environment. This situation very often ends up making the patient poorer, because it eventually forces the child to live through the body and the mind of the caregiver in an illusion of ability that prevents the individual from objectively becoming aware of his own limits. However, we must ask ourselves which psychomotor progress this child could autonomously achieve, if movement generates feelings of uneasiness, vertigo, fear of falling: if it allows him to overcome the boundary separating excitement from anguish, or if it leads to depression and ultimately to giving up.

The need for holding is often psychologically expressed:

- as uneasiness when the child goes to sleep (falling asleep is perceived as a change of state: from a controlled to an uncontrolled one)
- as difficulty to be separated from the mother's body (perceived as change in place)
- as uneasiness and unwillingness to remain alone, even for a short time
- as difficulty to be outside the hearing or visual range of caregivers.

Marzani (2005) calls this separation anxiety and assumes that the missing function may be phantasmal, because this disorder decreases with the simple physical presence of a family member or their voice which is used as a support to movement.

The falling child would like to be a mind without a body, able to direct a body without a mind of a consenting adult (usually the mother).

Drug treatment for the disperceptive disorders of the falling child includes antidepressants (tradozone) and anxiolytics (benzodiazepine, such as nitrazepam and clonazepam) that are anyway not always effective.

The falling child usually has a fairly good intellectual capacity and employs an adult language, sometimes overly elaborated, that is used to verbally express even experiences that the child has never been able to perform, preferring to imagine rather than to experiment, but showing knowledge of the mechanisms and processes underlying the actions. Usually, such children do not present with severe visual or oculomotor problems (see chapter 7) and can adequately coordinate eye and head movements. However, the child prolongs the optic defense (blinking reflex) for a longer period and employs gaze to map out his position within the surrounding space, aiming at nearby "targets", constantly substituting them each time he moves. Sometimes the child can face problems in orientating walking trajectory, that is to correctly direct the walking frame or the powered wheelchair, especially when helpful visual references are lacking. The child usually fails to achieve advanced manipulation skills but can be quite self-reliant for table sitting activities, such as using cutlery or computer keyboards. Under resting conditions, the upper limbs are usually kept adducted to the trunk with flexed elbows and wrists, semi-flexed metacarpus phalanx, and semi-extended interphalanx (hands in "drooping" position).

The generalized stiffness (muscle-like skin) exhibited in difficult situations or in conditions of uneasiness is usually proportional to the severity of the dysperceptive disorder still present.

Defensive spasticity in the falling child must be differentiated from the antigravity spasticity related to the organization of the support reaction. Tone changes generated in relation to an insufficient sensorial calibration (perception) are reduced whenever the patient learns to suppress them (see chapter 5) and is more organized from an emotional viewpoint, irrespective of the course of the antigravity behavior. Conversely, a pharmacological or surgical reduction of spasticity imposed on the child before solving the perception problem would only make the difficulties worse and force the child to give up or even refuse standing position and locomotion instead of improving them.

The motion prognosis of the falling child is not always the same. In many patients, the disperceptive disorder slowly fades away, allowing for the separation from adults during the second or third phase of childhood, so that the child can be left alone even to sleep before the beginning of adolescence. In this case, motor disorders progressively improve and patients can eventually move around with a walking frame or, in some rare cases, with four point canes. For other patients, independently of the therapeutic choices they have followed, there are no improvements in perceptive disorders, while better control of the state of anguish and development of the separation-individuation process can be achieved. The only attainable form of motion independence for such patients is obtained by the use of powered wheelchairs, which should also be applied early.

Functional orthopedic surgery should be proposed as late as possible due both to the risk of severe psychological regressions (return of fear of being undressed, touched, moved or left alone, etc.) and the possible occurrence of a secondary muscle failure and a definitive abatement of the support reaction in standing position (reappearance of astasia and abasia). Orthopedic surgery in fact upsets the whole control strategy previously developed through an enormous effort by the patient (i.e., the use of spasticity as perceptive defence).

2. The Stand-Up Child

The mechanism this child applies in order to limit the negative consequences of perceptive disorders is the suppression of sensations related to kinesthesis, bathyesthesis, and baresthesis (sense of movement, sense of position and sense of pressure), that is, all the information that initially is poorly tolerated by the child (see chapter 5). It is as if the child continuously repeats to himself: "You' re not falling and nothing' s happening to you", etc. By doing so, the child neglects to carry out the required posture corrections in order to orient, align and balance himself and in the end inevitably loses control of his position.

Some authors consider this phenomenon as a sign of "hypotonia" or "hypoposture" (Bobath and Bobath, 1975; Giannoni and Zerbino, 2000), misinterpreting the inability to perform posture corrections (motor aspects) as the inability to autonomously realize the need to urgently perform them (perception aspects). Marzani (2005) attributes this to a dysfunction of the body schema or sometimes to a problem of internal stability of the "physical self". Instead, for other children it could represent a primitive attention disorder (see chapter 8) which may explain why they are able to perform "voluntarily" (however usually "upon request") those posture corrections that otherwise they are not able to perform "spontaneously" or "automatically".

Perception elimination is a complex mental process which requires a certain degree of mental "maturity" by the individual. It usually emerges during the second part of childhood. Before then, the stand-up child presents many similarities with the perceptive and motor behavior of the falling child, even though, at the beginning, the clinical conditions overall appear less severe.

From the motion point of view, the stand-up child can produce an effective anti-gravity reaction, but is unable to do so automatically and stably because he suppresses the analysis of information required for this purpose. From the posture point of view, the child seems as if he is falling asleep in a chair, lowering his head while closing his eyes, then suddenly bolting up, as if "awakened" by the perception of the performed movement.

By not paying attention to self-perception, the stand-up child constantly needs additional external signals or advice and verbal support to control posture. The child realizes what is happening only when informed by other organs, mostly by sight, or more often by the caregiver who repeats sentences like "Stand-up, sit straight, don't slouch!".

Due to the inability to simultaneously perform different mental activities, the difficulty of posture control is increased if the child's attention is shifted to another task, for example, speaking, reading, or other cognitive activities.

Speech ability in this group of CP children is not particularly impaired, but it tends to become less understandable when the patient, due to the reduction of the support reaction, lowers the head and leans the trunk forward.

From the "motor" point of view, the stand-up child can appear diplegic, or in some rare cases even tetraplegic (with vertical trunk antigravity), able to reach and hold a standing position only with support and move around exclusively with a walker, tiring very quickly. When asked to stop, the child needs a considerably long time, taking additional steps in order to adjust the position upon hearing this request.

In the support reaction, the child tends to over-react at the beginning of the activity only to underperform after just a few minutes. The emotional state or motivation may prolong or strengthen the standing and walking ability, but it is difficult to quantify a real psychological determination for these activities.

On the ground, these babies can move by creeping like a seal (upper limbs pulling the trunk and lower limbs forward, the latter are held in flexion-adduction-intrarotation).

The risk of hip deformity is high due to flexion-adduction contractures, which sometimes are severe and accentuated by very intense emotional reactions.

Usually antispastic drugs generate over-reactions. Functional orthopedic surgery, even if well performed, often leads to an over-release of operated muscles. The application of AFO orthosis is justified even in sitting position, because it contributes to improve posture control. Posture systems instead have demonstrated not to be very successful because the trunk tends to lean forward and for this reason the belt system is often over-loaded and therefore uncomfortable.

The presence of perceptual disorders can be detected very early. In the first months of life there is already a reduced capacity by the infant to deal with and process perceptual information (indicated by startle reactions, frequent blinking and postural freezing). These are a consequence of emotional stress, have a low-threshold and maintain a constant response to sudden acoustic, tactile or proprioceptive stimulations. Afterwards, dysperceptive infants show a strong and persistent dependence on perceptual indexes for posture control (e.g., a constant need for visual cues, close support and external reference, a persistent lack of automated control, etc.). Preliminary results of a prospective study (Paolicelli and Bianchini, 2002) already reported in chapter 3, indicate that sense of motion disorders can be clinically detected in a follow-up study. The videotapes taken at 2 and 12 months of age in a group of 29 children, who went on to develop spastic tetraplegia or diplegia, as well a corresponding set of tapes of pre-term infants with normal outcome were scored for perceptual disorders by observers blind to the final outcome. The presence and severity of perceptual disorders were highlighted by a reduced capacity of the infant to deal with and process perceptual information. As reported in Table 14.1, children who already presented severe perceptual disorders between 2 and 6 months post-term, maintained a similar degree of severity afterwards. Postural and motor milestones such as sitting position, walking with support devices, and independent walking, were achieved much later when compared to controls, or even never. These were the same dysperceptive children who developed more severe motor disorders at subsequent stages of development, as indicated by the GMFCS score (Palisano et al. 1997). Such perceptual disorders were never observed in controls.

Table 14.1 Correlations between early signs of "sense of motion" disorders (at 2-12 months) and the severity of motor impairment, measured at greater than 4 years by *GMFCS*, Gross Motor Function Classification System (Palisano et al. 1997); *TP*, tetraplegia; *DP*, diplegia, (defined according to Hagberg et al. 1975) (modified from Paolicelli and Bianchini, 2002).

Case n.	CP type	Percentual disorders	GMFCS	Sitting position (months)	Walking with support devices (months)	Autonomous walking (months)
1	DP	-	1	16	30	36
2	DP	-	1	8	12	28
3	DP	-	1	8	12	18
4	DP	-	1	16	20	30
5	DP	-	1	9	20	30
6	DP	-	1	11	15	19
7	DP	+	1	9	21	22
8	DP	+	1	9	20	25
9	DP	+	1	10	15	18
10	DP	+	1	18	22	32
11	TP	++	5	/	/	/
12	TP	++	5	/	/	/
13	TP	++	3	36	54	/
14	DP	++	2	18	42	66
15	DP	++	3	13	84	/
16	DP	++	3	16	84	156
17	DP	++	2	/	48	96
18	TP	++	3	21	80	/
19	TP	++	5	/	/	/
20	DP	+++	2	18	30	72
21	TP	+++	5	/	/	/
22	TP	+++	5	/	/	/
23	DP	+++	3	19	/	/
24	TP	+++	4	84	/	/
25	TP	+++	5	/	/	/
26	TP	+++	4	72	/	/
27	TP	+++	4	/	/	/
28	TP	+++	4	48	/	/
29	TP	+++	3	48	108	/

These results seem to indicate that these types perceptual disorders can be detected early and are predictive of a later motor outcome.

_____

References

Adkin AL, Frank JS, Carpenter MG, Peysar GW (2002) How fear of falling modifies anticipatory postural control. Exp Bri Res 143:160-70

Berthoz A (1997) Le sens du mouvement. Odile Jacob Edition, Paris. English edition: Berthoz A (2000) The brain's sense of movement. Harvard University Press, Cambridge, Ma

Berthoz A, Viaud-Delmon I (1999) Multisensory integration in spatial orientation. Curr Opin Neurobiol 9:708-12

Bion WR (1962) Learning from experience. William Heinemann London

Bobath B, Bobath K (1975) Motor development in the different types of cerebral palsy. William Heinemann Medical Books Limited, London

Brown P (2002) Neurophysiology of the startle syndrome and hyperekplexia. Adv Neurol 89:153-9. Review

Brown P, Thomson PD, Rithwell JC et al (1991) The hyperekplexias and their relationship to the normal startle reflex. Brain 114:1903-1928

Ferrari A (2000) I problemi percettivi connessi ai disordini motori della paralisi cerebrale infantile. Giorn Ital Med Riab 4:17-24

Ferrari A, Muzzini S, Ovi A et al (2008) The influence of the sense of movement disorders on functionally independent walking in children with diplegia. EACD abstracts. Dev Med Child Neurol, Suppl. n°114, vol. 50, pp 11

Ferrari Ad, Muzzini S, Ferrari Al et al (2008) Functional reach and touch: how sense of movement disorders can influence anticipatory postural adjustments. Dev Med Child Neurol, suppl. n°114, vol 50

Ferrari Ar (1992) L'eclissi del corpo. Una ipotesi psicoanalitica. Borla editore

Fogassi L, Ferrari PF, Gesierich B et al (2005) Parietal lobe from action organization to intention understanding. Science Apr 29; 308:662-7

Giannoni P, Zerbino L (2000) Fuori schema. Springer-Verlag Italia, Milan

Koch M (1998) The neurobiology of startle. Prog Neurobiol 59, pp 107-128

Marzani C (2005) Psicopatologia e clinica dei disturbi mentali nella paralisi cerebrale infantile. In: Ferrari A, Cioni G (eds) Le forme spastiche della paralisi cerebrale infantile. Guida alla esplorazione delle funzioni adattive. Springer-Verlag Italia, Milan, pp 217-229

Meinck HM (2006) Startle and its disorders. Clinical Neurophysiology. 36, Issues -6, Sept-Dec, pp 357-364

Mirte J, Bakker MA, Gert van Dijk J et al (2006) Startle syndromes. The Lancet Neurology, pp 513-524, review

Nieuwenhujizen PH, Schillings AM, Van Galen GP, Duysens J (2000) Modulation of the startle response during human gait. J Nerophysiol 84:65-74

Palisano R, Rosenbaum P, Walter S et al (1997) Development and reliability of a system to classify gross motor function in children with cerebral palsy. Dev Med Child Neurol 39:214–223

Paolicelli PB, Bianchini E (2002) Perceptual disorders in children with cerebral palsy: implication for prognosis and treatment. Dev Med Child Neurol 44:9.

Weiner E Simpson (1989) J New Oxford English Dictionary, Oxford University Press

Forms of Diplegia

A. Ferrari, M. Lodesani, S. Perazza, S. Sassi

Literally, the word diplegia should refer to "any cerebral palsy distributed on any two limbs" (therefore including hemiplegia), but from Freud onwards (1897) this word has been commonly used to indicate "a cerebral palsy of both sides", therefore ranging from tetraplegia to diplegia and double hemiplegia, even including non-spastic syndromes. William Little (1862), considered the scientific father of cerebral palsy (CP), described clinical pictures that today could be defined as diplegia, but he never used this word, which was instead used by Sachs and Petersen (1890), together with the word paraplegia, in their proposal for CP classification. In Minear's interpretation table (1956), diplegia was presented as a form of bilateral CP "paralysis affecting like parts on either side of the body". However, starting from Ingram's interpretation (1955), the word diplegia has been used in the clinical field when the patient's homologous limbs are affected in a more or less symmetrical way and when the lower limbs are "significantly" more affected than the upper ones in relation to pathognomonic signs like "hypertonia", "hyper-reflexia", "weakness", etc., and to motor activities like standing, walking, and manipulating: "*Diplegia ... as a condition of more or less symmetrical paresis of cerebral origin more severe in the lower limbs than in the upper and dating from birth or shortly thereafter*". Another discriminatory criterion proposed by Milani Comparetti (1965), which is extremely practical and clarifying when trying to distinguish diplegia from tetraplegia, is to consider the patient's upper limbs' ability to express an efficient support reaction through the use of suitable orthopedic devices (*diplegia = tetraparesis functionally paraparesis*).

Therefore, diplegic individuals are generally less affected than tetraplegic ones, since they are always able to reach upright position and walk, and conserve this function for at least a certain period in their life.

The assessment of motor gestalt, however, is not sufficient to make a diplegia diagnosis. In fact, besides quantitative difficulties in comparing limbs that develop completely different activities, i.e. walking and manipulating, also individuals with biped antigravity tetraparesis (see chapter 13) can have the lower limbs that are more affected than upper ones and therefore they might be wrongly classified as diplegic, especially if they do not show any significant mental retardation. Conversely, it is also possible that real diplegic individuals, who are able to walk without orthopedic devices for the upper limbs, like

The Spastic Forms of Cerebral Palsy. Adriano Ferrari, Giovanni Cioni
© Springer-Verlag Italia 2010

15

walkers, canes, etc., are considered tetraplegic only due to the fact that their lower limbs are affected as much as their upper ones from a quantitative point of view. Therefore, we can find false diplegics who are not able to walk and false tetraplegics who can manage to walk without the need to use walking device for the upper limbs.

Hence, in order to set the limits of diplegia, it will be necessary to adopt other discriminatory criteria. Among the useful clinical signs which are more or less common to all types of diplegia, we can examine the following.

Controlling Central Pattern Generators

Regarding diplegic individuals, once the motor sequence has been activated, they have difficulty interrupting it in order to divide, separate, select, and reverse the movement. Conversely, tetraplegic individuals have more difficulty evoking and continuously carrying out the sequence without interruption, therefore avoiding its fractioning. As a consequence, kinetic rhythm and frequency, as well as sequential control are more accessible to diplegic individuals than to tetraplegic ones, while the opposite can occur when referring to the possibility of resetting the ongoing motor program.

Reducing Speed

Diplegic patients usually have fewer difficulties in learning to walk fast rather than slowly, and to keep on walking rather than standing in one spot. Their ground locomotion speed (creeping, crawling, walking on knees) and walking with devices (walkers, canes, etc.), as well as the greater difficulty to stop rather than to start walking, can be a significant discriminatory criterion when distinguishing diplegias from the tetraplegic form with biped antigravity.

Four Limb Coordination

Diplegic individuals find it difficult to coordinate the movements of the upper limbs with those of the lower ones during gait and, when using devices for the upper limbs, they find it difficult to correctly distribute the load among the four limbs (weight balancing). Tetraplegic children with biped antigravity are sometimes better at performing this than diplegic ones.

Stabilization and Achieving Proximal Fixation

Both diplegic and tetraplegic individuals with biped antigravity initially show difficulty in keeping a stable antigravity reaction, shifting from distal to proximal fixation, obtaining a correct alignment of the body in space (straight position), and maintaining the overall equilibrium (balancing), with consequent effects on posture control. However, only diplegic individuals manage to achieve sufficient proximal fixation and an adequate static equilibrium, at least in the sitting position.

Modules and Praxes

With regard to tetraplegic patients with biped antigravity, diplegics have more available modules, combinations, and motor sequences (see chapter 4), and make less use of pathological synergies in an adaptive way. Therefore, they have more freedom of choice, not to be interpreted as a residual normality sign, but rather as dependence from primitive and pathological patterns when different motor modules are associated. These aspects, together with the supposed existence of a "silent period" between birth and the 3rd-4th month of life, which is today disproved by modern neuro-developmental investigation systems (see chapter 3), could justify the clinical diagnostic delays of the past.

Some diplegic patients can have dyspractic aspects (sequentially organizing movements needed to achieve any specified motor activity) (see chapter 6) and other alterations of the upper cortical functions (see chapter 8).

Sensations and Perceptions

From the visual point of view, gaze paralysis is quite common, particularly in esotropy (convergent strabismus), which worsens the expressiveness of pathological motor patterns, especially during locomotion (scissor pattern) and manipulation (eye-hand-mouth interaction) (see chapter 7). Apart from balance, the other sensory functions are usually not affected. However, although without overgeneralizing, some dysperceptive problems are often present (orienting in space, correctly directing trajectory, especially when adequate visual targets are missing; coordinating gaze and head movements; dealing with void and surrounding depth, especially backwards; tolerating loss of balance; matching information coming from different reception systems, for example vision and proprioception, etc.) (see chapter 5). For these reasons, as well as for mental and emotional motivations (low self-esteem, delegation, renouncement, etc) (see chapters 9 and 10), by assessing the quality of motor control, regardless of the patient's repertoire, it is possible to make a distinction between diplegic individuals who are particularly able and others who are definitely inhibited and awkward. However, it is necessary to note that, the higher relative incidence of perceptive disorders and alterations of upper cortical functions in diplegia as compared to tetraplegia can be justified by the simple fact that tetraplegic children often cannot be adequately tested due to the severity of their motor disorders (see chapter 8). A comparison should rather be made with hemiplegia, even if it shows fewer dysperceptive disorders and a different involvement of other upper cortical functions and therefore is prognostically considered a less serious clinical form than diplegia.

Upper Cortical Functions

Diplegic individuals show mental retardation and epilepsy less frequently than tetraplegic ones (… the more affected the upper limbs, the lower is intelligence… Morrissy and Weinstein, 2001) (see chapter 8). Due to the low incidence of pseudobulbar paralysis, also hypersalivation and sialorrhea are less serious. Almost all diplegic children achieve a quantitatively acceptable speech, at least after infancy, but some of them can have phonetic problems which do not depend on respiratory function, or they make semantic mistakes (see chapter 8. However, as they can rely on a better cognitive ability, which is generally proportional to upper limbs functionality, diplegic children can have more psychopathological problems (exasperated conflict attitude, depression, anxiety, phobias, maniacal behaviors, etc.). Therefore, also the family's expectations become important (expecting a successful result according to the principle "if they want – they can"), (see chapters 9 and 10).

Manipulation

Diplegic children reach a quite satisfactory manipulation competence, especially in sitting position, apart from those cases in which also dyskinetic elements are present. Due to the difficulty in controlling their wrists (extensors deficiency), they can show some uncertainties when carrying out complex activities like using cutlery or other tools, writing, and drawing. Manipulation competence does not always mean acquiring a good level of autonomy since, as we have seen, there can be dyspraxic and dysperceptive problems which hamper the obtained results (see chapters 6 and 5).

Muscular Retractions and Articular Deformities

Differently from tetraplegia, in diplegic forms, functional surgery generally is performed after the acquisition of upright position and walking. It is necessary to remember that, compared to tetraplegics with biped antigravity, diplegics acquire these competences at a younger age and, as a consequence, there is a lower growth disproportion between long muscles and bones that is determined by spasticity (Mc Intosh et al. 2003). In diplegia, torsion deformities of long bones are quite frequent, with subsequent alterations of the step angle, which Gage (1991) has defined as "lever arm disease". The most common skeletal problems are femur intrarotation, tibia extratorsion, and break down of talus-scaphoid joint, with valgus adducted foot (Rodda and Graham, 2001).

It can be stated that all diplegic individuals manage to walk in a more or less functional way; however, due to the severity of secondary deformities, early fatigue, and poor motivation, many patients of the first and second form (see next paragraphs) give up walking, generally at the beginning of adolescence.

Clinical Forms of Diplegia

With regard to diplegia, similarly to what has already proposed by Sutherland and Davids (1993) in order to distinguish between clinical forms, we prefer the visual observation of gait (observational gait analysis), taking into account the relative age phase of gait development, and the changes provided by therapeutic interventions (physiotherapy, systemic antispastic drugs, district and focal, AFO and KAFO, functional surgery) on gait natural history.

The identification of clinical forms as proposed by our classification is first of all the result of longitudinal observations carried out for many years on a very large sample of diplegic children coming from all over Italy to the national children rehabilitation center of Reggio Emilia (highly specialized in neurological rehabilitation). After a clinical analysis of patient spontaneous gait during the different stages of his development, as well as before and after specific therapeutic interventions, a video-recording is made according to an agreed upon protocol (GIPCI: Italian group for cerebral palsy, 1998). The video is then examined, at normal and slow motion speeds, and the taxonomic analysis of the collected material is made. More recently, the reliability of clinically identified gait models has been subject to optoelectronic assessments (gait analysis) in the lab for motion study of IRCCS Stella Maris of Pisa (see enclosed DVD). The collaboration between students in physiotherapy and doctors specializing in Child Neuropsychiatry and Rehabilitation Medicine has allowed our group to test both the percentage of diplegic individuals that, starting from a random sample, could be assigned to one of our previously described forms, and the consensus among researchers on gait and clinical forms (Bianchini, 2003).

We are aware that no two palsied children can have an identical way of walking, as in normal individuals, therefore when talking generally about diplegia, if we refuse to distinguish between homogeneous macro-groups characterized by similar gait behavior, clinical research will become imprecise and above all it will also be impossible to measure the results obtained through therapeutic interventions (physiotherapy, drugs, orthosis, functional surgery) with any honesty and rigor.

Two legitimate questions are related to the stability of each clinical form, that is, the possibility of a diplegic child shifting, spontaneously or as result of a treatment, from one clinical form to another, and the existence of borderline forms, or/and of, "mixed forms".

Remembering that Hagberg (1989) stated that during development the taxonomic category of many spastic patients could even move from diplegia to tetraplegia and vice versa *"many children change categories as they grow older"*, we can affirm that clinical forms are stable categories, with internal differences, but which fundamentally do not modify gait strategy, which is mainly related to the action of top down components (see chapter 12). Instead, bottom up and especially coping solutions are responsible for the inter-individual differences that can be observed between individuals belonging to the same clinical form, and for intra-individual modifications that occur during development or after the most drastic therapeutic interventions (drugs and functional surgery) within the same compensating strategy (internal coherence). The differential signs between the various clinical forms are more or less apparent according to which aspects they are related to, namely, to main core aspects or accessory ones.

It is also necessary to notice that the gestalt we refer to is represented by "mature" gait and that during development the orientation towards one of the forms is not always supported by easily recognizable and sufficiently reliable predictive signs. We are sure that the possibility of periodically video-recording the patient and documenting his natural history will allow us to progressively obtain an early classifying capability, improving our predictive capacity to reach the final prognosis and, above all, to achieve therapeutic results.

Indeed, our declared goal is to be able to measure changes that have specifically occurred in each clinical form and not generally in diplegias, since the latter includes both individuals who have difficulties in walking with devices and others who can spontaneously learn how to run and jump without any limitations in terms of safety, speed and endurance.

In all honesty, we must point out that there is also a percentage of patients, no more than 10-15%, who cannot be correctly classified by our system.

To distinguish between the different clinical forms of diplegia, we have to analyze the features of the following elements with reference to gait architecture:
- Use of upper limbs and walking devices
- Head and trunk positioning
- Swinging movements of the trunk on frontal and sagittal planes
- Pelvis movements (horizontal translation and anterior-posterior swaying)
- Progression mechanisms
- Step sequence based on foot contact, stance and swing
- Choice of fulcra

According to these elements, it is possible to classify four main types of clinical diplegia (with some possible variants), which are summarized in Table 15.1 and appropriately described in the following pages of this chapter.

First form (forward leaning propulsion)
- With the use of orthopedic devices (four point canes) as a protective reaction
    - Flexed hip
    - Extended hip
- Without the use of orthopedic devices

Table 15.1 Main characteristics of diplegic clinical forms

Segments	1st form	2nd form	3rd form	4th form
Upper limbs	Devices used for protection 4 phases constant support	Devices used for direction 4 phases constant support	Tilted laterally used as stabilizers 2 phases, with no constant support	Lowered
Trunk	Forward leaning with or without lordosis	Vertical	Forward leaning with lordosis	Vertical or slightly forward leaning
Swing	Combined mainly sagittal	Combined, mainly sagittal	Frontal, related to shoulders and upper limbs or pelvis	Combined, mainly frontal Countertendency between shoulders and pelvis
Pelvis	Anteversed and unstable, translated toward the supporting limb with homolateral elevation	Sagittal swinging in anteversion/ retro-version and translation towards the supporting limb	Contralateral elevation, translation toward the lower limb in swing phase	Valid proximal fixation and slightly expressed inter-girdle rotation
Progression	Internal rotation on supporting hip	Flexion on supporting knee	Propulsion and pivot on foot	Hip intrarotation
Foot	Talipes equinus in contact, full support and swing phase Toe balancing	Contact talipes equinus/ dorsiflexion/ drop foot	Contact and push off talipes equinus, pivot/placing	Contact and push off talipes equinus, possible placing reaction Drop foot
Fulcrum	Hip/knee	Lumbar hinge/knee	Trunk/foot	Hip/foot
Distinguishing signs	Trunk forward leaning and toe balancing	Knee flexing in mid stance and pelvis swinging	Frontal trunk swinging	Increasing talipes equinus at start of walking

Second form (tight skirt)
- With the use of orthopedic devices (four point canes) as direction function
- Without the use of orthopedic devices

Third form (tightrope walkers)
- With the use of orthopedic devices (four point canes) as equalizer
- Without the use of orthopedic devices

Fourth form (daredevils)
* Generalized form
* Prevalent distal form
* Asymmetrical form (double hemiplegia)

For greater taxonomic completeness, it should be noted that atonic diplegia, that is, flaccid diplegia (Little Club Memorandum, 1959), and ataxic diplegia (Hagberg et al. 1975), which is characterized by coordination disorders, especially dyssynergy and intentional tremor of the upper limbs, are not included in this classification system, which is restricted to spastic forms of diplegia.

Instead, *double hemiplegia* and, more in general, the role played by asymmetry within the functional architecture (see chapter 12) deserve further comments. We encounter patients with significant bilateral differences in the fourth form, but also in the other forms of diplegia it is possible to detect that one side or one limb is more or less affected than the other, especially during walking at low speeds. Generally, the lower and upper limbs on the same side behave in a homogeneous way according to their degree of dysability, but it is not possible to cross-study the different situations. During faster walking, due to the increase of synkinetic and associated reactions, it is easy to observe higher symmetry, together with an increased expression of the pathological pattern. With regard to symmetry, during some developmental stages it can be difficult to clearly separate real hemiplegic forms from asymmetric bilateral ones (or double hemiplegia), especially if they do not include any dysperceptive disorders, due to the importance of recruiting and irradiating events. But if we tried to rule out all borderline situations, as proposed by Colver and Sethumanhavan (2003) with regard to tetraplegia and diplegia (see chapter 12), we would end up considering all forms of CP as one large clinical form, making it impossible to achieve a differential diagnosis, or to understand what can be modified, or to assess the outcomes of therapeutic treatment.

Validation of the Proposed Classification of Diplegia

In a recent paper (Cioni et al. 2008), we have attempted to validate the hypothesis of CP classification described in these pages. The subjects included in the study were all children, adolescent and young adults with CP admitted either to the Children's Rehabilitation Unit of S. Maria Nuova Hospital (Reggio Emilia, Italy) or the Department of Developmental Neuroscience of the IRCCS Stella Maris (Pisa, Italy) during the period from January 2005 to December 2006. Inclusion criteria were the diagnosis of CP according to international definitions (Bax et al. 1964; Bax et al. 2005), an age more than two years and the availability of data concerning possible associated disorders. An epidemiological chart to classify impairment which included an assessment according to SCPE (SCPE 2000), was administered to each subject. This chart was previously modified in order to further subdivide the spastic bilateral forms into diplegic and tetraplegic types, according to Hagberg et al. (1996) and Himmelmann et al. (2005). It also included the classification of walking in diplegia proposed by our groups (Ferrari et al. 2005; Ferrari et al. 2008) and listed below. Type of CP (various spastic types, dyskinetic, ataxic), severity of lower and upper limb impairment and other associated disorders (seizures, hearing and visual problems, mental retardation) were assessed for each patient. The overall motor impairment was classified using the gross motor function classification system (GMFCS) (Palisano et al. 1997) and the ability to handle objects was evaluated by means of two systems suitable to grade manual motor abilities: the bimanual fine motor function scoring system (BFMF) (Beckung et al. 2002), until early 2006, and subsequently the manual ability classification system (MACS) (Eliasson et al. 2006) until the end of the study.

The final sample group consisted of 467 subjects, aged 2.0-21.7 years (mean 7.8±4.1); 262 were male and 205 female. The CP distribution showed a large prevalence of spastic forms, 93% (434 subjects), versus dyskinetic, 5% (24 subjects), and ataxic 2% (9 subjects), ones (see Table 15.2). There were subjects with tetraplegia 115 (25% of spastic CP); 64 males, 51 females; mean age 7.8±4.5 (range 2.0-20.2) and 213 subjects with diplegia (46% of spastic CP); 115 were male, 98 female; mean age was 7.9±3.9 (range 2.0-21.7 years). These diplegic subjects were further divided into the four subgroups according to the proposed walking classification (see Table 15.1). Form IV (47% of diplegic sample, 89 subjects) prevailed over the other forms, followed by the form I (22%, 47 subjects) and then subsequently by forms III and II (15% and 12%, 33 and 26 subjects respectively). Also 18 subjects were not classified because they were too young to walk or they had just started (see Table 15.3). The results of the assessment for motor functions and associated impairments of subjects with tetraplegia and diplegia are described in Tables 15.2 and 15.4 respectively. As also reported in chapter 13, the subjects with tetraplegia were more severely impaired than those with diplegia; impairment differences were statistically significant (p<000). Generally, the sample of diplegic subjects had normal mental development and did not suffer seizures.

As indicated in Table 15.4, the greater involvement in visual and mental abilities was found in forms I and III; a significant correlation with severe mental impairment was found in form I (χ^2, p=.023). Moreover, GMFCS and MACS/BFMF levels showed a decreasing severity of impairment passing from form I to form IV. The GMFCS level distribution was statistically significant: form I and form IV had lower and higher values, respectively, II and III forms together had an intermediate position. BFMF level distribution showed a minor involvement in form IV. However, two subjects with form IV presented considerable manual impairment (BFMF level V): one had severe mental retardation (IQ < 20), whereas the other had no mental impairment but abnormal visual functions and an asymmetric distal involvement.

As indicated above, in our sample, among the spastic forms that included the largest group of CP children (93%), it was possible to distinguish children with diplegia and tetraplegia not only according to different levels of motor impairment, as demonstrated by the assessment scales (GMFCS, BFMF, MACS), but also according to other disabilities associated with the central paralysis (mental retardation, visual impairment, seizures). The GMFCS, according to Morris and Rosenbaum (2003), underlines the existence of two different categories, where diplegic subjects can be mainly found in levels I – III and tetraplegic ones in levels IV and V (see results shown in Table 15.2).

Table 15.2 Main features of 213 subjects with diplegia and 113 with tetraplegia

Type of Cerebral Palsy	Subjects	Diplegia n (%)	Tetraplegia n (%)	test	p
Mental development	Normal	105 (49%)	14 (12%)	Chi square	,000
	Abnormal	89 (42%)	95 (82,5%)		
	Missing	19 (9%)	6 (5,5)		
		Total ss 213	Total ss 115		
Epilepsy	Present	22 (10,5)	54 (47%)	Chi square	,000
	Absent	191 (89,5)	61 (53%)		
		Total ss 213	Total ss 115		
Visual abilities	Normal	94 (44%)	24 (21%)	Chi square	,000
	Abnormal	105 (49%)	89 (77,5%)		
	Missing	14 (7%)	2 (1,5%)		
		Total ss 213	Total ss 115		
GMFCS	Level 1	54 (25,5%)	2 (1,5%)		
	Level 2	51(24%)			,000
	Level 3	57(26,5%)	3 (2,5%)		
	Level 4	33 (15,5%)	34 (29,5%)		
	Level 5	4 (2%)	72 (62,5%)		
	Missing	14 (6,5%)	4 (3,5%)		
		Total ss 213	Total ss115		
BFMF	Level 1	41(33,5%)		ANOVA,	,000
	Level 2	68 (56%)	7 (10%)	Bonferroni	
	Level 3	9 (7,5%)	11(15%)	post hoc	
	Level 4	2 (1,5%)	22 (30%)		
	Level 5	2 (1,5%)	32 (45%)		
		Total ss 122	Total ss 72		
MACS	Level 1	18 (31%)			,000
	Level 2	22 (38%)			
	Level 3	15 (26%)	7 (17%)		
	Level 4	3 (5%)	13 (32%)		
	Level 5		21 (51%)		
		Total ss 58	Total ss 41		

BFMF, bimanual fine motor function; GMFCS, gross motor function classification system; MACS, manual ability classification system; ss, subjects

The distinction between diplegia and tetraplegia is important in order to measure appropriately the rehabilitation needs and the relative health and social costs due to different levels of motor impairment and consequent overall disabilities.

The possibility to distinguish different forms among the subjects with spastic diplegia by analyzing their walking pattern (guiding function) has been confirmed in our study. The 213 diplegic children of our series (46% of the whole sample) were classified with in the four clinical forms. In the past, Berta and Karel Bobath (1975) had already distinguished two categories of children with diplegia in reference to walking patterns, the so-called "pigeon walk" and the "duck walk". More recently, gait classification in children with CP has been the subject of several studies and proposals (see Dobson et al. 2007 for a review).

Table 15.3 Distribution of the subjects with diplegia according to the suggested classification

	n (%)
form I (forward leaning propulsion)	47 (22%)
form II (tight skirt)	26 (12%)
form III (tight rope walkers)	33 (15%)
form IV (dare devils)	89 (42%)
Unclassified	18 (9%)
Total	213

Table 15.4 Main features of the 213 subjects belonging to the four forms of diplegia

Forms of diplegia		Subjects n (%)				
		Form I	Form II	Form III	Form IV	Unclassified
Mental development (ss 213)	Normal	13(27.5%)	18(69%)	14(42%)	51(57.5%)	9(50%)
	Abnormal	29(62%)	5(19%)	16(48%)	31(34.5%)	8(44.5%)
	Missing	5(10.5%)	3 (12%)	3(10%)	7(8%)	1(4.5%)
Epilepsy (ss 213)	Present	6(13%)	3(12%)	1(3%)	12(13.5%)	
	Absent	41 (87%)	23(88%)	32(97%)	77(86.5%)	18(100%)
Visual abilities (ss 213)	Normal	16(34%)	13(50%)	16(48.5%)	40(45%)	9(50%)
	Abnormal	29(62%)	12(46%)	17(51.5%)	38(42.5%)	9(50%)
	Missing	2(4%)	1(4%)		11(12.5%)	
GMFCS (ss 213)	Level 1		5 (19%)	2 (6%)	46 (51.5%)	1 (5.5%)
	Level 2	2 (4%)	7 (27%)	11 (33.5%)	30 (33.5%)	1 (5.5%)
	Level 3	21 (45%)	8 (30%)	15 (45.5%)	6 (7%)	7 (39%)
	Level 4	22 (47%)	3 (12%)	2 (6%)	1 (1%)	5(28%)
	Level 5	2 (4%)				2 (11%)
	Missing		3 (12%)	3 (9%)	6 (7%)	2 (11%)
BFMF (ss 122)	Level 1	4 (13.5%)	8 (42%)	3 (15%)	26 (49%)	
	Level 2	21 (70%)	11 (58%)	15 (75%)	21 (39%)	
	Level 3	5 (16.5%)		2(10%)	2 (4%)	
	Level 4				2 (4%)	
	Level 5				2 (4%)	
MACS (ss 58)	Level 1		2 (50%)	2 (17%)	14 (48.5%)	
	Level 2	5(38.5%)	1 (25%)	6 (50%)	10(34.5%)	
	Level 3	8 (61.5%)	1(25%)	3 (25%)	3 (10%)	
	Level 4			1(8%)	2(7%)	
	Level 5					

BFMF, bimanual fine motor function; *GMFCS*, gross motor function classification system; *MACS*, manual ability classification; *ss*, subjects;

Our proposed classification system allowed us to easily allocate 91% of the diplegic subjects to one of the foreseen four forms, thus supporting the clinical existence of these forms and also determining their prevalence within a large hospital based sample.

The taxonomic system of the kinematic classification allowed us to assess and reliably classify the different clinical forms also through the use of videotapes (Pascale et al. 2008), based on the condition that these have been realized in accordance with standardized criteria (GIPCI, 1998).

We have compared the degree of limb impairment and other disabilities between tetraplegic and diplegic subjects and within the different forms of diplegia. Within the diplegic group, we were able to recognize a gradual increase in impairment and disability both for motor (GMFCS, BFMF, MACS) and non-motor disturbances, from I to form IV, enhancing the idea that among the subjects with diplegia there are different groups of patients. The GMFCS is able to distinguish the most severe form (I) and the least severe one (IV), but it cannot significantly separate the two intermediate forms. These two diplegic categories are in clinical practice very different, not only for their kinematic patterns of walking, but also for physiotherapeutic needs, most suitable types of AFO, modality of antispastic drug administration (i.e., timing and sites of botulinum toxin injections), and surgery planning. For example, the triceps surae release favors crouch gait in the second form (due to progressive weakness) and may delay walking acquisition and above all the ability to stop in the third form (due to the impossibility to adopt a velocity strategy). In addition the existence of four different diplegic categories was confirmed by gait analysis studies, which allowed us to outline the kinetic and kinematic features present in each clinical form.

In order to validate the kinematic classification system, the gait patterns of 50 children and adolescents with CP (23 M, 27 F; age range 3-17 years) were selected among patients whose videos were stored in the archives of the Reggio Emilia and Pisa Hospitals. Only videotapes of gait with homogeneous features (duration of at least 90 sec, simultaneous recordings on sagittal and frontal views, and other criteria) were taken into consideration. The videos were blindly scored, using an observational gait scale: firstly by two of the authors of the classification system (defined as "maximum" authorities), then by ten expert observers, and lastly by 206 rehabilitation professionals (physiotherapists, neuropsychiatrists, physiatrists, orthotists) after a one-day training session on the classification principles. The calculation of Cohen's kappa statistics (k) and intra class correlations (ICC) revealed an almost perfect agreement between the two maximum authorities and among the ten expert observers. Excellent results were also obtained in the group of one-day trained scorers (Pascale et al. 2008). Only a few cases in fact were assigned to the "unclassifiable" category. Profession of the observer (doctor or therapist) and previous knowledge of this classification system had no significant influence on the score reliability.

In the last part of this chapter we will describe in more detail the features of the four proposed forms of diplegia, reporting also data obtained by quantitative gait analysis.

Main Aspect of Each Form of Proposed Classification of Diplegia

1. First Form (Forward Learning Propulsion)

The prevailing aspects of the first form of diplegia are trunk antepulsion, with use of upper limb devices (four point canes) like a protective reaction, and toe balancing. Two subgroups of this form are represented by children who manage to bring the hip to extension at the end of the stance phase (extended hip variant) and by others, who are usually less compromised and able to temporarily abandon upper limbs devices ("holding onto air" variant) under special environmental conditions.

Upper Limb Devices (Four Point Canes) and Flexed Hip

During walking, the head is kept in vertical position or, more often, pulled forward and slightly retroflexed in comparison to the trunk. Gaze is directed downward and forward. The trunk is always forwardly inclined (antepulsion), often completely kyphotic, sometimes with lumbar lordosis compensating pelvic anteversion, which is frequently subsequent to an excessive surgical release of the hamstrings or to an unsolvable contracture/retraction of hip flexors, especially iliacus and psoas. During walking, the overall center of gravity tends to fall on the most anterior part of the support base and calls for lower limb advancement, mimicking a parachute reaction (Fig. 15.1). The "propulsive" feature of this gait derives from this aspect (it looks as if the individual is "pursuing" the projection of his center of gravity by making a series of subsequent steps and balancing himself on his toes by more or less flexing his knees) (Fig. 15.2). Also by wearing an ankle foot orthosis (AFO), the patient generally finds the point of balance on the shoe tip, therefore eluding the negative angle facilitation provided by the orthosis to the ankle joint (hence AFOs with flexible tips are better). Even after surgical correction of the talipes equinus and acquisition of a better foot dorsiflexion, the load continues to be projected onto the tip, sometimes also through a greater knee flexion. Four point canes are kept on the side and in front of the trunk. They are more useful as a protective tool rather than for real support, differently from tetraplegia with biped antigravity. Support on four point canes is constant, but the load on the upper limbs usually remains limited. It seems as if the patient is propped forward to improve the overall balance. Shoulders are depressed and slightly leaned forward, consistent with the kyphotic attitude of the upper trunk. Elbows are partially flexed (with consequent difficulties in correctly adjusting the device height), wrists are semi-extended, hands are clenched in a fist on the cane handles, with opposing thumb. The devices are moved forward in an alternate pattern, usually subdivided into four phases, with difficulties in balancing the progression and harmonizing the sequence of four limb alternate movements. If compared to the variability, speed, reliability and confidence shown when moving with a walker (a fundamental test for the differential diagnosis relative to the tetraplegic form with biped antigravity), walking with four point canes can be slow and tiring (Fig. 15.3). The patient's general resistance is however

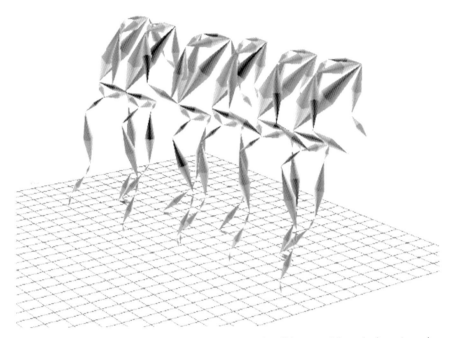

Fig. 15.1 *Propulsive diplegic patient.* Stick diagram of walking, semi-frontal plane (see also enclosed DVD)

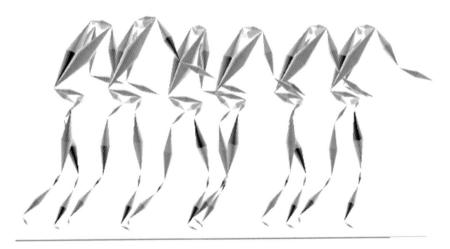

Fig. 15.2 *Propulsive diplegic patient.* Stick diagram of walking, semi-sagittal plane (see also enclosed DVD)

limited due to the exhaustion of the support reaction, especially if no AFOs are used.

Lower limbs present a pattern which is traditionally defined as "extension" (although none of the joint stations can be labeled as totally extended), with adductor interference (scissor pattern), evoked for stabilization purposes (search for proximal fixation, see

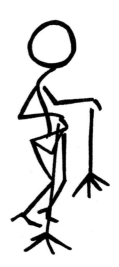

Fig. 15.3 *Propulsive diplegic patient with upper limbs devices (four point canes) with flexed hip.* Walking pattern

chapter 13) and with slight intrarotation of the thighs due to anteversion of the femoral necks. Knees remain semi-flexed during suspension and contact phases, and tend to extend, sometimes with accentuation of hip internal rotation, during the full support phase, especially when the contralateral lower limb crosses the zenith (jump gait with or without stiff knee according to rectus femoris behavior during swing phase of gait cycle, Rodda and Graham, 2001). Ground contact occurs in equinus-valgus-pronation, with the tibia sometimes slightly extrarotated; more rarely, it occurs in varus-supination, when thigh internal rotation due to femoral neck anteversion is very consistent and accompanied by tibia intratorsion (apparent equinus, according to Boyd et al. 1999: *semi-flexed hip, semi-flexed knee and plantigrade foot*). After talipes equinus correction, the foot evolves to flat-valgus-pronation, with clear adduction of the forefoot, leading to tibia extratorsion and progressive flexed valgus knee. In this situation, the talus dislocates medially, leading to the so-called "third malleolus", while the rotula tends to shift upward, due to subpatellar ligament failure, and therefore can be laterally displaced.

The diplegic individuals with the first form, due to over-reaction to the stretching of hip flexor muscles, especially iliopsoas, are not able to extend the hip of the lower limb that has to abandon the load at the end of supporting phase. In order to compensate for this defect, while the contralateral lower limb moves forward in suspension, they accentuate trunk internal rotation on the loaded limb (with subsequent torsion conflict on the knee, since the leg and foot are in external rotation) and homolateral translation on the frontal plane of the pelvis (which subsequently becomes unstable due to proximal fixation reduction). The pelvis is elevated on the loaded limb side.

> *"The children with a clear torsion of the dorsal column and anterior inclination of the pelvis lean the trunk backwards, lift the leg and place it forward in order to move a step. Therefore they launch their body forward to transfer the weight (pigeon gait)"*
> (Bobath, 1975).

Trunk intrarotation on the loaded limb influences the way the contralateral lower limb contacts the ground at the end of swing phase. The lower limb, although making an external rotation during swing phase, as a consequence of pelvis rotation, contacts the ground with the thigh already intrarotated in relation to the frontal plane (step angle usually closed or even negative). The effect of this movement on the overall alignment of the lower limb is often disguised by the relevance of flexed-valgus knee and valgus-pronated foot, which tend to keep the step angle open towards the external part. A contact talipes equinus is present, which then proceeds to one of full support. This is functionally advantageous to compensate for the foot drop of the contralateral limb, which generally becomes more pronounced. Before surgical correction, the supporting talipes equinus is more accentuated during the first phase (contact) and during zenith cross at mid stance, while it is reduced during late stance, with deformity increase in foot valgus-pronation (sometimes with collapse of the longitudinal arch). Foot valgus-pronation often masks the already existing talipes equinus deformity (the calcaneus dislocation creates a wide contact surface with the ground, while the Achilles tendon shifts externally, by medially dislocating the talus and keeping the calcaneus lifted and adducted). The foot of the suspended limb raises slightly off the ground and the toes drag along the surface. It is possible to see, if the patient wears ankle-foot orthosis (AFO) in order to limit foot valgus-pronation, during push off a pivot on the toes in external rotation or, more rarely, in internal one.

In case of loss of balance, patient belonging to this form have difficulties in evoking efficient parachute reactions with their lower limbs. Conversely, they rely rather on upper limbs, positioning the four point canes, even further forward and laterally if they fall sideways, or produce a startle reaction lifting the four point canes from the ground or abandoning them involuntarily if they fall backward. Indeed, the upper limbs cannot have a parachute reaction backwards, and due to girdle difficulty in reciprocal rotation, the lateral parachute reaction cannot be brought backwards beyond a certain point. The propulsive gait character of diplegic children belonging to the first form might derive from the need to defend themselves from falling backwards. For this reason, at least in the beginning, is important that the four point canes are not too light. Heavier four point canes, acting as counterweights, can indeed contribute to maintaining equilibrium in case of backward loss of balance.

If asked to walk backwards, the patient accentuates trunk antepulsion, increases load on the upper limbs and moves the lower limb by performing a rotation on the ground similar to skating.

Children usually start crawling within three years of age, after first learning to creep. For a long time they prefer to move horizontally, which allows them to move faster, usually without completely separating lower limb movements, and start walking relatively late, only after adequate physiotherapeutic treatment.

In sitting position, especially before surgical release of the hamstrings, patients adopt the so-called functional compromise, as defined by Milani Comparetti (1978): they sit on the sacrum and not on the ischium and prevalently keep an "extension pattern" of the lower limbs (semi-extended knees and feet in plantar flexion), while on the head, trunk and lower limbs the "flexion scheme" prevails (head antepulsion, large dorsal kyphosis, flexion of elbows and wrists). If the knees are forcibly flexed under the thighs, even before surgical release of the hamstrings, the head acquires a vertical position, the rachis straightens, and lumbar lordosis appears.

Manipulation activity can be effective even far from the body axis, as long as the sitting position becomes sufficiently stable (acquisition of a adequate proximal fixation or use of a chair with an appropriate pelvis blockage).

In this form of diplegia, functional surgery has to deal with adductors contracture and the medial hamstrings (but only when pelvis proximal fixation has become sufficiently stable) and later with contractures of the gastrocnemius and peroneus muscles (more rarely of the tibialis posterior muscle). The adductors though should not be excessively weakened due to their stabilizing role during control of horizontal translation of the pelvis (proximal fixation). Sometimes it can also be necessary to deal with the hip flexors, particularly iliopsoas. After surgery, leg-foot orthosis with anti-talipes calcaneus action (AFO) might be necessary to limit excessive reduction of the support reaction and to improve endurance. These individuals are more bound to a secondary failure of the triceps surae with foot valgus-pronation and knee flexed-valgus, in particular if the operation is done on the tendon portion of the muscle and not on the aponeurotic one, rather than to a recurrence of talipes equinus deformity resulting from residual spasticity and height growth.

Surgical operations on soft elements (adductors and medial hamstrings) lead to significant improvements also in sitting position: head and trunk straightening, support transferring from sacrum to ischium due to the reduction of pelvis retroversion, less tendency to keep knees semi-extended and feet lifted from the ground, better overall stability, and better use of the upper limbs, especially when moving away from the body axis (outgoing). It is however necessary to mention the negative effects that functional surgery can have on dysperceptive disorders in this form. In the months following surgery, a worsening of the previous disorders can reappear also in sitting position, especially with regard to control of backward space and tolerance to unbalance.

Failure of support reaction

Lengthening of triceps sure → shortening of neuromuscular spindles → reduced muscular recruitment → floppiness (favored by non-specific myopathic components which are generally present → involvement of the extension couple triceps-quadriceps → increase of knee flexion (crouch) → speed up of triceps failure and start of subpatellar ligament sagging → permanent loss of upright position and gait

Compared to the pre-surgery situation, surgical operations modify:

- talipes equinus but not foot valgus-pronation, which generally remains very marked
- knee flexion, with possible secondary increase of trunk antepulsion, if hamstrings have been released too much and lead to prevalence of the iliopsoas
- knee flexion with benefits for knees and hips, if the releases have been adequately performed
- thighs adduction but not intrarotation.

Flexed-valgus stress on the knee during monopodal load and the risk of rotula upward tilting are reduced after surgery.

Hoffer's classification (Hoffer et al. 1973)

> Walk everywhere, also outdoors
> Walk only in domestic environments (intramoenia)
> Walk only during physiotherapy (for exercise)
> Confined to wheelchair

In this form of diplegia, gait prognosis remains uncertain. A great majority of patients "only" achieves domestic walking (see Hoffer classification), or walking supported by a caregiver, and many of them abandon it in favour of the wheelchair, even before adolescence. The maintenance of a long-lasting support reaction and a gait assisted by orthosis and devices can already be considered as a success, especially in order to achieve autonomy for personal care activities.

First form of diplegia (propulsive)

> Upper limbs for defense with constant support on orthopedic devices
> Forward pulling of the trunk with or without lordosis
> Combined, mainly sagittal swinging
> Pelvis anteversion and instability, homolateral translation and elevation
> Progression: rotation on supporting hip
> Foot: contact and full support talipes equinus, balancing on toe tips, drop foot
> Fulcrum: hip/knee
> Distinguishing signs: trunk antepulsion and balancing on toes

Upper Limb Devices (Four Point Canes) and Extended Hip

The head is free to rotate, pulled forward and slightly moved backward in order to be vertical, since the trunk is steadily pulled forward. Gaze is often directed downwards. At each step, to transfer the load onto the front foot, the trunk is further inclined forward (propulsive pattern) and subsequently straightened, with hip extension and slight accentuation of lumbar lordosis, while the supporting lower limb becomes vertical. The pelvis remains aligned to the trunk, and the thigh of the loaded limb makes a complete excursion during late stance by extending from internal rotation or, more rarely, from external one. There is often pelvis instability, due to incomplete capacity to proximal fixation, with frontal translation towards the supporting limb. The baricenter remains projected forward and it seems to facilitate the start of lower limb suspension, which is about to be pulled forward (forward parachute reaction). The knee contributes to make the step longer by bending at the end of the monopodal support phase, and then it becomes suddenly flexed once the contralateral foot gets in contact with the ground. The vertical excursion of the baricenter is very accentuated, since during biped phase both knees are partially flexed and during monopodal phase the loaded knee tends to be hyperextended. With regards to trunk position in space, the hip and knee flexion movement starts late (stiff knee), as if the patient needed to support himself with a placing reaction starting from the trunk and extending through the hip and knee to the foot. Also the head and the shoulders, being inclined opposite to the limb to be advanced, seem to participate in the facilitating mechanism. The foot is talipes equinus-varus-supinated during suspension and when it contacts the ground. The talipes equinus is reduced during full support and rotates on its frontal-external border (pivot) during pre-swing phase. It can be pulled forward through a placing reaction when the suspension starts, but it generally scuffles on the ground during most of the swing phase. At mid stance, the suspended foot, forefoot dragging, literally has to overtake the supporting one.

The patients that have their hip extended by extrarotation show talipes equinus-valgus-pronation and can rub against the heel or ankle. Sometimes, patients also rub against the medial surface of the knee, despite hypertension tending to move this joint away. The crossing of the lower limbs can be more or less developed (scissor pattern). The point of balance is kept on the toes, which is a typical feature of the first form. In patients with extrarotation, the use of AFO protects the foot from longitudinal arch failure, but it does not improve walking performance compared to orthopedic shoes. In patients with intrarotation, it can contribute to limit tip dragging.

The upper limbs, semi-extended on the elbow, keep the orthopedic devices forward or on the trunk side, according to the patient's ability. Leaning on the devices is constant, but the load is kept moderate, since the patient is often able to lift or move the walking frame or four point canes and to momentarily detach one hand from the device. The walking pattern consists of four phases. To speed up walking, the child with this form of diplegia can push up on the devices and move the lower limbs forward (sagittal semi-swing). Walking with walking frame (possible also with four spinning wheels) is fast, a typical feature in diplegia, while speed with the use of four point canes or one-point crutches is usually reduced.

Without the Need for Upper Limb Device ("Grasping the Air")

The head is pulled forward and slightly retroflexed, free to rotate, but usually oriented in the direction of the advancing lower limb (Fig. 15.4). The upper limbs, flexed at the shoulders, are kept forward with semi-extended elbows and the hands, in a grasp position, are held about at shoulder height, as if the child wanted to grab the space in front of him in an attempt not to fall backwards ("I'm grasping the air"). A typical feature of patients with the first form is that during walking they show trunk inclination-antepulsion which is initially kyphotic, but which, after surgical stretching of the hamstrings, presents with a compensatory lumbar lordosis of the pelvis anteversion. At each step the pelvis shows a horizontal translation towards the supporting limb, which makes the gait acquire a slightly swinging behavior (pelvis swinging more than shoulders), which is generally not completely

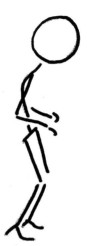

Fig. 15.4 *Propulsive diplegic patient without the need for upper limb devices.* Walking pattern

symmetrical. Advancing speed can be higher than that achieved by individuals with the same form who use orthopedic devices for the upper limbs. Hip extension of the loaded limb is limited by the huge reaction to iliopsoas stretching. The steps therefore are short and crowded, sometimes even fast, but interrupted by frequent stops (cluster). The patient keeps on walking until he finds something on which to grip in order to stop. In upright position, far from any possible support, he sometimes learns to achieve stability by leaning one knee against the other in flexed-adduction, with a strong internal rotation of the thighs, by exploiting femoral neck anteversion, which is usually present.

Walking without crutches frequently takes place in small areas or domestic environments, for example in a corridor, often with the hand occasionally touching on the wall. Outdoors, the patient prefers to hold hands or use crutches or walking frames, which are fundamentally important when the patient moves at low speed or must stand for a long time. Walking with crutches is not always so effective as could be imagined by observing the patients during walking without crutches, due to coordination problems in advancing the four limbs.

Sometimes, walking without supports is achieved after one or more surgical operations, but as a more or less temporary episode in the patient's history, linked to a particular period of his development and a particularly favorable muscular balancing.

According to the GMFCS for cerebral palsy (Palisano et al. 1997; Russell et al. 2002), diplegic children of the first form can be placed at the 2nd (4%), 3rd (45%), 4th (47%) and 5th (4%) levels (missing 0%) (Cioni et al. 2008).

2. Second Form (Tight Skirt)

Also the second form of diplegia can include individuals who, according to the severity of the clinical picture, walk with or without devices for the upper limbs. Compared to the first form, lower limbs are clearly more affected than trunk and upper ones.

With the Need for Devices Used by the Upper Limbs (Four Point Canes for Direction)

The head can be slightly pulled forward, but it is always held straighter than in the first form, while the trunk remains mainly vertical. Four point canes are usually kept forward and sometimes spun on the ground without being lifted. Although the load on the upper limbs is reduced, four point canes are constantly in contact with the ground. Walking occurs in a four-stage pattern. Once the individual reaches sufficient walking ability, he will be able to use two four point canes, bottom plate canes or one point crutches. If they use only one four point cane, the patients do not considerably change the characteristics of their walking, but they usually reduce their walking speed.

The gait pattern resembles that of a girl walking with a tight skirt (Fig. 15.5). Lower limbs show an increased knee flexion on the supporting limb between vertical shift and contact with the ground by the swinging limb, to facilitate its advancement.

The hamstrings muscles show an overreaction to stretching which, during anterior step, provokes pelvis retroversion. Like some first form patients (flexed propulsive hip), at the end of support phase, the hip is never completely extended but, differently from what happens in the first form, during swing phase its flexion is also limited. Therefore, the pelvis must sway at each step in anteversion/retroversion, increasing or reducing lumbar lordosis. It is as if the patient integrated the hip fulcrum with a knee fulcrum and a lumbar hinge fulcrum during gait. Pelvis frontal translation is frequent, and generally asymmetrical, on the supporting limb side. The adductor interference (scissor pattern) is not particularly marked and it is compensated by associating the trunk's predominantly sagittal swing to a frontal semi-swing towards the supporting limb. The internal rotation of the lower limbs is certainly prevailing, but external rotation is also possible. Suspension talipes equinus can be present (drop foot), followed by contact talipes equinus and full support talipes equinus. Pre-swing talipes equinus is missing. Gait is fast enough, but steps are short and crowded. The patient can usually stop immediately, without difficulty upon request.

To have the so-called "tight skirt" scheme, the tibia-tarsus complex or the forefoot will have to be available for dorsiflexion, which can occur due to an insufficient support reac-

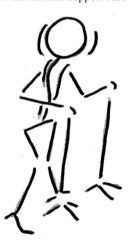

Fig. 15.5 *Tight skirt diplegic patient.* Walking patterns

tion (hypo-active or hyposthenic triceps), or due to foot deformity in valgus-pronation (contact talipes equinus and full support "disguised" talipes equinus), or after excessive surgical release of the Achilles tendon. Patients who tend to have retraction of the triceps surae and heel valgismus can show a reflexed foot, favored by hyposthenia and mesenchymal failure of the plantar muscles (plastic metaplasia). Both in case of talipes equinus and calcaneus, the load is on the forefoot. A previously talipes equinus that goes through a seemingly equinus while becoming reflex or talipes calcaneus can also occur (Miller et al. 1995; Boyd et al. 1997). Examining the sagittal plane, kinematics will show that the ankle has a normal dorsiflexion angle, while hips and knees are held in excessive flexion during the whole stance phase. The weakness of overextended triceps surae and badly oriented or "outbroken" foot can contribute to the crouch gait pattern (Rodda and Graham, 2001). The integrity of pelvis flexors/hip extensors coupling can be improved by correcting the foot deformity and the tibia extratorsion and by subsequently using an AFO leg-foot spring (Gage, 1991) calibrated to support body weight.

Although they have very thin muscles and tendons, these diplegic patients start to develop muscular retractions quite early, especially on the hamstrings and to a lesser degree on the adductors. During the first surgical phase, these muscle groups have to be treated and only later, due to the risk of secondary iatrogenic failure, are gastrocnemius and peroneus muscles addressed. The most frequent secondary deformity is foot valgus-pronation. Varus-pronation is less frequent, although it sometimes emerges unilaterally. Since after surgery the appearance of a secondary hyposthenia of the triceps surae is almost inevitable, with involvement of the support reaction, the post-surgery adoption of AFO is suggested to inhibit talipes calcaneus and for physiotherapy recovery of triceps surae activity. By wearing these splints, patients keep the knees semi-flexed and let the load pass through the metatarsophalangeals, submitting the feet to valgus-pronation stress. As well as talipes calcaneo-valgus, another very frequent deformity that determines long-term gait prognosis consists of rotula lifting due to progressive failure of the subpatellar ligament (crouch gait). This condition can require the use of long orthosis (KAFO) to stop knee flexion, or complex functional surgery (relaxation of suprapatellar tendon and recovery of subpatellar with rotula cerclage). If the rotula continues to rise, the gait prognosis becomes very uncertain.

As shown in the scheme, the motor solution adopted by these individuals to solve the walking problem is not so effective.

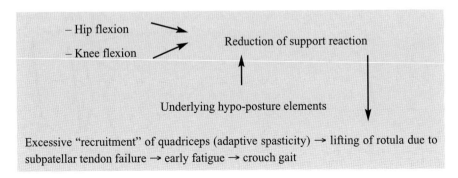

– Hip flexion

– Knee flexion   Reduction of support reaction

Underlying hypo-posture elements

Excessive "recruitment" of quadriceps (adaptive spasticity) → lifting of rotula due to subpatellar tendon failure → early fatigue → crouch gait

Perceptive tolerance, initially reduced, improves as the walking acquisition gets better. The presence of dysperceptive components can show up once the upright position is acquired or even later, especially immediately after functional surgery. However, it is more reduced than that observed in the first and third forms of diplegia.

In sitting position, patients with this form of diplegia make less use of the functional compromise observed by Milani Comparetti and described for the first form. The postural stages from and to the sitting position and the upright position are organized in a quite fast and effective manner.

On the ground, these diplegic children manage to move rapidly either by crawling on all fours or by leaping like a hare (one knee forward and the other backward). An excessively prolonged horizontal locomotion can favor rotula raising due to the subpatellar ligament sagging.

Manipulation quite rapidly achieves good levels of efficiency since the upper limbs are less affected.

Second form of diplegia (tight skirt)

> Use of upper limb canes for direction
> Vertical trunk
> Combined swing, mainly sagittal
> Pelvis in anteversion/retroversion,
> Advancement: flexion on supporting knee
> Foot: contact talipes equinus/talipes calcaneus/drop foot
> Fulcrum: lumbar hinge/knee
Connotative element: flexion of loaded knee

Without the Need for Devices Used by the Upper Limbs

Walking characteristics are: slightly forward tilted head, relatively vertical aligned trunk, and reciprocal mechanical relation between lumbar-sacral hinge and knee, which is necessary in order to avoid the abnormal reaction to hamstring stretching. If dysperceptive disorders are present, arms are tilted upward and adducted at each step with semi-extended elbows and hands ready to grip. If these disorders are not present, or if they are mild, hands are dropped alongside the hips and elementary swinging movements can occur (usually asymmetrical). In the first case, as soon as walking starts, upper limbs are laterally inclined to the right and left to improve the overall balance. At each step, as well as in a sagittal direction, the trunk is laterally inclined towards the supporting limb (frontal semi-swing), to facilitate, in the contralateral one, the lifting of the foot from the ground and the suspension phase, since it is not possible to adequately support talipes equinus (Fig. 15.6). Then, the pelvis rotates both on the anteroposterior axis that goes through the supporting hip (frontal semi-swing), and on the transversal axes that go through the coxofemorals and lumbar-sacral hinge (sagittal swing). If, due to the presence of adductor interference, which is

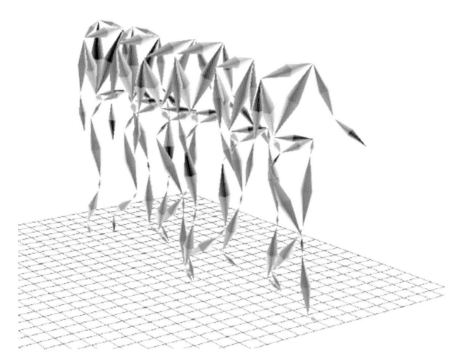

Fig. 15.6 *"Tight skirt" diplegic patients.* Stick diagram of walking, semi-frontal plane (also see enclosed DVD)

usually not severe, during monopodal phase the pelvis translates towards the supporting limb, swinging movements between shoulders and pelvis can occur in countertendency on the frontal plane. Between girdles, no more rotations can occur, not even when the upper limbs acquire basic swinging movements. Despite the increased joint mobility of hip and pelvis, steps generally remain short and rushed. Pivoting on the ground occurs on the forefoot, where most of the load is concentrated, with the possible appearance of a deformity in valgus-pronation or, more rarely, in varus-supination (Fig. 15.7). It is not rare to see the early appearance of valgus deformity on the great toe. Support talipes equinus, with a tendency to reflexed foot, and suspension talipes equinus can coexist. Sometimes this can be quite significant. Pre-swing talipes equinus is missing. When dysperceptive disorders are present, if requested to stop, children show a partial startle reaction on the upper limbs and need to make quick adjustment steps for some time after receiving the order. When walking without shoes, these patients keep the toe grasp reaction for a long time (plantar grasp).

To stabilize themselves in upright position, patients asymmetrically lean one knee against the other in adduction, intrarotation, and semi-flexion. The internal rotation of the lower limbs resulting from anteversion of the femoral necks, useful from the kinesiologic point of view to increase knee stability during monopodal support, can be slowly progressive. When they start to abandon four point canes, children can strategically increase gait speed. During this stage it is better if they abandon AFO and use wrap around orthopedic shoes with anti-slip flexible soles.

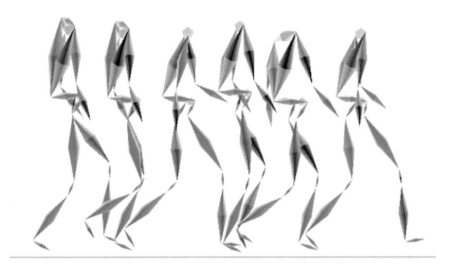

Fig. 15.7 *"Tight skirt" diplegic patients.* Stick diagram of walking, lateral plane (also see enclosed DVD)

Walking is usually achieved after three years of age.

Postural stages from and to the upright position without supports for the upper limbs are quite difficult but not impossible.

The sitting position is quite easily acquired and does not show any significant alteration.

Even without excessive talipes equinus surgical correction, a progressive hyposthenia of the triceps surae, with secondary accentuation of knee flexion and subsequent rotula upward tilting (crouch gait), often appears. Under these conditions, to "preserve" walking, the use of knee-ankle-foot orthosis (KAFO), which is blocked at the knee, and a return to the use of four point canes is inevitable, unless a complex surgical rotula correction is performed, although this operation is not always successful.

According to the GMFCS for cerebral palsy (Palisano et al. 1997; Russell et al. 2002), diplegic children of the second form can be placed at 1st (19%), 2nd (27%), 3rd (30%), and 4th (12%) levels (missing 12%).

3. Third Form (Tightrope Walker)

In the third form of diplegia, differently from previous ones, the number of children who walk without orthopedic devices for the upper limbs is significantly higher than the number of childer emploing them. Usually, these diplegic patients are less severe from the motor point of view, and often show important dysperceptive disorders. The acquisition of independent walking can require a long time and remain unstable, depending on the current emotional state of the patient, the environmental characteristics, and above all on caregiver behavior.

15

The head is tilted forward or upright and the trunk is slightly pulled forward, with pelvis anteversion and mild increase of lumbar lordosis. The rotation between girdles is sufficiently free, especially in sitting position. Hips are quite extended with poor adduction interference (scissor pattern). Conversely, there can be thigh intrarotation, usually asymmetrical, that results from a progressive accentuation of femoral necks anteversion.

With regard to walking, these children remain borderline for a long time, between the need to use orthosis for the upper limbs and the capacity to walk independently. They usually start with a quite heavy two front wheel and two back point walking frame, by which they jump from one foot to the other, even if it would be better if they used a posterior trolley with backward block mechanisms for its better perceptive containment. When they shift to mobile devices, such as four point canes or crutches, these almost never contact the ground in a rhythmic and periodic way during forward walking (four stage pattern), apart from when they stop and stand. These patients have many difficulties to stop walking and remain upright if they are far from any support. When they are young, they almost always prefer long crutches, sometimes real shepherd sticks or broom sticks, to guarantee a forward projection of the baricenter, a defense from falling forward and, above all, a protection against falling backward (control of posterior space). Some even manage to use one crutch. Before advancing, they swing the trunk once or twice on the frontal plane, as if they had to "load" the pendulum. As soon as they leave, they lift the four point cane from the ground and, keeping it on the side of their body, with the upper limbs adduced and semi-extended, they use it in a way similar to a tightrope walker. The trunk keeps swinging on the frontal plane. In difficult conditions, these individuals may use a simplified strategy (coping solution, see chapter 12) like progressive gait acceleration, especially when they approach the point of arrival. To speed up, they use pre-swing talipes equinus, pivoting on the forefoot. With time they manage to walk without crutches, provided a person behind them keeps a hand on their shoulder thus creating a "screen" against backward space (perceptive facilitation). Hand contact (one finger is sufficient) reassures the child about the acceptance conflict generated by the information on the body-space relation and in particular about the body moving in space (see chapter 5). In a well-known environment, these children move by leaning on furniture and walls, and in the end do not use four point canes. For them, walking with devices can represent a prolonged transitory phase leading to walking without devices.

This clinical form of diplegia often includes coordination disorders which partly generate the difficulties emerging from the upper limb/lower limb joint movement (four stages gait). The simplification strategy adopted (coping solution, see chapter 12) consists either of simultaneous advancement of the upper limbs (two stages gait) or advancement with alternated upper limb-lower limb according to the homolateral pattern.

The step sequence is usually short (cluster steps). Between one sequence and the next, at least one of the two crutches is used for support. Despite the poor fluency, the speed of gait is quite good.

If an opportune support for at least for one upper limb is present, the child can manage to stand up by using a half kneeling maneuver, otherwise he leans with both hands on a fixed, suitably high support and simultaneously extends both knees.

Without the Need for Devices Used by the Upper Limbs

When they walk, these children frontally swing their trunk, keeping their upper limbs semi-extended and adducted in order to achieve balance, as if they ideally wanted to lean on the lateral space. During swinging movements, which are often not perfectly rhythmic, hands, more or less open, can rise and go above the shoulder level. Pelvis and shoulder swing in countertendency (lateral pulsion and frontal translation on the loaded limb) with a prevalence of shoulder movement, before surgical lengthening of the medial hamstrings (frontal pendulum), and pelvis, maybe due to a reduction in the adduction component. Shoulder movement and swinging of the upper limbs (pendulum) are more noticeable than in the individuals with the same form who use crutches. If the child keeps an object in his hand, arm movements are reduced, revealing a good control capacity of associated reactions, as long as the achieved perceptive tolerance allows for this (see chapter 5). The head, quite straight, is pulled forward and backward at each step in order to find a better balance on the sagittal plane, together with the variation of pelvis position. At the start, the upper limbs can become stiff, with clenched hands, or lift up in startle position. Advancement occurs in a propulsive and quite fast manner. They start swinging on the frontal plane and subsequently accelerate in a sagittal direction, as if they were following a continuous forward baricenter projection (Fig. 15.8). They have difficulties in stopping; they acquire

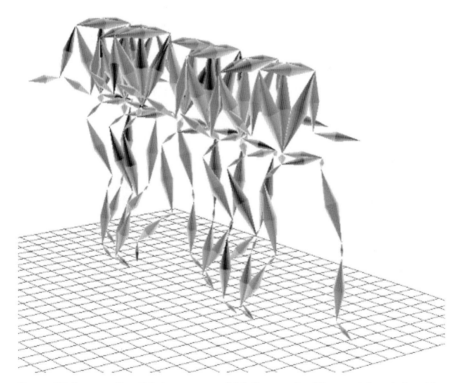

Fig. 15.8 *"Tightrope walking" diplegic patients.* Stick diagram of walking, semi-frontal plane (also see enclosed DVD)

15

this ability later and most of the times they need three or four adjustment steps to stop the trunk's swinging movement on the frontal plane. Often patients, in order to stop walking, grip onto someone or lean against something, ending up being always a bit too "heavy or abrupt". Over time, the step length increases and they manage to stop upon request. During walking, they look for a lateral support, occasionally a wall or whatever they find, especially if they need to change their forward direction. During longer "routes", the lower limbs acquire a pattern based on a moderate hip flexion (sometimes resolving at the end of stance), thigh internal rotation (often asymmetrical), with knee flexion (sometimes hyperextended, in an attempt to have a complete foot contact with the ground) and foot varus-supination. One hemiside may be positioned more forward than the other, and a lower limb may result more intrarotated, with subsequent asymmetry in anterior steps length. When standing still, they manage to extend or hyperextend their knees. The foot contacts the ground with its tip (suspension talipes equinus and inversion of gait sequence), and it accentuates plantiflexion at the end of stance (pre-swing talipes equinus). Foot drop during swing can be reduced by a placing reaction at the moment of detachment, which can facilitate the contraction of dorsiflexors and toe extensors, recruited in reversed kinetic chain. The compensation is increased by wearing orthopedic shoes as when thigh internal rotation occurs. The pivoting takes place on the forefoot, at least until skeletal functional surgery (derotation of femoral necks) is performed . Speed acceleration, which serves to overcome fear but leads to step overcrowding, is a compensatory strategy that should be respected at least at the beginning (therefore avoiding a too early functional surgery and AFO adoption). These patients lack posterior parachutes for upper limbs, but they can manage to shift lateral ones backwards, rotating their shoulders on the pelvic girdle.

The final gait pattern can display the upper limbs, usually held below the shoulder level, swinging together in the direction of the supporting lower limb (Fig. 15.9).

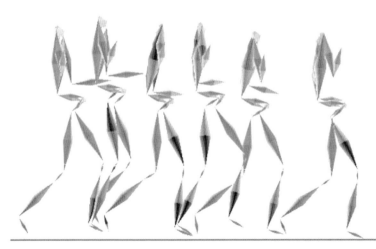

Fig. 15.9 *"Tightrope walking" diplegic patients.* Stick diagram of walking, lateral plane (also see enclosed DVD)

Adduction is never excessive and achieving a standing position is possible, even spontaneously, starting from a half kneeling or a "starter block" position as in a foot race, especially if an opportune support for both or at least for one hand is not immediately present.

> *"The children who have a straight and upright dorsal column with lumbar lordosis (due to flexor spasticity of the hips, especially iliopsoas) will alternate the lateral flexion of the trunk from the belt upward in order to move their stiff legs forward. While a normal person has ductile motoricity of the legs and relatively stable trunk, these children show excessive trunk mobility and stiff legs (goose gait)"*
> (Bobath, 1975).

Patients show a significant change in gait pattern (Fig. 15.10) when they are subject to medial hamstrings and adductors surgery (first stage): the hip shows a slight adduction with accentuation of intrarotation, the knee is curved, and the foot displays varus-supination, with a tendency to pivot on the anterior-external part of the foot. Therefore, in this form early surgery and, above all, excessive reduction of spasticity are detrimental. To correct femur intrarotation (second stage, through proximal subtrochanteric skeletal derotation or distal juxta-epiphyseal), it is advisable to wait until adolescence.

From the perceptive point of view, these diplegic patients have significant problems in controlling posterior space. At the beginning of gait they require the constant presence of a person who walks behind them. When they become more confident, the caregiver can also walk at their side or in front of them, provided she constantly looks at them and talks to them (visual-verbal contact). Patients usually start out with low self-esteem and gradually become aware of being able to walk autonomously, relying on the opinion of the adult caregiver.

The propulsive characteristic of gait and the arm position are due more to dysperceptive disorders (see chapter 5) rather than to a lack of balance and coordination. When these children detach from adult contact, perceptive control improvement can be signald by the lowering of upper limbs and the increasing degree of swinging movements of head, neck, shoulder, and pelvis.

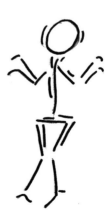

Fig. 15.10 *"Tightrope walking" diplegic patient.* Walking pattern

A very long time may elapse between gait appearance and acquisition of independent walking when compared to expectations; this can seem frustrating because the patient often seems on the verge of acquiring independent walking.

If they are trained and able to use crutches, they can adopt the four-stage pattern quite rapidly and become sufficiently confident, but they will still have the problem of synchronizing upper and lower limb movements.

However, not all patients present significant dysperceptive disorders or retain them until school age. Those who do not have dysperceptive problems manage to walk quite early by hyperextending the knee and resolving the hip flexion at the end of stance.

On the ground, these individuals learn how to move by crawling on all fours or by leaping like a hare quite early, often by simultaneously advancing the upper limbs but with a poor lower limb movement synchronization.

Children with dysperceptive disorders move slower, although their girdles rotate quite well, and they even prefer assisted walking to horizontal locomotion. Also when sitting, children with dysperceptive disorders remain quite still, preferring to talk rather than to act (see chapters 9 and 10).

Third form of diplegia (tightrope walkers)

> Upper limbs laterally tilted upward
> Slightly pulled-forward trunk with lumbar lordosis
> Frontal pendulum
> Pelvis: contralateral elevation, frontal translation towards loaded lower limb
> Progression: propulsive scheme and pivot on the foot
> Foot: contact and pre-swing talipes equinus
> Fulcrum: trunk/foot
Connotative element: trunk frontal swinging

According to the GMFCS for cerebral palsy (Palisano et al. 1997; Russel et al. 2002), diplegic children of the third form can be placed at 1st (6%), 2nd (33.5%), 3rd (45.5%) and 4th (6%) levels (missing 9%).

4. Fourth Form (Daredevil)

This form is characterized by the complete absence of dysperceptive disorders (space control and tolerance to unbalancing), at least from the moment when walking is acquired onwards. Also motor impairment is less serious and therefore children show a substantially favorable gait evolution. They do not need crutches or any other devices for the upper limbs, since they achieve good proximal fixation and quite good balance, especially considering the reduction in support base due to stance talipes equinus.

The fourth form of diplegia consists of two subgroups with decreasing severity depending on how the motor impairment is distributed: either homogeneous or mainly distal. A third subgroup is represented by the forms with significant asymmetry, which are frequently indicated as "double hemiplegia".

Generalized

The distribution of motor disorders can still display a proximal-distal accentuation, but, differently from purely distal forms, it is possible to note adduction interference (scissor pattern). During gait, the pelvis is in anteversion and the patient is forced into a lumbar lordosis accentuation or to keep the trunk in slight antepulsion. Shoulders and hips swing in countertendency and slight rotations between girdles are possible. Upper limbs are slightly adduced to maintain balance, with semi-extended elbows, and dropped wrists and hands. Lower limbs can present slight asymmetries, in particular during flexion and intrarotation, which make gait seem slightly oblique with respect to the body progression plane (Fig. 15.11). In upright standing, patients have difficulties in finding a balance, and end up keeping the load more on one limb than on the other and thus become asymmetrical. In the attempt to put the heel on the ground, generally in valgus-pronation, some individuals can bend their hips, with trunk antepulsion, and stress their knees in hyperextension (hidden equinus, Miller et al. 1995). Before starting to walk, children stand on tiptoe (starting talipes equinus). During gait suspension, talipes equinus is common, followed by contact talipes equinus (with some varus foot components), while support talipes equinus is reduced when stopping, similar to in the upright position. Therefore, AFO, chemical spasticity inhibition, and surgical correction, especially if very early, are not advisable. Suspension talipes equinus worsens when the Achilles tendon is surgically treated due to the reduction of ankle joint stiffness with an unexpected subsequent increase in free joint excursion. To facilitate foot dorsiflexion during swing phase, patients can use placing

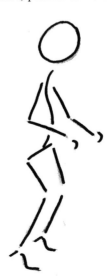

Fig. 15.11 *"Daredevil" diplegic patient.* Walking pattern

reactions, favored by the internal rotation of the lower limb. Knee stiffening at the beginning of swing phase and the appearance of a snap extension movement during load transfer is possible. It is also possible to see abnormal reactions to stretching of the triceps surae and intrinsic muscles, which anticipates the appearance of pre-swing talipes equinus immediately after vertical passing. At the beginning of walking, children can show floppiness ("low tone") elements, with frequent recruitment. However, the overall gait endurance is good.

Diplegic children of this form refuse support quite early and are happy to walk "as they can". At the beginning, since they do not know how to stop, they tend to fall on their knees, with intrarotated and adducted thighs. They are not scared of falling or hurting themselves. Due to rather good balance, they are just as fast at falling down as getting up and starting again. They can soon manage to stop the gait without having to adopt subsequent adjustment steps after receiving the order. They are also very good at running (a performance from which they eventually work out the coordinates for walking) and in obstacle jumping. Some of them stiffen their knees when running, therefore they run as if they were walking fast with little steps. When they get up from the ground, they can use the half kneeling maneuver; otherwise, they tend to lean forward by simultaneously extending both knees and immediately starting to walk (Figg. 15.12 and 15.13).

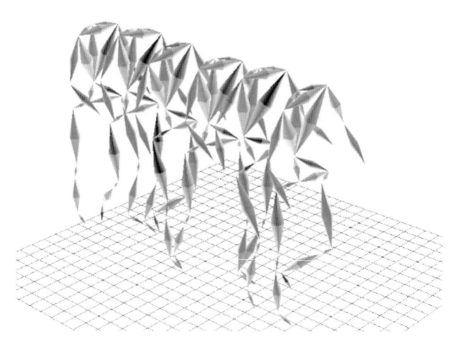

Fig. 15.12 *"Daredevil" diplegic patient.* Stick diagram of walking, semi-frontal plane (also see enclosed DVD)

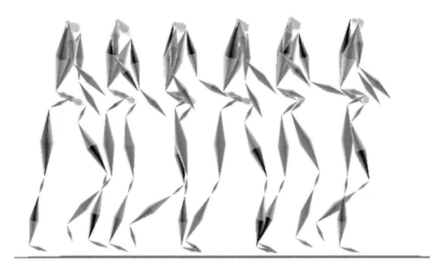

Fig. 15.13 *"Daredevil" diplegic patient.* Stick diagram of walking, lateral plane (also see enclosed DVD)

Distal

These children have difficulties in standing still, especially in a symmetrical position, but they have no problem with proximal fixation. They usually load one foot more than the other, frequently alternating the load. The unloaded limb can display a semi-flexed knee and a heel lifted from the ground; the loaded limb maintains an extended knee, in internal rotation, and the whole foot plant is in contact with the ground. This pattern increases when the child is barefoot. The child has particular difficulties in balancing the support reaction between the two lower limbs (equilibrium), perceptively tolerating the load and bearing the triceps surae tension (over-reaction to stretching).

When standing still, patients stress the foot in valgus-pronation, while during walking they load it more in talipes equinus-varus, pivoting the toe tip on the ground.

The gait pattern, which is achieved rapidly, displays an inversion of step pattern (contact talipes equinus, full stance, and pre-swing) and internal rotation of the thighs, but no adduction interference. Also, hip and knee flexion are more limited than in the general form, and lumbar lordosis consequently is mild. Instead of using placing, these diplegic individuals usually step forward by lifting the knee and scuffling the front-external part of the shoe tip on the ground as an effect of dynamic varus-supination. They can also snap-hyperextend the knee during monopodal support (over-reaction to triceps surae stretching), and display, at the beginning of the swinging phase, the so-called "stiff knee" sign. Since they benefit from speed, these patients generally do not take any advantage from the use of AFOs, which should however be flexible at the tip or, as suggested by Buckon et al. (2001), articulated at tibia-tarsus level.

Some children can have elements of asymmetry, however without ever separating the lower limbs (differently from what happens in asymmetrical diplegia or double hemiplegia). Upper limbs are kept in a good position and during gait they show swinging movements that can be reduced as speed increases. This is a consequence of the influence of associated movements. Girdles rotations are almost completely free. The overall balance is good and the gait rhythm is fluent (Fig. 15.14).

These children are able to walk backward, run, and jump. They have no difficulties in stopping upon request. They soon learn how to get up from the ground using a half kneeling maneuver, without any need for further adjustment steps after the first one.

When they are on the ground, they learn to creep and roll over quite early and within the first two years they are able to crawl very fast. They rarely move by creeping on their bottom; in this case it takes them a bit longer to move.

The word "distal" refers to the distribution of the motor disorder, which is present on foot or knee, forearm or hand.

The progressive extension of the defect in a proximal way, in an initially distal diplegic patient, makes us suspect the presence of a familiar spastic paraparesis or other forms of genetic etiology.

According to the GMFCS for cerebral palsy (Palisano et al. 1997; Russel et al. 2002), diplegic children of the fourth form can be placed at 1st (51.5%), 2nd (33.5%), 3rd (7%), and 4th (1%) levels (missing 7%).

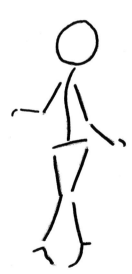

Fig. 15.14 *"Daredevil" diplegic patient.* Walking pattern

> ## Fourth form of diplegia (daredevils)
>
> › Upper limbs lowered
> › Vertical trunk, in slight antepulsion
> › Combined frontal swing between shoulders and pelvis
> › Pelvis with good proximal fixation
> › Progression: hip intrarotation
> › Foot: start and pre-swing talipes equinus, drop foot, possible placing
> › Fulcrum: hip/foot
> Connotative element: talipes equinus increase at gait start

Asymmetric (Double Hemiplegia)

These diplegic patients are best at postural change, balance, and upright position (often possible in monopodal load), gait start and stop, fast running, inter-girdles rotation, and swinging movements of the upper limbs, at least on the less impaired side. They can manage to stop walking upon request without difficulties, because they do not have any disorders related to space perception and movement intolerance. One hemiside is decidedly more affected than the other, the lower limb is more intrarotated, the knee more flexed, and the foot in a more pronounced varus-supination, more rarely in valgus-pronation. The hip, especially on the more impaired side, does not resolve the flexion at the end of its stance phase, therefore keeping the pelvis in anteversion and lumbar rachis in compensatory lordosis. The pelvis is usually more tilted upward on the more impaired side, without developing scoliosis. The knee of the more affected lower limb remains slightly flexed also in mid stance; more rarely, it can be recurved, generally in intrarotation. Drop foot can be present, to justify the placing reaction at the end of stance. It can become more apparent after talipes equinus surgical correction, due to the increased range of ankle motion. During swing phase, there can be an over-reaction to hamstring stretching, favored by pelvis anteversion, which limits the anterior step length.

When standing still, these patients prefer to balance themselves in anasymmetrical way, while when gait starts, they tend to become more symmetrical, increasing talipes equinus on the less affected side. During fast running, they reinforce associated reactions, especially on the more affected upper limb (elbow flexion, forearm pronation, tendency to more hand closure) (Fig. 15.15).

The children get up from the ground by spontaneously separating their lower limbs (half kneeling) even without physiotherapy training, since adductors interference is always very limited or completely absent.

Gait is acquired early. There is no resistance problem. Many patients can even manage to jump on one foot.

Sitting position does not display significant changes. Sometimes, there is a slight obliquity with pelvis retroversion, usually proportional to the higher tension of the hamstrings on the more affected side.

15

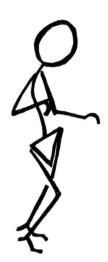

Fig. 15.15 *"Asymmetrical" diplegic patient.* Walking pattern

During manipulation, one upper limb can show dyskinesic elements that can become clinically more apparent on the Fog test.

When crawling, children can present an asymmetry in lower limb advancement and dyssynchrony between lower and upper limb displacement. Usually, they prefer to adopt hare-like movements. Shuffling or the three-quarter movement is rarely preferred. The latter is typical of hemiparesis.

According to the GMFCS for cerebral palsy (Palisano et al. 1997; Russel et al. 2002), diplegic patients of this form can be placed at 1st (5.5%) 2nd (5.5%), 3rd (39%), 4th (28%), and 5th (11%) levels (missing 11%).

References

Bax M (1964) Terminology and classification of cerebral palsy. Dev Med Child Neurol 6:295-297

Bax M, Goldstein M, Rosenbaum P et al (2005) Proposed definition and classification of cerebral palsy. Dev Med Child Neurol 47:571-6

Beckung E, Hagberg G (2002) Neuroimpairments, activity limitations, and participation restrictions in children with cerebral palsy. Dev Med Child Neurol 44:309-16

Bianchini E (2003) Tesi di Dottorato in Neuroscienze dell'Età Evolutiva, Università di Pisa.

Bobath B, Bobath K (1975) Motor development in the different types of cerebral palsy. William Heinemann Medical Books, London

Boyd R, Graham HK (1997) Botulinum Toxin A in the management of children with cerebral palsy. Indication outcome. Eur J Neurol 4:15-22

Boyd RN, Griaham JEA, Nattrass GR, Graham HK (1999) Medium-term response characterization and risk factor analysis of botulinum toxin type A in the management of spasticity in children with cerebral palsy. Eur Journ Neurol 6:S37-S46

Buckon CE, Thomas SS, Jakobson-Huston S et al (2001) Comparison of three ankle-foot orthosis configurations for children with spastic hemiplegia. Dev Med Child Neurol 43:371-378

Campbell AGM, McIntosh N (1998) Forfar & Arniel's textbook of pediatrics, 5th ed. Churchill Livingstone

Cioni G, Lodesani M, Coluccini M et al (2008) The term diplegia should be enhanced (II): contribution to validation of a new classification system. Eur J Physic Rehab Med 44:203-211

Colver AF, Sethumanhavan T (2003) The term diplegia should be abandoned. Arch Dis Child 88:286-290

Davis RB, Ounpunn S, Tyburschi D, Gage JR (1991) A gait analysis data collection and reduction technique. Journal of Human Movement Science 5, vol. 10. Newington Connecticut

Dobson F, Morris ME, Baker R, Graham HK (2007) Gait classification in children with cerebral palsy: a systematic review. Gait Posture 25:140-152

Eliasson AC, Krumlinde-Sundholm L, Rosblad B et al (2006) The Manual Ability Classification System (MACS) for children with cerebral palsy: scale development and evidence of validity and reliability. Dev Med Child Neurol 48:549-54.

Ferrari A, Alboresi S, Muzzini S et al (2008) The term diplegia should be enhanced (I): around the problem of classification of cerebral palsy. Eur J Physic Rehab Med 44:195-201

Ferrari A, Cioni G (2005) Le forme spastiche della paralisi cerebrale infantile. Guida all'esplorazione delle funzioni adattive. Springer-Verlag Italia, Milan

Freud S (1897) Die Infantile Zerebral Laehmung. In: Notnagel ab Specielle Pathologie und Therapie. A Holder Inc, Wien 2:1

Gage JR (1991) Gait analysis in cerebral palsy. Mac Keit

Gruppo Italiano Paralisi Cerebrale Infantile (GIPCI) (1998) Protocol of videorecording. Giorn Neuropsich Età Evol 2:52-57

Hagberg B (1989) Nosology and classification of cerebral palsy. Giorn Neuropsich Età Evol, suppl. 4:12-17

Hagberg B, Hagberg G, Orlow I (1975) The changing panorama of cerebral palsy in Sweden 1954-70. 1 Analysis of general changes. Acta Paediatr Scand 64:187-92

Hagberg B, Hagberg G, Orlow I (1996) The changing panorama of cerebral palsy in Sweden, VII. Prevalence and origin during the birth period 1987-1990. Acta Paed 85:954-960

Himmelmann K, Hagberg G, Beckung E et al (2005) The changing panorama of cerebral palsy in Sweden, IX. Prevalence and origin in the birth-year period 1995-1998. Acta Paed 94:287-94.

Hoffer MM, Feiwell E, Perry R et al (1973) Functional ambulation in patients with myelomeningocele. J Bone Joint Surg Am 5:137-148

Ingram TTS (1955) A study of cerebral palsy in the childhood population of Edinburgh. Arch Dis Child 30:85-98

Little WJ (1862) On the influence of abnormal parturition, difficult labours, premature birth and asphyxia neonatorum on the mental and physical condition of the child, especially in relation to deformities. Transactions of the Obstetrical Society of London

MacKeith RC, Mackenzie ICK, Polani PE (1959) The Little Club memorandum on terminology and classification of cerebral palsy. Cerebral Palsy Bulletin 5:27-35

Mc Intosh N, Helms PJ, Smyth RL (2003) Forfar & Arniel's Textbook of Paediatrics, 6th ed. Churchill Livingstone, London

Milani Comparetti A (1965) La natura del difetto motorio nella paralisi cerebrale infantile. Infanzia Anormale 64:587-628

Milani Comparetti A (1978) Classification des infirmités motrices cérébrales. Médicine et Hygiène 36:2024-2029

Miller F, Dabney K, Rang M (1995) Complications in cerebral palsy treatment. In: Epps CH, Bowen JR (eds) Complications in paediatric Orthopaedic Surgery. Lippincott JB, Philadelphia, pp 498-500

Minear WL (1956) A classification of cerebral palsy. Paediatrics 18:841-52

Morris C, Rosenbaum PL (2003) Describing impairment and disability for children with cerebral palsy. Electronic Letter to editor. Arch Dis Child 2003

Morrissey RT, Weinstein SL (2001) Lovell and Winter's pediatric orthopaedics, 5th ed. Lippincott Williams & Wilkins, Philadelphia

Palisano RJ, Rosenbaum PL, Walter S et al (1997) Development and reliability of a system to classify gross motor function in children with cerebral palsy. Dev Med Child Neurol 39:214-223

Pascale R, Perazza S, Borelli G et al (2008) The term diplegia should be enhanced (III) Reliability of a classification of spastic diplegia: inter-observer agreement in 50 cases. Eur J Physic Rehab Med 44:213-220

Rodda J, Graham HK (2001) Classification of gait patterns in spastic hemiplegia and diplegia: a basis for a management algorithm. Eur J of Neurol, vol. 8 issue 5, pp 98-110

Rosenbaum PL, Walter SD, Hanna SE et al (2002) Development and reliability of a system to classify gross motor functions in children with cerebral palsy. JAMA 288:1357-1363

Russell D, Rosenbaum P, Avery LM et al (2002) Gross motor function measure (GMFM-66 and GMFM-88) User's manual. Clinics in Developmental Medicine. Mac Keith Press, Cambridge

Sachs B, Petersen F (1890) A study of cerebral palsies of early life. J Nerv Ment Dis 17:295-332

Surveillance Cerebral Palsy in Europe (SCPE) (2000): a collaboration of cerebral palsy register. Dev Med Child Neurol 42:816-24

Sutherland DH, Davids JR (1993) Common gait abnormalities of the knee in cerebral palsy. Clin Orthopedics Related Res 288:139-149

Forms of Hemiplegia

16

G. Cioni, G. Sgandurra, S. Muzzini, P.B. Paolicelli, A. Ferrari

---

Definition and Prevalence

Traditionally, hemiplegia or hemiparesis, is defined as a central "unilateral" palsy that only affects one side of the body, almost always of "spastic" type (Aicardi and Bax 2009), while the word "hemidystonia" is more adequately used to define the dyskinesic form. With respect to cerebral palsy (CP), a distinction is made between a *congenital form* of hemiplegia, when the lesion occurs before the end of the neonatal period (within the first four weeks of life), and an *acquired form*, when the lesion provoking hemiplegia occurs later, within the first three years of life. According to the main case studies published (Hagberg and Hagberg, 2000), congenital forms amount to 70-90% of childhood hemiplegia, while acquired forms only amount to 10-30%. In a recent review conducted by the SCPE (Surveillance of Cerebral Palsy in Europe) working group, the prevalence of unilateral spastic hemiplegia accounted for about 0.6 per 1000 live births and it did not change significantly over time (Krägeloh-Mann, 2009). Hemiplegic forms are the most common expression of CP (more than 38 % of cases) and the second in terms of frequency, after diplegia, in premature infants (around 20% of cases) (Hagberg et al. 1996; Himmelmann et al. 2005).

In many cases of hemiplegia (around 30-40%, according to Hagberg) it is not possible to trace back, in the infant's personal or family history, the etiopathogenic factors that determined the cerebral lesion. This can be confirmed for normal term infants, while for premature infants, who later develop hemiplegia, pre- or perinatal factors are frequently and significantly correlated to the lesion (Cioni et al. 1999). In both normal term infants and premature infants multiple genetic and environmental factors can play an important role in lesion etiopathogenesis, acting in a negative way ("detrimental" elements) and in a positive way ("protective" elements). Among them are thrombophilic factors, which are particularly relevant in the outbreak of cerebral infarction in normal term infants (Mercuri et al. 2001). However, it is difficult to establish a linear correlation between a genetic factor of the coagulation chain (for example Leiden factor V), and a complex syndrome like hemiplegia, determined by many factors and containing multiple and different clinical pictures (Smith et al. 2001). The lesion has long been thought to be driven by nonhemato-

The Spastic Forms of Cerebral Palsy. Adriano Ferrari, Giovanni Cioni
© Springer-Verlag Italia 2010

331

logic maternal and perinatal events. Conversely, recent studies have indicated that plasma-phase risk factors, such as Leiden factor V, elevated lipoprotein (a), and mutations in MTHFR, may have an important role in the pathogenesis of perinatal stroke, if not always in the risk of recurrence. The latter is only about 2% according to the largest follow-up study to date. Nonetheless, when strokes do recur, they tend to be associated with the presence of plasma-phase risk factors in the affected child. Authors are therefore suggesting that a small percentage of children with a first perinatal stroke may benefit from anticoagulation therapy, both to prevent stroke recurrence as well as occurence of a second, non cerebral thrombotic event (Grabowski et al. 2007).

Neuroimaging, especially magnetic resonance imaging (MRI), enabled, also in the field of childhood hemiplegia, very encouraging studies on the natural history of the lesion and the factors determining it, although this section of neurology is only at the beginning of its development. Negative MRI in children with congenital hemiplegia, as reported by some authors (Wiklund, 2000; Krägeloh-Mann, 2004, 2007, 2009; Korzeniewski et al. 2008; Robinson et al. 2008), is rare (Cioni et al. 1999). The scanning may probably be judged as normal due to a mistake in MRI execution, timing, or to poor quality of the images obtained (Korzeniewski et al. 2008). The most frequent lesions of hemiplegia in children can be subdivided into malformation groups (cysts of different nature, schizencephaly, other disorders of neuronal migration, etc.), periventricular lesions (leukomalacia), atrophy and dilatations of the lateral ventricle, especially at the level of the atria, cortico-subcortical lesions (porencephalic cysts, areas of perilesional gliosis), diencephalic lesions (affecting basal ganglia, thalamus, internal capsule) and diffuse lesions, as a result of infant cranial trauma. The above-mentioned lesions can be grouped according to the type observed by pathologists, through neuroimaging and timing, that is to say the development stage during which they become patent (pre-, peri- or postnatal).

Krageloh-Mann (2004, 2007, 2009) classified MRI results according to the etiopatho-genetic patterns in four groups:

1: brain maldevelopments, or "1st and 2nd trimester patterns", presumed to occur in utero, such as lissencephaly, pachygyria, polymicrogyria, focal cortical dysplasia or unilateral schizencephaly, accounted for 16%;

2: periventricular white matter (PWM) lesions related to the early 3rd trimester of pregnancy and the pre-term infant, such as periventricular leukomalacia (PVL) defects following intraventricular hemorrahage (IVH) or periventricular hemorrhagic infarctions, accounted for 36%;

3: cortical or deep gray matter lesions that occur towards the end of gestation "late 3rd trimester patterns" and peri or neonatally, such as basal ganglia/thalamus lesions, parasagittal injury, multicistic encephalomalacia and middle cerebral artery infarcts, were noted in 31%;

4: miscellaneous patterns considered abnormal but not meeting the above criteria were seen in 7%. Again, there was a clear difference between pre-term and term infants: PWM lesions occurred significantly more often in pre-term than in term (86% vs 20%, $p<0.001$) infants and cortical gray matter lesions significantly less often (0 vs 41%; $p<0.01$). Brain maldevelopments occurred in pre-term nearly as often as in term infants (14% vs 16%, $p>0.05$).

Bax et al. (2006) conducted a population-based investigative study in eight European centers and compared clinical findings with information available from MRI studies. They developed a standardized scoring system for MRI scans that were grouped according to the primary pattern of damage: malformation, white-matter damage of immaturity, focal infarct, cortical/subcortical damage, basal ganglia damage, miscellaneous, and normal.

So, MRI has a high potential to elucidate etiology, or at least pathogenesis, in hemiplegic CP. Also, investigation of the relation between structure and topography of the brain lesions and clinical function in children with CP is an important prerequisite for studying the reorganization and plasticity of the brain. Moreover, a better understanding of these relations may contribute to early diagnosis, and therefore to early intervention.

Although the above reported studies have consistent overlaps, a consensus on the classification of MRI results is not yet established.

Considering the criteria of type and timing of the lesion, the classification proposed by our group (Cioni et al. 1999) identifies the following four archetypes of childhood hemiplegia:

- Type I (early malformative)
- Type II (prenatal)
- Type III (connatal)
- Type IV (acquired)

The specific characteristics of lesions belonging to the four groups are listed in Table 16.1 (Cioni et al. 1999). As described later, the main factors that determine both the clinical characteristics of hemiplegia with its natural history, and the possibility, modality, and efficacy of post-lesion reorganization of the central nervous system (CNS) are the type of lesion and its timing. Obviously, some other individual factors, like lesion size and, detrimental and protective genetic and environmental factors also play an important role in determining the variability of the clinical pictures. Clinical signs altogether, even those that are not strictly motor and perceptive, determine the characteristics of the hemiplegic form and its evolution over time to a larger extent than for other types of CP.

The validity of our classification, previously reported in a group of 91 hemiplegic patients (Cioni et al. 1999), has been confirmed in a larger hospital-based population of 165 children with hemiplegia (Petacchi, 2008).

The classification approach of hemiplegia based on the study of the lesions' characteristics on MRI has clear limits, mostly for children with type II, or prenatal hemiplegia, often presenting with periventricular bilateral lesions, usually asymmetrical, although sometimes seeming symmetrical.

Modern neuroimaging techniques, like tensor diffusion, and perfusion, and in vivo studies of post-lesion functional re-organization with functional imaging techniques will probably enable us to better understand the correlation between lesions and functions, also for this group of individuals.

Table 16.1 Classification of forms of hemiplegia in children according to brain lesion type and timing (Cioni et al. 1999)

	TYPE I: MALFORMATIVE Lesion of the 1st and 2nd trimester	TYPE II: PRENATAL Lesions of the 3rd trimester	TYPE III: CONNATAL Perinatal lesion at term	TYPE IV: ACQUIRED Early acquired lesions
Lesion type	Often complex malformative cerebral pictures, especially related to early migration disorders (cortical dysplasia, schizencephaly, areas of heterotopia, arachnoid cysts, etc). Sometimes encephaloclastic cysts, mostly extended.	Hemorrhage of the periventricular white substance, mostly unilateral, or asymmetrical, resulting from a periventricular venous infarction; hemorrhagic periventricular leukomalacia; at MRI during chronic stage, frequent encephaloclastic cysts inside dilated lateral ventricle and possible gliotic areas also in contralateral periventricular white matter. In some cases, periventricular gliotic areas are symmetrical or almost symmetrical	Frequent cortico-subcortical lesions due to the infarction of a major cerebral artery (mostly the main branch or one main cortical branch of the median cerebral artery). Sometimes the lesion affects the deeper branches with involvement of diencephalic structures (especially the upper arm of the internal capsule), thalamus and basal ganglia affection of putamen especially in dystonic forms.	Malacic and/or gliotic results mainly due to thrombotic occlusion of intracranial arteries in the area of median cerebral distribution (as a result of trauma, infections, vascular malformations, or others).

(RE) - Organization of the Sensory-Motor System

The developing CNS possesses greater capacities of post-lesional compensation than the mature adult brain and the term "re-organization" is applied in a broader sense to indicate "lesion-induced deviations from normal organization".

TMS (Transcranial Magnetic Stimulation) is the "gold standard" for the identification of corticospinal pathways. When TMS elicits short-latency motor-evoked potentials (MEP) in a target muscle, this demonstrates that monosynaptic fast-conditioning cortico-spinal fibers to the motoneurones of this target muscle originate from the stimulation site. Thus, the stimulated cortical area is identified as the primary motor representation (M1) of this muscle (Staudt, 2007). In humans, like in other mammals, corticospinal projections develop transient ipsilateral projections early in development that are predominantly elim-inated when maturity is reached (Eyre et al. 2001, 2007a). In neonates, focal TMS of the motor cortex evokes ipsilateral responses with similar threshold and amplitude as obtained for contralateral responses; this indicates a bilateral innervation of the spinal cord from each motor cortex. In longitudinal studies of normal infants, the findings are consistent with withdrawal in significant numbers of ipsilateral corticospinal projections so that responses at two years are less frequent and significantly smaller. By contrast, the contralateral projections are enhanced so that responses at two years are stronger (Eyre et al. 2001, 2007a, 2007b). Functional and anatomical evidence in animal models and in humans demonstrates that this type of organization depends on activity and on environmental experience (Martin, 2004, 2005; Friel and Martin, 2007).

After brain damage, there are two main types of (re)-organization: perilesional and contralesional (Staudt et al. 2002). In adults with stroke and in some children, the main mechanism for a reconnection of the motor cortex to the spinal cord consists of a (re)-organization within the ipsilesional cortex, based on partial sparing of the primary motor cortex or on the possibility that functions may be taken over by intact non-primary motor areas within the damaged hemisphere (*perilesional or contralateral (re)-organization*). This type of (re)-organization is based on the multiple representation of the body inside M1 or on the possibility that functions, formerly assumed by the primary motor cortex, may also be taken over by remote and intact non-primary motor areas within the damaged hemisphere (Staudt et al. 2004, 2005; Guzzetta et al. 2007). However, when the lesion occurs at an early stage of development, either during intrauterine life or soon after birth, a different mechanism can be observed. It is based on the persistence of a significant component of monosynaptic fast-conducting ipsilateral motor projections, normally withdrawing within the first months of life, that may be permanently maintained if brain damage occurs early in life (Eyre, 2001, 2007a, 2007b; Guzzetta et al. 2007). In this case, the unaffected hemisphere directly controls both upper limbs, giving rise to a pattern of reorganization unknown in adult pathologies (*contralesional or ipsilateral (re)-organization*). Also, there is an intermediate (re)-organization that shows both types of projections (Staudt et al. 2002).

This variability in the types and efficacies of CNS (re)-organization following early brain lesions has been attributed to several factors influencing it. The extent and location of the lesion, the presence or absence of epilepsy, and the maturational stage of the CNS at the time when the insult occurred are important factors, particularly in patients with periventricular damage. Staudt et al. (2002, 2007) detected a strikingly clear relationship between lateral extent of the periventricular lesion and type of reorganization: patients with small lesions showed preserved contralateral corticospinal projections to the paretic hand, whereas a majority of patients with large lesions possessed fast-conducting ipsilateral corticospinal pathways originating in the contralesional hemisphere. However, this finding has not been confirmed with other types of brain lesions, such as cortico-subcortical infarctions or malformations.

An increasing volume of data suggest that an important role in determining the pattern of reorganization may also be played by the activity of the affected limb in the very early stages of development (Friel and Martin, 2007). The quality and quantity of movement, with its associated sensory feedbacks, may be relevant in the early competition between the ipsilateral fibers of the unaffected hemisphere and the contralateral fibers of the affected side (Eyre, 2003). In this respect, the integrity of the somatosensory system may be considered an important factor.

16

Our group (Guzzetta et al. 2007) investigated the reorganization of the somatosensory system in patients with congenital hemiplegia due to a wide spectrum of brain lesions with different times of origin using TMS and functional magnetic resonance imaging (fMRI) during sensory stimulation. Sensory feedback such as the location and extent of the lesion and the amount of early motor activity is a key factor in determining the type of motor (re)-organization. There are general differences in the (re)-organization capabilities of the motor and sensory system following different types of early brain lesions. Following early damage, the sensory function is consistently reorganized in the affected hemisphere. The possible scenarios are shown in Figure 16.1.

A child with hemiplegia may show ipsilesional representation of both primary sensory and primary motor function of the paretic hand, or ipsilesional representation of primary sensory function and contralesional representation of primary motor function (interhemispheric sensory-motor dissociation) or ipsilesional representation of primary sensory function and bilateral representation of motor function.

A contralesional shifting is uncommon and poorly efficient in function restoration. The degree of sensory impairment, ranging from normal to severe deficits, seems to be related to the extension of the cortical representation of sensory stimulation. A recent study (Wilke et al. 2009) using fMRI, TMS and MEG (magnetoencephalography) confirmed that in both models of motor reorganization no interhemispheric reorganization of somatosensory functions occurred.

Eyre et al. (2007b) performed a longitudinal neurophysiological study of corticospinal tract development in healthy subjects and in patients with unilateral and bilateral lesions. The findings of TMS soon after perinatal stroke were not predictive, because the presence of response was equally associated with good and poor motor outcomes. Conversely, at two years the maintenance of response from the infarted cortex (perilesional reorganization) was associated with grasping and manipulation skills of the contralateral hand

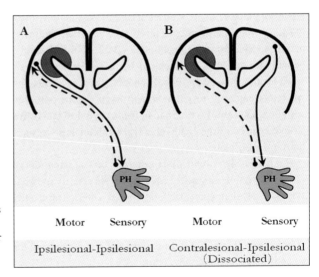

Fig. 16.1 Two basic patterns of reorganization of hand sensorimotor function after early focal brain lesion. *PH*, paretic hand

whereas the lack of response (contralesional (re)-organization) was associated with no use of the hand.

These data confirm the hypothesis that ipsilesional reorganization is more effective in the restoration of good motor function as opposed to contralesional reorganization (Eyre et al. 2007b; Guzzetta et al. 2007). However, the presence of fast-conducting ipsilateral projections is not sufficient for preservation of function; rather, as in adult-onset stroke, good function of the paretic limb is observed only if responses after TMS of the infarcted contralateral motor cortex are preserved. Now, the limitations of efficacy of contralesional (re)-organization are quite apparent, showing this pattern to be potentially maladaptive. This contrasts strongly with the superior efficacy of this type of (re)-organization in the language system, where left-sided lesions can induce (re)-organization of speech production in the right hemisphere with normal language functions (Staudt, 2007).

These findings support the hypothesis that the degree of motor impairment suffered after perinatal stroke depends not only on the size of the lesion (Martin et al. 2004, 2005), but also on the competitive-activity-dependent refinement of bilateral corticospinal projections. Progressive displacement of surviving corticospinal projections from the intact hemisphere with development may provide an explanation for the clinical observation that signs of hemiplegia are often not established in some children until well into the second year of life. Such changes would be analogous to the progressive development of amblyopia in the visual system in a child with strabismus. For this reasons, in the quoted study, this particular process was called "amblyopia of the corticospinal system" (Eyre et al. 2007b).

Assessment Instruments for Hand Function

Several assessment instruments are available to quantify and monitor developmental milestones and skills of manual function and to assess the quality of life of patients with CP. When making the decision about which assessment instrument to use, an organizing framework may be useful to guide the process. Many authors have proposed the framework outlined in the International Model for Classification of Functioning, Disability and Health (ICF; WHO, 2001) which can be used to clarify focuses of measurements. The ICF classification is structured in a hierarchical scheme and the main components are: Body Function and Structure, Activities (related to tasks and actions by an individual) and Participation (involvement in life situations). Problems in these domains are denoted as impairments, activity limitations and restricted participations, respectively. There is additional information on severity and environmental factors. However, no one measure provides the perfect assessment tool for children with hemiplegic CP; therefore, clinicians must pick the tools that best meet their needs for evaluating the upper extremities of children over time (Majnemer, 2006; Eliasson and Burtner, 2008).

Body functions comprise basic components of motor and sensory functions, e.g. range of motion, grip strength, spasticity and tactile sensibility. The modified Ashworth scale is a 6-point rating scale that is used to measure muscle tone (Bohannon and Smith, 1987). The Modified House Functional Classification (MHC) system is designed to evaluate changes in hand function following hand surgery and may be useful to document specific unilateral hand changes at the ICF Body Structure and Function levels (House et al. 1981; Koman, 2000). Range of motion is measured using a goniometer and may be active or passive (Eliasson and Burtner, 2008). The Shriners Hospital for Children Upper Extremity Evaluation scale (SHUEE, Davids et al. 2006) is a new tool which incorporates different subscales of traditional measures of range of motion and muscle tone, dynamic position analysis and spontaneous functional analysis, for grasp and release. Administration of the SHUEE requires comprehensive training and ongoing practice by evaluators to ensure proper assessment. However, this scale is a comprehensive tool that allows the assessment of several ICF components (Davids et al. 2006; Eliasson and Burtner, 2008). The Quality of Upper Extremity Skills Test (QUEST) concerns arm-related movement and hand manipulative skills, the latter to a lesser extent. The QUEST evaluates four domains of upper extremity function: dissociated movements, grasp patterns, weight bearing, and protective extension (DeMatteo, 1992, 1993).

The Activity and Participation domains can be measured with the Melbourne Assessment of Unilateral Upper Limb Function (Randall et al. 1999, 2001). This test provides objective measures of upper extremity functions (e.g. pointing, grasping and reaching) and quantifies their quality. Also, Assisting Hand Assessment (AHA; Krumlinde-Sundholm and Eliasson, 2003), designed for children with unilateral disabilities (e.g., hemiplegic CP, obstetric brachial plexus palsy), measures how effectively these children use the affected hand in bimanual performance. However, while the Melbourne scale evaluates the capacity (the person's ability to execute a task or an action on the highest probable level of functioning that a person may reach in a standardized environment), AHA measures performance (the person's ability to execute a task or an action in a real-life environment, e.g. semi-structured play session). Another example of capacity measurement is the Jebsen & Taylor Test of Hand Function (Jebsen et al. 1969; Taylor et al. 1973) which provides objective measurements of standardized tasks with norms against which patient can be compared. The objects included in the assessment are commonly used in daily activities and the test evaluates hand use and speed of performance with them.

Participation in daily life can be assessed with questionnaires, administered to parents and /or to caregivers. For example, PEDI (Pediatric Evaluation of Disability Inventory) is a standardized test that includes three measurement dimensions: ability in functional skill (self-care, mobility and social function), the amount of caregiver assistance, and the equipment and modifications needed for function (Berg et al. 2004). Another option is ABIL-HAND-Kids (Arnould et al. 2004), a questionnaire developed to assess manual ability as perceived by children with CP or their parents. Both unimanual and bimanual activities are included.

Lastly, individualized measures can be built. The Goal Attainment Scale (GAS) is an individualized assessment suitable for evaluation of goal specific training and for addressing child and family needs (Kiresuk and Sherman, 1968; Ottenbacher and Cusick, 1990). The Canadian Occupational Performance Measure (COPM) is a semistructured interview in which participants (children or caregivers) rate the most important issues in the areas of self-care, work and leisure (Law, 2000).

Recently, Eliasson et al. (2006) proposed a new classification with a functional approach for the use of the hands based on the ICF model. The test Manual Ability Classification System (MACS) is designed to classify how children with CP use both hands together when handling objects in daily activities (Eliasson and Burtne, 2008).

Clinical Signs of Hemiplegia

The main clinical characteristic of hemiplegia certainly is **reduction of the motor repertoire** of the affected hemiside in *module acquisition* (meant as the elementary components of movement the child is provided with), *combinations* (possibility to subdivide the individual modules into different patterns according to space relations), and *sequences* (ability to assemble the individual modules according to different time relations). These early clinical signs allow a prompt diagnosis of hemiplegic CP (see chapter 3 on early diagnosis).

The assessment of the motor repertoire shown by the infant's spontaneous motility during the first weeks of life has contributed to make obsolete the traditional concept regarding the existence of a "silent period" for the appearance of the first clinical signs, traditionally considered to last up to the first year of life and sometimes even longer (Goutieres et al. 1972; Bouza et al. 1994).

The clinical history of the four hemiplegic forms testifies how early the motor repertoire is altered. Motor abnormal signs occur generally on both sides during the first weeks after the damage, especially for premature infants affected by the second form, and can also further worsen with time. In particular, a further reduction of the residual motor repertoire, especially of the upper limb, is possible when new postural and displacement competences are organized (sitting position, upright standing position, horizontal locomotion, start of walking). After the first years of life, the patient's residual motor repertoire is usually considered as scarcely likely to be modified (concept of gate closure).

Examples of the classification of motor patterns of hemiplegic children's walking, in particular by the American Gillette Hospital (Winters et al. 1987; Novacheck, 2000), and examples of classification for manipulation by our group, are reported in Tables 16.2 and 16.3.

Another clinical sign that is often reported in hemiplegic CP is the presence of **associated movements** that express the relation and mutual influence among the preserved hemiside, the plegic hemiside and the different segments of the plegic hemiside. They are traditionally classified into *synergies* (activation of a motor module at a distal level allows complete expression of the combination and sequence inside the limb) and *synkinesis* (involuntary movements produced by plegic hand when voluntary movements are made by the preserved hand). One of these particular components is imitation synkinesis or "mirror movements", with opposite direction. These movements are also highly indicative of re-organization of hand control in the intact hemisphere, which then guides both hands.

Sensory and perceptive defects (tactile, thermal, pain, proprioceptive, etc.) certainly occur more rarely and less seriously in childhood hemiplegia than in adult hemiplegia. Conversely, stereognosia disorders are quite frequent (Brown and Walsh, 2000) and

Table 16.2 Locomotor patterns in hemiplegia according to Winters et al. (1987)

Pattern type 1	Pattern type 2	Patter type 3	Pattern type 4
• Equinus foot during swing due to hyperactivity of triceps and/or failure of foot dorsoflexors	• Equinus foot both during swing and stance due to significant contracture or retraction of sural triceps, posterior tibia or toe flexor	• Co-contraction of femoral rectum and ischiocrural	• Proximal involvement of hip and adductor flexors
• Initial flatfoot contact with the ground or with pattern inversion		• Walking with stiff knee	• Equinus foot both during stance and swing, stiff knee flexion, anteversion and pelvis sideshifting
• Absent first fulcrum, almost normal second fulcrum due to the absence of limitation to dorsoflexion during stance	• Early interruption of the second fulcrum with a resulting extension (2a) or curved knee (2b) and stance hip	• Limited flexion of the knee during swing with difficult foot clearance	
• Compensations:	• Hyperactivity of the pair composed of knee extensors and foot plantar flexors	• Use of contralateral (inclination) or homolateral (circumduction, hip hyperflexion) compensations	• Reduced sagittal movement of the knee
- increased knee flexion at swing end, initial contact and load acceptance	• reduction in walking speed	• Hyperactivity of the foot plantar flexors/knee	• Contracture during flexion / adduction / intrarotation of the thigh and pelvis moving back
- hip hyperflexion during swing			• Compensation with lumbar hyperlordosis at stance end.
- increased hip anteversion			

according to some authors they are present in more than half of hemiplegic children (Fedrizzi et al. 2003).

Attention disorders certainly represent useful data for the expression of the clinical picture in time and for the results of the rehabilitation treatment (neglect, which is related both to vision, to be distinguished from hemianopia – see chapter 7 – and to other components of the perceptive area – see chapter 5). These attention disorders can cause the child not to use the plegic limb, with a consequent lack of functional use of a motor repertoire still preserved. Hence, the presence of sensory and perceptive disorders is a fundamental element in the assessment of children with CP since it is able to determine, especially for the upper limbs, the quality of their residual motor ability and therefore their functional use, separately and, with the aid of the other hand, during bimanual activities.

According to the traditional neurological definition, the alteration of **muscle tone** with spasticity occurs quite late, in most cases taking place more than a year after the lesion (Bouza et al. 1994) and is scarcely useful from a diagnostic point of view or in understanding its correlation with the functional disorder (Brown and Walsh, 2000). In connatal forms (form III) with involvement of basal ganglia (hemidystonia), the picture can be dominated by dyskinesia, with major differences also at the motion pattern level.

Among the other possible signs of hemiplegia, **muscle retractions** and (early or late) **bone growth alterations** are more or less frequent according to the different clinical forms of hemiplegia (see later).

Table 16.3 Hemiplegia: proposal of classification of manipulation patterns in hemiplegia (Ferrari, 2005)

Class	Integrated	Semi-functional	Synergic	Imprisoned	Excluded
Hand	Semi-opened with almost completely extended fingers.	Semi-opened with quite extended fingers.	Semi-opened with semi-extended metacarpophalangeal joints, semi-flexed and slightly abducted fingers.	Frequently closed fist enclosing thumb, or flexed wrist, semi-flexed fingers and adducted thumb (placed almost underneath palm).	Semi-opened with generally flexed wrist and semi-extended or more or less flexed fingers.
Thumb	Slightly abduced. Subterminal terminal opposition with index and/or middle finger.	Aligned or almost abducted. Subterminal/ terminal or subterminal lateral opposition with index and or middle finger.	Adducted or sometimes positioned underneath other fingers, but never imprisoned.	Imprisoned in the palm between index and middle finger or between middle and ring finger.	Aligned or fairly abducted. Can be adducted but functionally not opposed.
Finger movements	Possible selective finger movements, especially of index finger, with good variability.	Still possible selective finger movements, especially of index finger, but with reduced variability.	Only possible combined finger movements. Possible independent index activity.	Impossible independent finger movements, index autonomy is sometimes still present.	Very difficult independent finger movements, except for overall adduction.
Pinch or grasp	Subterminal/ terminal bi- or tripodal distal pinch.	Subterminal/lateral bi o tripodal distal pinch.	Still possible the tripodal pinch, but with poor thumb adaptation.	Indirect digit-palmar or interdigital grasping through passive placement of object by unaffected hand.	Inefficient or absent lateral thumb/index pinch.
Wrist	Rather extended and sufficiently mobile.	Slightly flexed but sufficiently mobile.	More or less semiflexed with an ulnar deviation. Generally not very mobile.	Flexed with an ulnar deviation. Active and passive stiffness.	In flexion. Passively mobile.
Forearm	Neutral or slightly pronated. Possible active supination	Semipronated with limited possible supination.	Semi pronated with reduced or completely absent supination.	Pronated with reduced or completely absent supination (also passive).	Semipronated or in neutral position. Difficult or very limited active supination.
Elbow	Slightly flexed, generally mobile	Semiflexed, generally mobile.	Semiflexed and still sufficiently mobile.	Frequently flexed with poor mobility.	Usually semiflexed, generally with acceptable mobility.
Arm	Aligned	Slightly intrarotated.	Slightly abducted and intra rotated.	Abducted and intrarotated.	Positioned near trunk.
Shoulder	Good general mobility in neutral pattern	Mobile, only slightly lowered and antepulsed.	Mobile, slightly lowered and antepulsed.	Poor mobility, somewhat lowered and antepulsed.	Mobile, sometimes slightly lowered and antepulsed.
Grasping modality	Grasping of medium or small size objects through good hand adaptation. Grasping is not influenced by the activity of the unaffected hand.	Grasping of medium size objects through acceptable hand adaptation. Grasping is somewhat possible also if unaffected hand is performing another task.	Simple synergy of grasping triggered through controllable elbow and shoulder movements and under visual control. No hand adaptation to object. Grasping is possible only if unaffected hand takes part in the same action.	Indirect grasping (passive placement with thumb imprisoned or positioned underneath palm). Possibilities: - interdigital grasping or hooklike with second and third finger - positioning of fist on flat surface in order to hold, push, press, hit, etc. - bimanual grasping through opposition of the wrist against unaffected hand - fixation of the object between wrist and thorax. Sometime neglect.	Neglect. Inefficient or absent grasping. Sometimes, after several attempts, momentarily grasping of a thin and light object, through an inferior grasp between thumb and palm. Upon request, possibility to fix between flexed wrist and flat surface under constant visual control and without any hand adaptation. Usually the hand is open with extended fingers.

(cont ➤)

(*cont*)

Class	Integrated	Semi-functional	Synergic	Imprisoned	Excluded
Reaching	Orientation, anticipation, pre-adaptation. Motor pattern combinations without restrictions.	Orientation, anticipation and pre-adaptation possible, but more uncertain. Restricted motor pattern combinations.	Orientation, anticipation and pre-adaptation with insufficient motor pattern modulation. Reaching dependent on flexion and extension synergies.	Orientation without modulation. Impossible anticipation and pre-adaptation of the hand. Difficult reaching due to freezing of elbow and wrist.	Reaching very difficult or absent.
Visual-motor integration	The object can be spontaneously passed from one hand to the other without visual control.	The object can still be passed from one hand to the other. Necessity of non continuous visual control.	The object is passed with difficulties from the affected hand to unaffected one, better vice versa. Necessity of visual control.	The object is held in the affected hand through the placement by the unaffected one (passive loading). Necessity of constant visual control.	Usually there is no visual attention towards the hand, which is often outside visual field. The object can be picked up by the affected hand only after insistent requests and with continuous visual control.
Releasing	The object is readily released, without difficulty, without necessity of visual control.	The object is readily but roughly released. Necessity of frequent visual control.	The object is released slowly and with difficulty, often using servomotor movements.	Difficult hand opening. The object is released only with great difficulty. Generally it is pulled out by the unaffected hand.	Poor capacity to hold the object in the hand, frequently unintentionally dropping it. Object is preferably pulled out rather than voluntarily released by hand opening. In any case poor timing of release.
Manipulation	Mastery of intrinsic motricity for manual exploration	Scarce/absent intrinsic motricity. The hand still adapts to the object, but performs complex movements with difficulty.	Extremely limited. The manipulation is possible only if the object possesses suitable dimensions, weight and consistency.	No manipulation of the object is possible.	Impossible.
Bimanual activity	Good collaboration between hands also for complex manual activities. There is a discreet part of lateral hemispace in which the affected hand can be spontaneously used first.	Good cooperation between two hands. Positioning of affected hand near trunk during complex activities. There is only an extreme part of lateral hemispace in which the affected hand can be spontaneously utilised first.	Possible collaboration in achieving the same aim. Affected hand is used to support unaffected one. There is no part of lateral hemispace in which the affected hand can be spontaneously utilised first.	Cooperation, if strictly necessary, through passive loading of the affected hand. Possibility to load the affected hand only in the immediate and paramedian space. Use of alternative grasping solutions.	Hyper specialization of unaffected hand and absence of bimanual activity. Use of the affected hand only upon insistent and explicit external request. Use of alternative grasping solutions.
Main core	Subterminal terminal pinch. Intrinsic motricity.	Subterminal lateral pinch with basically adduced thumb.	Stereotypically expressed grasping and releasing within flexion and extension synergies. Active loading of object.	Indirect grasping (passive loading) Imprisoned thumb or positioned underneath palm.	Functionally ineffective or negligible grasping.

Epilepsy and **disorders of cognitive functions** (the latter more as alterations of specific functions rather than as global mental delay, a rare condition in this type of CP) are frequent and have a major relevance on the clinical picture, with a different distribution on the different forms (see later and compare with chapter 8).

Motor repertoire, perceptive alterations, neuropsychological aspects, and epilepsy are all factors strongly affecting the child's **learning** ability ("motor learning") and cause motor organization defects, especially at the praxic level. These defects are also obviously reported for the hemiplegic children's preserved side (Eliasson et al. 1991, 1995).

Acknowledging the variability of the clinical picture between one individual and the other, due to the variable size of the main lesion, the presence of associated lesions, individual factors, the environment, etc, Table 16.4 shows the distribution of the main disorders, and Table 16.5 the most frequent motor patterns that can be observed in the upper and lower limbs in the four forms of spastic hemiplegia and hemidystonia. A detailed insight of such aspects will be presented in the next paragraphs, to emphasize the importance of lesion type and timing.

Classification of Manipulation

In recent years we have attempted to validate a recent classification of manipulation in children with spastic hemiplegia (see Table 16.3). It describes five patterns of manipulation in hemiplegic children by analyzing hand kinematic profile and functional use (Ferrari et al. 2005). We started by checking the inter-rater reliability of different scorers (either expert or trained observers) in assigning subject manipulation performance to one of the five patterns described in the classification. The manipulation patterns of 35 children and adolescents (age range 4-15 years) with hemiplegic CP were selected among patients whose videos were stored in the archives of the Department of Developmental Neuroscience of the IRCCS Stella Maris (Pisa, Italy) and of the Children Rehabilitation Unit of S. Maria Nuova Hospital (Reggio Emilia, Italy). Only video recordings of manipulation with homogeneous features were taken for examination. Subjects were included if 4 to 15 years and affected by hemiplegic CP, with lesions documented by MRI. The videos had to last a minumun of 3 and a half minutes and to include some items of the Melbourne Assessment of Unilateral Upper Limb Function and of spontaneous use on bimanual activity (spontaneous play and activity of daily living). They were blindly scored at first by two of the authors of the classification (defined as "maximum experts), then by ten expert observers who performed test-retests (after 4 months). Finally, the 35 videos in which the highest agreement was reached by the ten scorers were later classified by 124 professionals of rehabilitation (medical doctors, physical therapists, students, orthopedic technicians) after a training course on the classification. For internal reliability, chance-corrected agreement between observers was measured using Fleiss' kappa statistics (K). Kappa values were interpreted according to conventional groups (0.0-0.20=slight agreement; 0.21-0.40=fair; 0.41-0.60=moderate; 0.61-0.80=substantial; 0.81-1=almost perfect). High K values (range 0.836-0.982) were obtained for test-retests of the 10 expert observers,

16

Table 16.4 Main clinical characteristics for the whole group and for each different form of hemiplegia in a group of 165 subjects with hemiplegic cerebral palsy (Petacchi, 2008)

	Whole group n=165 n (%)	Form I n=23 (14%) n (%)	Form II n=63 (38%) n (%)	Form III n=58 (35%) n (%)	Form IV n=21 (13%) n (%)
Clinical side*	R=77 (47) L=88 (53)	R=8 (35) L=15 (65)	R=27 (43) L=36 (57)	R=35 (60) L=23 (40)	R=7 (33) L=14 (67)
Site of main impairment**	UL=86 (52) LL=51 (31) EQ=29 (17)	UL=15 (65) LL=3 (13) EQ=5 (22)	UL=18 (29) LL=35 (55) EQ=10 (16)	UL=39 (67) LL=10 (17) EQ=9 (15)	UL=14 (67) LL=3 (14) EQ=4 (19)
Severity of UL motor impairment**	Mild=61 (37) Mod=82 (50) Severe=21 (13) Unknown=1	Mild=5 (22) Mod=14 (61) Severe=4 (17) Unknown=0	Mild=39 (62) Mod=21 (33) Severe=3 (5) Unknown =0	Mild=12 (21) Mod=38 (65) Severe=7 (13) Unknown =1 (2)	Mild=5 (24) Mod=9 (43) Severe=7 (33) Unknown =0
Cognitive level*	N=128 (78) Mild=21 (13) Mod=8 (5) Severe=7 (4) Unknown =1	N=13 (57) Mild=4 (17) Mod=3 (13) Severe=3 (13) Unknown =0	N=51 (81) Mild=7 (11) Mod=4 (6) S=1 (2) Unknown =0	N=46 (79) M=8 (14) Mod=1 (2) S=2 (3) Unknown =1 (2)	N=18 (86) M=2 (9) Mod=0 S=1 (5) Unknown =0
Seizure**	Yes=46 (28) No= 117 (72) Unknown =3	Yes=14 (61) No= 9 (39) Unknown =0	Yes=11 (17) No=51 (81) Unknown =1 (2)	Yes=14 (24) No=43 (74) Unknown =1 (2)	Yes=7 (33) No=13 (62) Unknown =1 (5)
EEG abnormalities**	Yes=90 (60) No= 66 (40) Unknown =9	Yes=21(91) No=2 (9) Unknown =0	Yes=25 (40) No=35 (55) Unknown =3 (5)	Yes=32 (55) No=21 (36) Unknown =5 (9)	Yes=12 (57) No=8 (38) Unknown =1 (5)
Language delay	Yes=59 (36) No= 105 (63) Unknown =1	Yes=11(48) No=12 (52) Unknown =0	Yes=19 (30) No=43 (68) Unknown =1 (2)	Yes=21 (36) No=37 (64) Unknown =0	Yes=8 (38) No=13 (62) Unknown =0
Language disorder	Yes= 25 (15) No= 90 (85) Unknown =50	Yes=3 (13) No=14 (61) Unknown =6 (26)	Yes=8 (13) No=35 (55) Unknown =20 (32)	Yes=8 (14) No=29 (50) Unknown =21 (36)	Yes=6 (29) No=12 (57) Unknown =3 (14)

* $0.05 < p < 0.1$, ** $p < 0.05$; *R*, right; *L*, left; *UL*, upper limbs; *LL*, lower limbs; *EQ*, equally

whereas a substantial agreement (K=0.70) was found in the group of 124 trained scorers. The agreement of trained scorers with the gold standard (expert scorers) was calculated to assess the facility index (f), i.e., the ratio between correct responses and total number of scorers. In three cases trained observers agreed completely with the gold standard (f=1), in four cases the agreement was low (f=0.41-0.59) and in the remaining cases (28 videos) the agreement was more than 0.6. However, the discordance was between contiguous classes of manipulation. Also, we calculated the item discrimination index, which is the difference between the proportions of high and low scorers answering a dichotomous item correctly. In the majority of cases the discrimination index was very low, denoting the feasibility of this manipulation's classification. The profession of the observer and previous knowledge

Table 16.5 Most frequent motor profiles in the different forms of hemiplegia in children

	Form I	Form II	Form III	Form IV	Form V
Neuromot or pattern: Lower limb	- support with intratorsion - aligned knee - detachment of foot in varus-supination - suspension equinism	- sometimes incomplete resolution of hip flexion - predominating distal expression - talipes equinus-valgus-pronation - talipes equinus-varus-supination	- sometimes incomplete resolution of hip flexion - flexed and intrarotated knee - talipes equinus-valgus-pronation	- proximal-distal involvement - stepping or plodding gait - variable pattern in presence of dyskinesia	- lifted hemipelvis, adduction-extrarotation of the thigh - extended or hyperextended knee - detachment of the foot in supination
Neuromot or pattern: Upper limb	- depressed shoulder - semi-extended elbow - flexed wrist - semi-extended fingers - adduced but not underlying thumb. Thumb aligned with other fingers - fingers in fork-back position	- free shoulder - semi-extended elbow - difficult supination - sometimes semi-flexed wrist - open hand - possible isolated finger movements (opposition)	- forward-pulled shoulder - adduced arm - flexed elbow - pronated forearm - flexed wrist, ulnar deviation - fist-closed hand - thumb lying under the fingers	- flexed shoulder -adduced elbow - flexed elbow - semi-pronated forearm - flexed wrist with falling hand - underlying thumb, sometimes imprisoned under fingers	- backward-pulled shoulder - flexed-adduced arm - flexed elbow - supinated forearm - semi-open hand

of the classification had no significant influence on reliability scores. These preliminary results suggest that the proposed classification can be reliably applied, even utilizing short video recordings, to arrange manipulation by hemiplegic children into different patterns.

In the same sample of 35 cases, the external validity was also determined by correlating hand manipulation classes with scores of the Melbourne Assessment of Unilateral Upper Limb Function. The regression coefficient was very high (R=0.86), indicating a significant correlation between the two scales as previous reported in a smaller sample (Sberveglieri, 2005).

Also, our group performed another preliminary study to test the external validity by correlating hand manipulation classes with the House modified classification (Perazza et al. 2008). The sample was composed of 45 children with hemiplegic CP (23 males, mean age: 7.73 yrs, age range: 3-12) selected among patients whose videos were stored in the archives of the Department of Developmental Neuroscience of the IRCCS Stella Maris (Pisa, Italy) from September 2007 to November 2008. The videos included items of the Melbourne Assessment of Unilateral Upper Limb and/or Assisting Hand Assessment (AHA). Exclusion criteria were acquired hemiplegia (timing of lesion after 3 years), mild or severe mental retardation, drug resistant seizures and behavioral disorders. Two independent scorers (a physical therapist and a physiatrist) with experience in the field of CP classified each video according to pattern of manipulation and to the House modified scale. A gold standard of scoring the same videos came by maximum expert classification score. Internal reliability of the two scales was calculated by Intraclass Correlation Coefficient (ICC), and by the Fleiss Kappa and Spearman rho coefficients. External reliability was calculated by the coefficient of determination (R square) between the two scales. A high concordance for classification of manipulation (ICC 0.996; Fleiss kappa 0.93, Spearman rho coefficient intraoperator 0.986, Spearman rho coefficient between two operators and gold standard .996 and .989 respectively, $p<0.01$) and for the House modified scale (ICC 0.994; Fleiss'kappa 0.86, Spearman rho coefficient intraoperator 0.981, Spearman rho coefficient between two operators and gold standard 0.982 and 0.986 respectively, $p<0.01$) was found. Lastly, R square between the two scales was 0.887 indicating a high linear correlation.

Main Features of the Four Clinical Forms of Hemiplegia

In this final part of the chapter some of the characteristics of the four forms of hemiplegia in children, classified according to our proposal on the basis of timing and type of the lesion, will be presented. The reported incidence of the different signs refers to our recent hospital based series of 165 cases with congenital or early acquired hemiplegia (Petacchi, 2008).

Form I (Early Malformative)

In this form of hemiplegia, the damage occurs early, generally at the end of the first or during the second three months of pregnancy. Most of the times the pregnant woman does not notice any symptom and the pregnancy progresses without problems until term. Therefore, this form of hemiplegia is not accompanied by a premature delivery. The lesion is frequently of vascular or infective origin, sometimes malformative due to early disorders of cell proliferation and migration, also of genetic origin (cortical dysplasia, schizencephaly, heterotopic areas, pachygyria areas, hemimegalencephaly, arachnoid cysts, etc.). It can affect one or both cerebral hemispheres (50% of the cases).

In this hemiplegic form, as an effect of after-lesion functional re-organization, speech and the other upper cortical functions are quite preserved despite the presence of wide areas of parenchymal destruction. A mental retardation, usually mild, can be present in about half cases (10/23, 43%). Sensory disorders are sometimes limited to tactile discrimination between two points (lack of tactile attention) and to morphosynthesis (tactile asymbolia, tactile agnosia, astereognosis). However, more complex neuropsychological disorders can also be present (see chapter 8).

Independent walking tends to occur later than in other forms, with a mean age of 19.8 months.

More than half of these children have convulsions (61%)s. Anomalies at EEG are even more frequent, showing alterations in more than 91% of cases.

At birth, there can already be a clear asymmetry in terms of length and trophism between homologous limbs, hands and feet included. The overall trunk alignment with respect to its median longitudinal axis is good. Hypometria and hypotrophy are directly proportional to CNS damage size and not to limb functionality, which is generally quite good.

The absence of signs of CNS disorders at birth and during the perinatal period and the lack of a reduction in the quantity (but not in the quality) of motor activity in the plegic hemiside explain the diagnostic delay.

The child's ability to develop suitable compensations and efficient functional substitutions tends to achieve excellent results since the mistakes made are stable and the individual is able to learn and acquire. The overall balance is good, unlike in the other forms of hemiplegia. The patients learn how to achieve balance also on the plegic lower limb. When walking and running they manage to reach quite a high speed.

The gait generally shows contact with the ground with an intrarotated leg, while the knee remains aligned, even if slightly flexed (Fig. 16.2). If an abnormal reaction to the stretching of triceps surae occurs, the knee can be stressed by curved snapping. During the last stance phase, the hip of the plegic limb manages to extend enough, but the pelvis keeps the anteversion. There is a frequent increase of foot varus-supination during detachment. A suspension equinus foot is often present, being compensated, during vertical passage, by a functional equinus foot of the preserved foot. For this reason, the hypometry of the plegic foot is at least partially useful and must be maintained. Synkinetic and associated reactions are clearer than the pathological pattern and tend to be prominent during fast walking, running and postural passages. During fast gait, running, and when the upper plegic limb

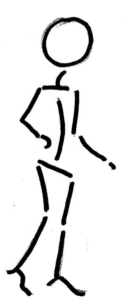

Fig. 16.2 *Form I of hemplegia.* Walking pattern

has to perform praxic activities, mirror movements are likely to be observed on the preserved limb.

Upper limbs are often affected in the same way or more than the lower limbs. Shoulders are slightly depressed, arms are a bit intrarotated, elbows are flexed, forearms are partially pronated, and wrists are flexed, unless dyskinesic components are present. Hands are slightly open, fingers can have a fan behavior or a fork-back behavior (flexion of the first phalanx and extension of the first and third ones). Patients can be very good at supporting themselves, and also at handling small objects (buttons, caps) or tools (scissors). Opposition between the thumb and the index can be achieved, but not complete forearm supination.

Form II (Prenatal)

This form generally follows a hypoxic-ischemic lesion that occurred during the third trimester of pregnancy for normal term infants and during the perinatal period for premature infants (before the 37th week). Pre-term birth is predominant (63%) with a medium gestational age of 34.7 weeks. The clinical picture can vary according to the lesion extension; it is generally located near the white periventricular substance and it consists of (according to the frequency order) secondary venous infarctions and intraventricular hemorrhages (Volpe, 2008), parenchymal hemorrhages secondary to anoxic processes, periventricular leukomalacia, etc. At the chronic stage, unilateral ecenphaloclastic cysts can be observed, associated to a widening of the lateral ventricle. Ventricular walls can have irregular borders. In some cases, a symmetrical or asymmetrical periventricular gliosis, with normal size ventricles can be detected. Bilateral lesions are present mostly in PVL and these were asymmetrical in the majority of our sample, but the side of the more severe lesions is not always contralateral to the hemiplegic side. Left side lesions seem to prevail. A slight prevalence of females is observed. Intellective abilities are mostly preserved. In most cases, these clinical forms are not severe and the prognosis is in general better than in the other forms. Indeed, mild impairment of the upper limb, a low incidence of mental retardation, epilepsy and EEG abnormalities are found, probably due to the sidedness of the lesion which rarely involves the cortex.

The patient's lower limbs almost always are more affected than the upper limbs. Until motility becomes generalized (in the incubator until the second month of normal term birth), no major differences between the two sides can be observed, but a bilateral reduction in the range and variability of the repertoire can be noticed. When motility becomes more restricted, asymmetry emerges. Therefore, pathological signs of hemiplegia become more evident only at three-six months of age, especially by analyzing distal movements. No major differences can be observed in terms of length and trophism in the development of plegic limbs as compared to contralateral limbs, in particular if dyskinesic components are present. Feet mainly make a distal effort (pattern 1 of Winters et al. 1987): the most frequent contact with the ground is talipes equinus-valgus-pronation, rarely talipes equinus-varus-supination. Thighs are slightly flexed and adducted, while the pelvis is pulled forward with compensatory lumbar hyperlordosis. At the end of stance, hip keeps a certain flexion angle, sometimes also on the preserved hemiside (flexed-adduction interfer-

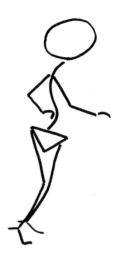

Fig. 16.3 *Form II of hemplegia.* Walking pattern

ence). The hand can appear free ("integrated hand") or with minor impairments ("semi-functional hand"), generally flexed at the wrist and extended at the fingers, which appear crowed and without an underlying thumb (Fig. 16.3). Single movements of the fingers are often possible, for example using them to point at things, and to perform a digito-digital grip. Elbows are extended and shoulders are free to allow a sort of swinging movement during fast walking. Supination movements of the forearm are allowed, both voluntary and associated (detected by Fog's test). The latter can be accompanied by a stronger fist clenching.

The overall balance is generally satisfactory.

Dispraxic elements can be present, both manual and visual, especially if the lesion even partially affects the homolateral hemisphere of the palsy.

Form III (Connatal)

In this form, the lesion often occurs on the left side and most of the time it occurs inside the uterus, around the end of the pregnancy (after the 37th week of pregnancy), or during the perinatal period. Generally, it is of anoxic-ischemic origin (infarction of a major artery, especially of the median cerebral artery, in particular of the main branch or one of the cortical branches), sometimes hemorrhagic. Sometimes the deepest branches of the median cerebral artery are affected, alone or associated to other lesions, with subsequent involvement of diencephalic structures, in particular of the internal capsule, thalamus, basal ganglia (the posterior branch of the internal capsule and the putamen) are often affected, the latter being especially affected in dyskinesic forms; see below.

The cortico-subcortical involvement is higher than in the other forms of childhood hemiplegia and in one fourth of cases it is bilateral due to the presence of hypoxic lesions, mostly mild ones, also on the other hemisphere. The functional re-organization process mostly occurs perilesionally and more rarely in the preserved hemisphere (ipsilateral sites).

16

The lesion size, often extended, and the involvement of cortical and subcortical structures make the resulting disability level quite significant, especially the hand. At birth there is no significant difference in terms of trophism and length between homologous limbs, although later they can develop without growing enough and with a different motility between the two lower limbs and a reduced functional use of the plegic hand.

Associated problems are frequent such as dyspraxia and intellectual disability (15-20% of the cases); EEG abnormalities are frequent (55%) but seizures are rare.

Motor integration of the plegic hemiside, balance and the overall abilities of the patient are certainly lower than in form II (prenatal), in particular with regard to the upper limb. A low error stability is present, with subsequent higher difficulties in finding compensation and a lower central representation of segments and their operating possibilities. On the lower limbs, the pathological pattern is important and can often be traced back to patterns 2, 3 or 4 of Winters et al. (1987): if equinus foot is significant, the limb is flexed at the knee and intrarotated, otherwise, it is extended or hyper-extended; the foot has talipes equinus-valgus-pronation or talipes equinus-varus-supination especially if dyskinesic components are present. Usually the rotation only affects the leg-foot segment (tibiae in intratorsion). The hip never abandons flexion, not even at the end of the stance phase; it can however be reduced it if the knee curves. Upper limbs very often are highly affected (with a severity which is not always related to the lesion severity); shoulders are pulled forward, elbows are flexed and adduced, forearms show pronation, wrist are ulnarly deviated, and the hands are clenched in a fist with underlying thumb ("imprisoned" hand). The associated reactions make the upper limbs stiff, with strongly clenched fist and flexed elbow (Fig. 16.4). Sensory disorders are generally severe, especially on the hands. When a bimanual action is

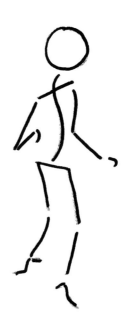

Fig. 16.4 *Form III (spastic) of hemplegia.* Walking pattern

required, the plegic hand is "loaded" by the preserved hand under a careful visual control, as if it was a tool (interdigital or digitopalmar grasp). Sometimes the only hand portion to be used is the wrist (radial surface) or the third distal part of the forearm, and sometimes even the elbow or the shoulder. In less severe cases, the hand is more open, with the underlying but not clenched thumb. More proximal patterns generally show a reduced level of stiffness.

Sensory and perceptive disorders (even if not as severe as in acquired forms or in adult forms) and attention disorders (neglect) are frequent. When carrying out a bimanual task, some individuals completely neglect the upper plegic limb and use their thighs, chin or mouth to create a forceps function.

Form IV (Infantile or Acquired)

In this form of hemiplegia, the lesion occurs later (suckling age or first-second year of childhood) and generally has a vascular, infectious, tumor or traumatic origin. Conceptually, the lesion produces a loss of previously acquired functions rather than a missed functions acquisition: it is therefore closer to adult hemiplegia than to the other forms of hemiplegia in children. Upper limbs are generally more affected than lower limbs, with a mild to medium-severe motor impairment. Often, it involves significant learning problems, complex perceptive disorders and attention disorders (visual hemiagnosia, hemisomatoagnosia, and hemineglect - see chapter 7). EEG abnormalities are frequent (57%) but seizures are rare, as in form III.

As far as motor functions are concerned, pattern types 3 or 4 (Winter et al. 1987) prevail on the lower limbs. Frequently, stiff patterns like sickle gait (with adduction-extrarotation when the hip starts moving) are observed, especially if the lesion appears after the second year of age, or stepping gait with hemipelvis being lifted, accentuated hip flexion, and secondary flexion of the knee. Hands are often engaged like in form III (connatal) ("excluded" or "imprisoned" hand). Associated reactions are very intense: shoulder flexion, slight adduction of the arm, elbow flexion, forearm pronation, wrist and finger flexion, adduced thumb or thumb lying under the other fingers, or clenched between the index finger and the middle finger. Other times the elbow and the wrist are flexed, while the hand appears loose and totally inactive (Fig. 16.5). Perceptive disorders of the upper limbs, especially related to stereognosis and discrimination between two points, are frequent in the most severe cases (O'Malley and Griffith, 1977; Yekutiel et al. 1994).

To fix objects, the child can use the plegic hand by placing it as it is; conversely, to manipulate the child will have to prepare the plegic hand together with the contralateral, hand under careful visual control. Very often patients prefer to use the wrist or the forearm instead of the hand, which is poorly centrally represented.

Trophic disorders do not generally become severe. The shortening of the lower limbs is often due to pelvis obliquity such that the pelvis tilts upwards on the plegic limb side, rather than real dysmetria, also leading to the reduction of foot length.

Unlike other forms, patients may also present with central palsy of the facial nerve, usually homolateral and mainly lower, which is often not visible at rest. On the plegic side,

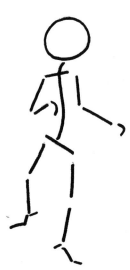

Fig. 16.5 *Form IV of hemplagia.* Walking pattern

the corrugation of the forehead is maintained, as well as eyelids closure and the lifting of the eyebrow angle.

Dystonic Form (Hemidystonia)

The lesion occurs at the perinatal or postnatal stage (first three years of life), almost always with vascular origin, mainly infarctions and hemorrhages of the median cerebral artery, with involvement of terminal branches (lenticular-striatal arteries). In many cases the lesion is bilateral, but asymmetrical (more severe on one side).

Motor patterns are extremely variable: the most typical one is characterized by shoulder retropulsion, flexed and adduced arm, flexed elbow, supinated forearm, semi-open hand. During fast walking the hand can reach higher than the shoulder line. Other times the shoulder is pulled forward, the arm is flexed-adduced and intrarotated, the elbow is semi-extended, the wrist is slightly flexed and the fingers are extended with underlying thumb. The upper limb can also be posteriorly moved away (hyperextended), with the shoulder being pulled forward and intrarotated and the elbow extended. The hemipelvis is tilted upward, with adduction-extrarotation of the thigh, the knee is extended or hyperextended or semi-flexed, the tibia is often intrarotated, the foot has varus-supination. Use of the hands for manipulation tasks is better than what can be observed in postural tasks. During walking, the detachment of the foot is typically characterized by an accentuation of varus-supination (dystonic detachment), and the contact with the ground can also happen on the toe back, especially during fast walking and barefoot.

In upright position, the knee can be stressed by curved snapping with the hemipelvis moving backward and a position of the trunk oblique to the walking direction (Fig. 16.6).

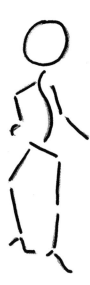

Fig. 16.6 *Hemidystomia.* Walking pattern

Involuntary movements are more frequently related to the upper limb than to the lower limb. The patient learns soon how to "block" the plegic hand with the preserved hand in order to hide, or at least to retain, hyperkinesias.

References

Aicardi J, Bax M (2009) Cerebral palsy. In: Aicardi J (ed) Diseases of the nervous system in childhood, 3nd ed. MacKeith Press, London

Arnould C, Penta M, Renders A, Thonnard JL (2004) ABILHAND-Kids: a measure of manual ability in children with cerebral palsy. Neurology 63:1045-1052

Bax M, Tydeman C, Flodmark O (2006) Clinical and MRI correlates of cerebral palsy: the european cerebral palsy study. JAMA 296:1602-1608

Berg M, Jahnsen R, Froslie KF, Hussain A (2004) Reliability of the Pediatric Evaluation of Disability Inventory (PEDI). Phys Occup Ther Pediatr 24:61-77

Bohannon RW, Smith MB (1987) Interater reliability of a modified Ashworth scale of muscle spasticity. Phys Ther 67:206-207

Bouza H, Dubowitz LM, Rutherford M, Pennock JM (1994) Prediction of outcome in children with congenital hemiplegia: magnetic resonance imaging study. Neuropediatrics 25: 60-66

Brown JK, Walsh EG (2000) Neurology of the upper limb. In: Neville B, Goodman R (eds) Congenital hemiplegia. Clinics in developmental medicine. Cambridge University Press, Cambridge, pp 113-149

Carswell A, McColl MA, Baptiste S et al (2004) The Canadian Occupational Performance Measure: a research and clinical literature review. Can J Occup Ther 71:210-222

Cioni G, Sales B, Paolicelli PB et al (1999) MRI and clinical characteristics of children with hemiplegic cerebral palsy. Neuropediatrics 30:249-255

Davids JR, Peace LC, Wagner LV et al (2006) Validation of the Shriners Hospital for Children Upper Extremity Evaluation (SHUEE) for children with hemiplegic cerebral palsy. J Bone Joint Surg Am 88:326-333

DeMatteo C, Law M, Russel DJ et al (1992) Quality of upper extremity skill test manual. Canchild, McMasters University, Hamilton, Ontario

DeMatteo C, Law M, Russel DJ et al (1993) The reliability and validity of the quality of upper extremity skill test. Phys Occup Ther Pediatr 13:1-18

Eliasson AC, Gordon AM, Forssberg H (1991) Basic coordination of manipulative forces in children with cerebral palsy. Dev Med Child Neurol 33:661-670

Eliasson AC, Gordon AM, Forssberg H (1995) Tactile control of isometric fingertip forces during grasping in children with cerebral palsy. Dev Med Child Neurol 37:72-84

Eliasson AC, Krumlinde-Sudholm L, Rosblad B et al (2006) The Manual Ability Classification System (MACS) for children with cerebral palsy: scale development and evidence of validity and reliability. Dev Med Child Neurol 48:549-554

Eyre JA (2003) Development and plasticity of the corticospinal system in man. Neural Plast 20:93-106

Eyre JA (2007) Corticospinal tract development and its plasticity after perinatal injury. Neurosci Biobehav Rev 31:1136-49

Eyre JA, Smith M, Dabydeen L et al (2007) Is hemiplegic cerebral palsy equivalent to amblyopia of the corticospinal system? Ann Neurol 62:493-503

Eyre JA, Taylor JP, Villagra F et al (2001) Evidence of activity-dependent withdrawal of corticospinal projections during human development. Neurology 57:1543-54

Fedrizzi E, Pagliano E, Andreucci E, Oleari G (2003) Hand function in children with hemiplegic cerebral palsy: prospective follow-up and functional outcome in adolescence. Dev Med Child Neurol 45:85-91

Ferrari A, Cioni G (2005) Le forme spastiche delle paralisi cerebrali infantili. Springer-Verlag Italia, Milan

Friel KM, Martin J (2007) Bilateral activity-dependent interactions in the developing corticospinal system. J Neurosci 27:11083-11090

Goutieres F, Challamel MJ, Aicardi J, Gilly R (1972) Les hémiplégies congenitales: sémeiologie, étiologie et prognostic. Arch Fr Pediatr 29: 839-851

Grabowski EF, Buonanno FS, Krishnamoorthy K (2007) Prothrombotic risk factors in the evaluation and management of perinatal stroke. Semin Perinatol 31:243-249.

Guzzetta A, Bonanni P, Biagi L et al (2007) Reorganisation of the somatosensory system after early brain damage. Clin Neurophysiol 188:1110-21

Hagberg B, Hagberg G, Olow I (1996) The changing panorama of cerebral palsy in Sweden, VII. Prevalence and origin during the birth period 1987-1990. Acta Paediatrica 85:954-960

Hagberg G, Hagberg B (2000) Antecedents. In: Neville B, Goodman R (eds) Congenital hemiplegia. Clinics in developmental medicine. Cambridge University Press, Cambridge, pp 5-17

Himmelmann K, Hagberg G, Beckung E et al (2005) The changing panorama of cerebral palsy in Sweden, IX. Prevalence and origin in the birth-year period 1995-1998. Acta Paediatr 94:287-94

House JH, Gwathmey FW, Fidler MO (1981) A dynamic approach to thumb-in-palm deformity in cerebral palsy. J Bone Joint Surg Am 63:216-225

Jebsen RH, Taylor N, Trieschmann RB et al (1969) An objective and standardized test of hand function. Arch Phys Med Rehabil 50:311-319

Kiresuk TJ, Sherman RE (1968) Goal attainment scaling: a general method for evaluationg community mental health programs. Community Men Health J 4:442-453

Koman LA (2000) Cerebral palsy: house classification modified. In: Orthopedic care: medical and surgical management of musculoskeletal disorders: a comprehensive, peer-reviewed internet textbook. J South Orthop Ass

Korzeniewski SJ, Birbeck G, DeLano MC et al (2008) A systematic review of neuroimaging for cerebral palsy. J Child Neurol 23:216-227

Krägeloh-Mann I (2004) Imaging of early brain injury and cortical plasticity. Exp Neurol 190:84-90

16

Krägeloh-Mann I (2007) The role of magnetic resonance imaging in elucidating the pathogenesis of cerebral palsy: a systematic review. Dev Med Child Neurol 49:144-151

Krägeloh-Mann I, Cans C (2009) Cerebral palsy update. Brain Dev, in press

Krumlinde-Sudholm L (2008) Choosing and using assessments of hand function. In: Eliasson AC, Burtner PA (eds) Improving hand function in children with cerebral palsy: theory, evidence and intervention. Mac Keith Press, Cambridge, pp 176-197

Krumlinde-Sudholm L, Eliasson A (2003) Development of the Assisting Hand Assessment, a Rasch built measure intended for children with unilateral upper limb impairments. Scand J Occup Ther 10:16-26

Kulak W, Sobaniec W, Kuzia J-S, Bockowski L (2006) Neurophysiologic and neuroimaging studies of brain plasticity in children with cerebral palsy. Exp Neurol 198:4-11

Majnemer A (2006) Assessment tools for cerebral palsy. Future Neurol 1:755-63

Martin JH (2005) The corticospinal system: from development to motor control. Neuroscientist 11:161-173

Martin JH, Choy M, Pullman S, Meng Z (2004) Corticospinal system development depends on motor experience. J Neurosci 24:2122-2132

Mercuri E, Cowan F, Gupte G et al (2001) Prothrombotic disorders and abnormal neurodevelopmental outcome in infants with neonatal cerebral infarction. Pediatrics 107:1400-1404

Niemann G (2000) A new MRI-based classification. In: Neville B, Goodman R (eds) Congenital hemiplegia. Clinics in developmental medicine. Cambridge University Press, Cambridge, pp 37-52

Novacheck TF (2000) Management options for gait abnormalities. In: Neville B, Goodman R (eds) Congenital hemiplegia. Clinics in developmental medicine. Cambridge University Press, Cambridge, pp 98-112

O'Malley PJ, Griffith JF (1977) Perceptual–motor dysfunction in the child with hemiplegia. Dev Med Child Neurol 19:172-178

Ottenbacher KJ, Cusick A (1990) Goal attainment scaling as a measure of clinical service evaluation. Am J Occup Ther 44:519-525

Perazza S, D'Avino C, Scapazzoni P (2008) Lesion and function: which relationship? Thesis Master in Research in Rehabilitation, University of Modena and Reggio Emilia

Petacchi E (2008) Reorganization of hand function in subjects with an early lesion of the corticospinal system. PhD thesis, University of Pisa

Randall M, Carilin JB, Chondros P, Reddihough D (2001) Reliability of Melbourne assessment of unilateral upper limb function. Dev Med Child Neurol 43:761-767

Randall MJ, Johnson LM, Reddihough DS (1999) The Melbourne assessment of unilateral upper limb function. Royal Children's Hospital, Melbourne

Robinson MN, Peake LJ, Ditchfield MR et al (2008) Magnetic resonance imaging findings in a population-based cohort of children with cerebral palsy. Dev Med Child Neurol 51:39-45

Sberveglieri N (2005) The upper limb in childhood emiplegia: perceptual-motor disorder and functional classification. Thesis for degree in Physical Therapy, University of Modena and Reggio Emilia

Smith RA, Skelton M, Howard M, Levene M (2001) Is thrombophylia a factor in development of hemiplegic cerebral palsy? Dev Med Chid Neurol 43:724-30

Staudt M (2007) (Re-)organization of the developing human brain following periventricular white matter lesions. Neurosci Biobehav Rev 31:1150-1156

Staudt M, Gerloff C, Grodd W et al (2004) Reorganization in congenital hemiparesis acquired at different gestational ages. Ann Neurol 56:854-863

Staudt M, Grodd W, Gerloff C et al (2002) Two types of ipsilateral reorganization in congenital hemiparesis. A TMS and fMRI study. Brain 125:2222-2237

Staudt M, Krägeloh-Mann I, Grodd W (2005) Ipsilateral cortico-spinal pathways in congenital hemiparesis on routine magnetic resonance imaging. Pediatr Neurol 32:37-39

Taylor N, Snad PL, Jebsen RH (1973) Evaluation of hand function in children. Arch Phys Med Rehabil 54:129-135

Volpe JJ (2008) Neurology of the newborn, 5rd ed. Saunders Elsevier Science, Philadelphia

Wiklund LM (2000) Neuroradiology. In: Neville B, Goodman R (eds) Congenital hemiplegia. Clinics in developmental medicine. Cambridge University Press, Cambridge, pp 26-36

Wilke M, Staudt M, Juenger H et al (2009) Somatosensory system in two types of motor reorganizazion in congenital hemiparesis: topography and function. Hum Brain Mapp 30:776-788

Winters Jr TR, Gage JR, Hicks R (1987) Gait patterns in spastic hemiplegia in children and young adults. J Bone and Joint Surg 69:438

World Health Organization (2001) International classification of hand functioning, disability and health. World Health Organization, Geneva

Yekutiel M, Jariwala M, Stretch P (1994) Sensory deficit in the hands of children with cerebral palsy: a new look at assessment and prevalence. Dev Med Child Neurol 36:619-624

Subject Index